Vector-Borne Diseases

Editor

LINDA KIDD

VETERINARY CLINICS OF NORTH AMERICA: SMALL ANIMAL PRACTICE

www.vetsmall.theclinics.com

November 2022 • Volume 52 • Number 6

ELSEVIER

1600 John F. Kennedy Boulevard • Suite 1800 • Philadelphia, Pennsylvania, 19103-2899
http://www.vetsmall.theclinics.com

VETERINARY CLINICS OF NORTH AMERICA: SMALL ANIMAL PRACTICE Volume 52, Number 6
November 2022 ISSN 0195-5616, ISBN-13: 978-0-323-96149-3

Editor: Stacy Eastman
Developmental Editor: Axell Ivan Jade Purificacion

Photocopying

Single photocopies of single articles may be made for personal use as allowed by national copyright laws. Permission of the Publisher and payment of a fee is required for all other photocopying, including multiple or systematic copying, copying for advertising or promotional purposes, resale, and all forms of document delivery. Special rates are available for educational institutions that wish to make photocopies for non-profit educational classroom use. For information on how to seek permission visit www.elsevier.com/permissions or call: (+44) 1865 843830 (UK)/(+1) 215 239 3804 (USA).

Derivative Works

Subscribers may reproduce tables of contents or prepare lists of articles including abstracts for internal circulation within their institutions. Permission of the Publisher is required for resale or distribution outside the institution. Permission of the Publisher is required for all other derivative works, including compilations and translations (please consult www.elsevier.com/permissions).

Electronic Storage or Usage

Permission of the Publisher is required to store or use electronically any material contained in this periodical, including any article or part of an article (please consult www.elsevier.com/permissions). Except as outlined above, no part of this publication may be reproduced, stored in a retrieval system or transmitted in any form or by any means, electronic, mechanical, photocopying, recording or otherwise, without prior written permission of the Publisher.

Notice

No responsibility is assumed by the Publisher for any injury and/or damage to persons or property as a matter of products liability, negligence or otherwise, or from any use or operation of any methods, products, instructions or ideas contained in the material herein. Because of rapid advances in the medical sciences, in particular, independent verification of diagnoses and drug dosages should be made.

Although all advertising material is expected to conform to ethical (medical) standards, inclusion in this publication does not constitute a guarantee or endorsement of the quality or value of such product or of the claims made of it by its manufacturer.

Veterinary Clinics of North America: Small Animal Practice (ISSN 0195-5616) is published bimonthly by Elsevier Inc., 360 Park Avenue South, New York, NY 10010-1710. Months of issue are January, March, May, July, September, and November. Business and Editorial Offices: 1600 John F. Kennedy Blvd., Ste. 1800, Philadelphia, PA 19103-2899. Customer Service Office: 3251 Riverport Lane, Maryland Heights, MO 63043. Periodicals postage paid at New York, NY and additional mailing offices. Subscription prices are $369.00 per year (domestic individuals), $980.00 per year (domestic institutions), $100.00 per year (domestic students/residents), $465.00 per year (Canadian individuals), $1029.00 per year (Canadian institutions), $503.00 per year (international individuals), $1029.00 per year (international institutions), $100.00 per year (Canadian students/residents), and $220.00 per year (international students/residents). To receive student/resident rate, orders must be accompanied by name of affiliated institution, date of term, and the *signature* of program/residency coordinator on institution letterhead. Orders will be billed at individual rate until proof of status is received. Foreign air speed delivery is included in all *Clinics* subscription prices. All prices are subject to change without notice. **POSTMASTER:** Send address changes to *Veterinary Clinics of North America: Small Animal Practice*, Elsevier Health Sciences Division, Subscription Customer Service, 3251 Riverport Lane, Maryland Heights, MO 63043. Customer Service (orders, claims, online, change of address): Elsevier Periodicals Customer Service, Elsevier Health Sciences Division Subscription **Customer Service 3251 Riverport Lane Maryland Heights, MO 63043. Tel: 1-800-654-2452 (U.S. and Canada); 314-447-8871 (outside U.S. and Canada). Fax: 314-447-8029. E-mail: journalscustomerservice-usa@elsevier.com (for print support); journalsonlinesupport-usa@elsevier.com (for online support).**

Reprints. For copies of 100 or more of articles in this publication, please contact the Commercial Reprints Department, Elsevier Inc., 360 Park Avenue South, New York, NY 10010-1710. Tel.: 212-633-3874; Fax: 212-633-3820; E-mail: reprints@elsevier.com.

Veterinary Clinics of North America: Small Animal Practice is also published in Japanese by Inter Zoo Publishing Co., Ltd., Aoyama Crystal-Bldg 5F, 3-5-12 Kitaaoyama, Minato-ku, Tokyo 107-0061, Japan.

Veterinary Clinics of North America: Small Animal Practice is covered in *Current Contents/Agriculture, Biology and Environmental Sciences, Science Citation Index, ASCA, MEDLINE/PubMed (Index Medicus), Excerpta Medica, and BIOSIS.*

Contributors

EDITOR

LINDA KIDD, DVM, PhD
Diplomate, American College of Veterinary Internal Medicine (Small Animal Internal
Medicine); Professor, Small Animal Internal Medicine, Western University of Health
Sciences, College of Veterinary Medicine, Pomona, California, USA; Current Employment
Zoetis US Diagnostics

AUTHORS

KELLY ALLEN, MS, PhD
Department of Veterinary Pathobiology, Oklahoma State University College of Veterinary
Medicine, Stillwater, Oklahoma, USA

GAD BANETH, DVM, PhD
Diplomate, European College of Veterinary Clinical Pathology; The Koret School of
Veterinary Medicine, The Hebrew University of Jerusalem, Rehovot, Israel

ADAM BIRKENHEUER, DVM, PhD
Diplomate, American College of Veterinary Internal Medicine (Small Animal Internal
Medicine); Professor and Andy Quattlebaum Distinguished Chair in Infectious Disease
Research, Department of Clinical Sciences, College of Veterinary Medicine, North
Carolina State University, Raleigh, North Carolina, USA

LEAH A. COHN, DVM, PhD
Diplomate, American College of Veterinary Internal Medicine (Small Animal Internal
Medicine); Professor, Small Animal Medicine, Department of Veterinary Medicine and
Surgery, University of Missouri College of Veterinary Medicine, Columbia, Missouri, USA

AUDREY K. COOK, BVM&S, MRCVS, MSc Vet Ed
Diplomate, American College of Veterinary Internal Medicine (Small Animal Internal
Medicine); Diplomate, European College of Veterinary Internal Medicine–Companion
Animals; Diplomate, American Board of Veterinary Practitioners–Feline Practice;
Professor of Small Animal Internal Medicine, Department of Small Animal Clinical
Sciences, College of Veterinary Medicine and Biomedical Sciences, Texas A & M
University, College Station, Texas, USA

JONATHAN D DEAR, DVM, MAS, DACVIM (SAIM)
Department of Medicine and Epidemiology, School of Veterinary Medicine, University of
California, One Shields Avenue, Davis, California, USA

PEDRO PAULO V.P. DINIZ, DVM, PhD
Professor in Small Animal Internal Medicine, Director of Outcomes Assessment, Western
University of Health Sciences, College of Veterinary Medicine, Pomona, California, USA

SARAH A. HAMER, MS, PhD, DVM
Diplomate, American College of Veterinary Preventive Medicine (Epidemiology);
Department of Veterinary Integrative Biosciences, College Station, Texas, USA

MAGGIE JENSEN, BSE
Student, School of Veterinary Medicine, University of Wisconsin-Madison, Madison,
Wisconsin, USA

LINDA KIDD, DVM, PhD
Diplomate, American College of Veterinary Internal Medicine (Small Animal Internal
Medicine); Professor, Small Animal Internal Medicine, Western University of Health
Sciences, College of Veterinary Medicine, Pomona, California, USA

ERIN LASHNITS, MS, DVM, PhD
Diplomate, American College of Veterinary Internal Medicine (Small Animal Internal
Medicine); Department of Medical Sciences, School of Veterinary Medicine, University of
Wisconsin-Madison, Madison, Wisconsin, USA

ALLISON L. LUDWIG, BS
NIH Predoctoral Fellow, Department of Comparative Biomedical Sciences, School of
Veterinary Medicine, University of Wisconsin-Madison, Waisman Center, Madison,
Wisconsin, USA

VERONICA MAGSAMEN, BS
Student, School of Veterinary Medicine, University of Wisconsin-Madison, Madison,
Wisconsin, USA

DANIEL MOURA DE AGUIAR, DVM, PhD
Professor in Infectious Disease of Animals, Laboratory of Virology and Rickettsiosis,
Faculty of Veterinary Medicine, Federal University of Mato Grosso State - UFMT, Cuiabá,
Mato Grosso, Brazil

ANNE PANKOWSKI, BS
Student, School of Veterinary Medicine, University of Wisconsin-Madison, Madison,
Wisconsin, USA

ASHLEY B. SAUNDERS, DVM
Diplomate, American College of Veterinary Internal Medicine (Cardiology); Professor of
Cardiology, Department of Small Animal Clinical Sciences, College of Veterinary Medicine
and Biomedical Sciences, College Station, Texas, USA

LAIA SOLANO-GALLEGO, DVM, PhD
Diplomate, European College of Veterinary Clinical Pathology; Departament de Medicina i
Cirurgia Animal, Facultat de Veterinària, Universitat Autònoma de Barcelona, Bellaterra,
Spain

RACHEL TABER, DVM
Student, School of Veterinary Medicine, University of Wisconsin-Madison, Madison,
Wisconsin, USA

SéVERINE TASKER, BSc (hons), BVSc (hons), DSAM, PhD, FHEA, FRCVS
Diplomate, European College of Veterinary Internal Medicine–Companion Animals; Chief
Medical Officer, Professor, Honorary Professor of Feline Medicine, DSAM is RCVS
Diploma in Small Animal Medicine, Linnaeus Veterinary Limited, Bristol Veterinary School,
University of Bristol, Langford, Bristol, United Kingdom

Contents

Preface: Changes   xi

Linda Kidd

How Changing Tick-Borne Disease Prevalence in Dogs Affects Diagnostic Testing   1153

Linda Kidd

Ixodes scapularis (the deer tick), Amblyomma americanum (the lone star tick) and Rhipicephalus sanguineus (the brown dog tick) are ticks that commonly parasitize dogs in the United States. In the first part of this article, we will examine their changing epidemiology to illustrate how being aware of their distribution and adapting diagnostic testing to include a broad range of pathogens may improve our ability to identify and help infected patients, especially those with suspected idiopathic immune-mediated disease. We will then discuss how to optimize testing for these pathogens using available panels.

Bartonellosis in Dogs and Cats, an Update   1163

Rachel Taber, Anne Pankowski, Allison L. Ludwig, Maggie Jensen, Veronica Magsamen, and Erin Lashnits

The unique virulence factors of Bartonella spp make them stealth pathogens that evade the immune system and cause persistent infections that are often difficult to diagnose and treat. Understanding these pathogenic mechanisms allows clinicians to recognize when to pursue diagnostics, how to optimize diagnostic testing and treatment, and ultimately can lead to improved outcomes.

Babesia in North America: An Update   1193

Jonathan D. Dear and Adam Birkenheuer

Canine babesiosis results from infection of 1 of 5 identified protozoal species in the United States (Babesia conradae, Babesia sp. "coco," Babesia gibsoni, Babesia vogeli, and Babesia vulpes). They are part of the Apicomplexa family of protozoa and are obligate intraerythrocytic parasites. Domestic and wild canids are suspected of being intermediate hosts. This updated article aims to provide practical guidance about the clinical manifestations of disease, treatment options, and outcomes. In addition, the authors hope to provide some clarity about the taxonomy and nomenclature of these organisms, as they have undergone multiple changes since their initial discovery.

Cytauxzoonosis   1211

Leah A. Cohn

Cytauxzoon felis is a hematoprotozoan parasite with a complex life cycle involving a tick-vector and a mammalian host. The mammalian hosts are all felidae but in the bobcat reservoir host, the parasite typically causes only a brief, self-resolving illness followed by a prolonged subclinical infection. In domestic cats, however, infection often leads to an acute febrile illness characterized by severe morbidity and mortality. Diagnosis is based on microscopic identification of parasites or molecular testing. Treatment for ill cats is expensive, difficult, and often unsuccessful. Prevention is quite possible and depends on avoidance of feeding by vector ticks.

Ehrlichiosis and Anaplasmosis: An Update   1225

Pedro Paulo V.P. Diniz and Daniel Moura de Aguiar

Canine ehrlichiosis and anaplasmosis are zoonotic tick-borne diseases with broad distribution in the United States and abroad. Advances in serologic and molecular-based diagnostics have enhanced the understanding of the species of rickettsial organisms involved; their expanding geographic distribution; and their impact on the health of dogs, cats, and people. Although clinical remission is achieved with appropriate antimicrobial therapy, optimal treatment modalities for the elimination of infection remains uncertain. Protection through vaccines for ehrlichiosis or anaplasmosis remains elusive. This review provides practicing veterinarians with the most current information about transmission, diagnosis, and management of ehrlichiosis and anaplasmosis in dogs and cats.

Veterinary Chagas Disease (American Trypanosomiasis) in the United States   1267

Sarah A. Hamer and Ashley B. Saunders

Veterinary Chagas disease is a persistent threat to humans, dogs, and other wild or domestic mammals that live where infected triatomine "kissing bug" insect vectors occur across the Americas, including 28 states in the Southern United States. Animals infected with the Trypanosoma cruzi parasite may be asymptomatic or may develop myocarditis, heart failure, and sudden death. It is difficult to prevent animal contact with vectors because they are endemic in sylvatic environments and often disperse to domestic habitats. Challenges for disease management include imperfect diagnostic tests and limited antiparasitic treatment options.

Schistosomiasis in the United States   1283

Audrey K. Cook

Canine schistosomiasis is a well-established cause of a granulomatous enteropathy and hepatopathy in dogs. In a small subset of patients, infection triggers significant hypercalcemia. Clinical signs and clinicopathologic findings are fairly nonspecific but ultrasonographic evidence of heterogenous small intestinal wall layering and pin-point hyperechoic foci in bowel, nodes, and liver is highly suggestive of infection. A sensitive, commercially available, fecal polymerase chain reaction test can be used to establish the diagnosis. Treatment protocols rely on praziquantel with fenbendazole. Most dogs will recover, although retreatment may be necessary in a substantial proportion. Housemates should be screened as infection can be asymptomatic.

Emerging Spotted Fever Rickettsioses in the United States   1305

Linda Kidd

Spotted fever rickettsioses are important causes of emerging infectious disease in the United States and elsewhere. Rocky Mountain Spotted

Fever, caused by R. rickettsii causes a febrile, acute illness in dogs. Because it circulates in peripheral blood in low copy number and because of the acute nature of the disease, dogs may test PCR and seronegative at the time of presentation. Therefore, therapy with doxycycline must be initiated and continued based on the clinician's index of suspicion. Combining PCR with serologic testing, repeat testing of the same pre-antimicrobial blood sample, and testing convalescent samples for seroconversion facilitates diagnosis. The prognosis can be excellent if appropriate antimicrobial therapy is begun in a timely fashion. It is well established that dogs are sentinels for infection in people in households and communities. Whether R. rickettsii causes illness in cats is not well established. The role of other spotted fever group rickettsia in causing illness in dogs and cats is being elucidated. Veterinarians should keep in mind that novel and well characterized species of SFG Rickettsia are important causes of emerging infectious disease. Veterinarians can play an important role in detecting, defining, and preventing illness in their canine patients and their human companions.

Hemotropic Mycoplasma   1319

Séverine Tasker

Hemoplasma infections are erythrocytic infections in both cats and dogs but are more common, and more often associated with disease, in cats. Mycoplasma haemofelis is the most pathogenic species in cats, causing hemolytic anemia and fever in immunocompetent hosts, whereas Mycoplasma haemocanis usually only results in hemolytic anemia in splenectomized or immunocompromised dogs. Diagnosis is by polymerase chain reaction on blood samples because cytology is unreliable. Prompt treatment of clinical disease with supportive care and at least 2 weeks of doxycycline is usually successful. Transmission pathways have not been confirmed, but indirect, via vectors, and direct via bites/fights/predation are likely.

Hepatozoonosis of Dogs and Cats   1341

Gad Baneth and Kelly Allen

Hepatozoon canis and Hepatozoon americanum are tick-borne infections of dogs transmitted by different tick species, with dissimilar geographic distributions, target organs, and clinical syndromes. H canis is transmitted mostly by the brown dog tick Rhipicephalus sanguineus sensu lato, affects hemolymphoid organs, is associated with anemia and other hematologic abnormalities, and is widely prevalent globally, whereas H americanum is transmitted by the Gulf Coast tick Amblyomma maculatum, causes severe myositis, and is an emerging parasite in the southern United States. Treatment of these 2 infections decreases the parasitic load without elimination. Domestic cats are infected with 3 Hepatozoon species.

Leishmaniasis   1359

Gad Baneth and Laia Solano-Gallego

Leishmaniasis caused by Leishmania infantum is an important zoonotic disease transmitted by sand flies with a high prevalence of infection in dogs and cats in regions whereby transmission occurs. Clinical disease is systemic with variable presenting signs and degrees of severity. It affects the skin, lymph nodes, eyes, bone marrow, kidneys, and other organs. The clinical findings in dogs and cats with L. infantum infection are generally similar. Subclinical infection of canines and felines in endemic areas is frequent. Long-term treatment of the disease with allopurinol, or combination of allopurinol with meglumine antimoniate or miltefosine, is needed, and clinical relapse is probable.

VETERINARY CLINICS OF NORTH AMERICA: SMALL ANIMAL PRACTICE

FORTHCOMING ISSUES

January 2023
Clinical Pathology
Maxey L. Wellman and M. Judith Radin, *Editors*

March 2023
Ophthalmology in Small Animal Care
Bruce Grahn, *Editor*

May 2023
Diabetes Mellitus in Cats and Dogs
Thomas K. Graves and Chen Gilor, *Editors*

RECENT ISSUES

September 2022
Telemedicine
Aaron Smiley, *Editor*

July 2022
Small Animal Orthopedic Medicine
Felix Duerr and Lindsay Elam, *Editors*

May 2022
Hot Topics in Small Animal Medicine
Lisa L. Powell, *Editor*

SERIES OF RELATED INTEREST

Advances in Small Animal Care
https://www.vetexotic.theclinics.com/
Veterinary Clinics: Exotic Animal Practice
https://www.vetexotic.theclinics.com/

THE CLINICS ARE NOW AVAILABLE ONLINE!
Access your subscription at:
www.theclinics.com

Preface

Changes

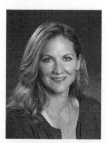

Linda Kidd, DVM, PhD, DACVIM
Editor

The geographic distribution and prevalence of vector-borne disease are changing. Changes in disease prevalence have resulted from shifts in the geographic distribution of vectors and global movement of dogs and people. Advances in molecular and other diagnostic techniques have increased our ability to detect and differentiate disease-causing agents. These and other factors have contributed to an increased recognition of vector-borne disease in the United States and other parts of the world. This issue of the *Veterinary Clinics of North America: Small Animal Practice* highlights changes in the distribution, diagnosis, and treatment of select "classic" vector-borne disease agents, such as *Ehrlichia*, *Anaplasma*, *Rickettsia*, and *Bartonella*. It also highlights those that are less well known to practitioners in some regions due to their previously restricted geographic distributions. It is important for clinicians in every region of North America (and beyond) to be familiar with the clinical and laboratory abnormalities associated with these organisms because their geographic distributions are expanding and because, like many vector-borne agents, their clinical manifestations mimic other disease. For example, schistosomiasis is an important differential for a dog with protein-losing enteropathy with heterogenous small intestinal wall layering and pinpoint hyperechoic foci in the bowel on ultrasound, and trypanosomiasis is a differential for a dog with dilated cardiomyopathy and arrhythmias. I hope that readers enjoy reading and learn as much as I did from this issue. The authors are thought-leaders in their fields, and, by writing these articles, it is my hope that the task of diagnosing and treating

Vet Clin Small Anim 52 (2022) xi–xii
https://doi.org/10.1016/j.cvsm.2022.08.004
0195-5616/22/© 2022 Published by Elsevier Inc.

these sometimes elusive infectious diseases will be more straightforward for busy practicing veterinarians.

Linda Kidd, DVM, PhD, DACVIM
Past Affiliation
Professor Small Animal Internal Medicine
Western University of Health Sciences
College of Veterinary Medicine
309 East Second Street
Pomona, CA 91766, USA

Present Affiliation
Veterinary Field Specialist Zoetis US Diagnostics

E-mail addresses:
lkidd@westernu.edu; linda.kidd@zoetis.com

How Changing Tick-Borne Disease Prevalence in Dogs Affects Diagnostic Testing

Linda Kidd, DVM, PhD*

KEYWORDS

- PCR • Serology • *Ehrlichia* • *Anaplasma* • *Rickettsia* • *Bartonella* • *Borrelia*
- *Babesia* • Hemotropic *Mycoplasma*

KEY POINTS

- The geographic distribution of ticks and tick-borne disease is changing.
- Awareness of the current distribution of ticks and tick-borne disease is essential to accurately prevent and diagnose disease in dogs.
- Coinfections from multiple organisms infecting ticks or exposure to more than one tick species are common and complicate diagnosis and treatment.
- Combining polymerase chain reaction (PCR) and serology and repeat testing using PCR and convalescent serologic testing can facilitate diagnosis.

INTRODUCTION

The geographic distribution and prevalence of tick-borne disease is changing. Changes in disease prevalence have resulted from shifting geographic distributions of tick vectors and global movement of dogs and people. In addition, improvement in molecular and other diagnostic techniques have increased our ability to detect well-known organisms, new species, and to determine that organisms thought to be nonpathogenic may cause disease in some individuals. Technological advances have also led to the discovery of coinfecting agents in ticks and hosts. These and other factors have likely contributed to an increased recognition of tick-borne disease in the United States and other parts of the world.

CHANGES IN TICK AND TICK-BORNE DISEASE PREVALENCE IN THE UNITED STATES
Ixodes spp

Historically, dogs in the Northeastern United States are commonly exposed to *Borrelia burgdorferi* and *Anaplasma phagocytophilum*, organisms that are transmitted by

Western University of Health Sciences, College of Veterinary Medicine, 309 East Second Street, Pomona, CA 91766, USA
* Corresponding author.
E-mail address: lindabkidd@gmail.com

Vet Clin Small Anim 52 (2022) 1153–1161
https://doi.org/10.1016/j.cvsm.2022.06.005
0195-5616/22/© 2022 Elsevier Inc. All rights reserved.

vetsmall.theclinics.com

Ixodes scapularis, which is endemic to the region. *I scapularis* and *Ixodes pacificus* also expose dogs in the upper Midwest and Northwestern United States, respectively, to these organisms. The geographic distribution of *Ixodes* ticks overall is expanding.[1] Accordingly, in recent years, the geographic distribution of seroprevalence of *A. phagocytophilum* and *B. burgdorferi* in dogs has also expanded.[2–4] That said, in some regional endemic areas, the seroprevalence of these organisms in dogs has declined, possibly due to the prevention and testing efforts by veterinarians.[4,5] A novel *Ehrlichia* species, *Ehrlichia muris*, thought to be transmitted by *I scapularis* has also been amplified from an ill dog in Minnesota.[6]

Amblyomma americanum

Amblyomma americanum is a tick vector for multiple organisms including *Ehrlichia chaffeensis* and *Ehrlichia ewingii*. *Ehrlichia ewingii* is the most seroprevalent *Ehrlichia* species in dogs in the United States.[3] The seroprevalence for *E. ewingii* and *E. chaffeensis* in dogs is highest in the Southern and Mid-Atlantic United States.[3] The geographic distribution of this tick is expanding and includes large portions of the South, Central, and Eastern United States (https://www.cdc.gov/ticks/maps/lone_star_tick.pdf).[7] This tick has also been implicated as a novel vector in the United States for *Rickettsia rickettsii*, the cause of rocky mountain spotted fever (RMSF) in a people.[8] Other spotted fever group *Rickettsia* associated with *Amblyomma* species have been recently amplified from dogs in the Southern United States.[9,10] In addition, infection with an *E ewingii*-like agent has been described in dogs in California.[11]

Rhipicephalus sanguineus

The geographic distribution of *Rhipicephalus sanguineus*, a tick that prefers dry, hot environments, is also expanding as are exposures to, and infections with the many organisms it carries. *Rhipicephalus sanguineus* is commonly found in the Southwest United States but overall, its distribution in the United States is considered ubiquitous (https://www.cdc.gov/ticks/maps/brown_dog_tick.pdf). *Rhipicephalus sanguineus* is a known or suspected vector for *E. canis*, *Babesia vogeli* (formerly *B. canis vogeli*), spotted fever group *Rickettsia*, *Bartonella* species, hemotropic *Mycoplasma*, *Anaplasma platys* and in some locales, *Hepatozoon canis*.[12–17] *Rickettsia rickettsii* provides an interesting example of changes in tick borne disease prevalence due to *Rh. sanguineus*. Historically, the geographic distribution of RMSF in people in the United States has primarily followed that of the tick vectors *Dermacentor variabilis* and *Dermacentor andersoni*. Accordingly, the area of highest prevalence of RMSF is the Southcentral and Southeastern United States. However, in the early 2000s, *Rh. sanguineus* caused a recent fatal outbreak of RMSF in people in a Native American community in a previously nonendemic area of Arizona. Retrospectively, it was shown that infection existed in the free roaming dog population before the fatal outbreak in people. *Rhipicephalus sanguineus* is also the primary vector of *R. rickettsii* in Mexico, and a recent outbreak in people in Mexicali Mexico, which borders southern California was also associated with this tick species and exposure to dogs. Southern California dogs living close to the border are more likely to be seropositive to spotted fever group *Rickettsia* than those living further from the border.[18]

Dogs with heavy exposure to *Rh. sanguineus* are infected with and exposed to other organisms for which *Rh. sanguineus* is the suspected or proven vector. For example, exposure to spotted fever group *Rickettsia* was demonstrated in more than 50% of dogs on a Hopi reservation in Arizona with heavy *Rh. sanguineus* infestation.[19] Active infection with *E. canis* was demonstrated in greater than 36% of dogs. Coinfections and coexposures also occurred (see later discussion). Infection with or exposure to

A. platys, *B. canis* (vogeli), and *Bartonella* species was also documented. Similarly, retired racing greyhounds, commonly exposed to *Rh. sanguineus* in racing kennels, are frequently exposed to *B. canis (vogeli)*, and infection with this organism is more common than in other breeds.[20–22] Exposure to *E. canis* has also historically been reported in retired racers.[21,23] Recently, we showed that healthy retired racing greyhounds were also exposed to *Bartonella* species and actively infected with hemotropic *Mycoplasma*.[24] It is important to note that for *Bartonella* and hemotropic *Mycoplasma*, flea exposure, and other means of transmission are thought to occur. *Rh. sanguineus* has also been implicated in transmitting novel species of vector-borne disease agents to dogs in the southwest United States. For example, a focal re-emergence of *Babesia conradae* and suspected illness due to *Rickettsia massiliae* in dogs in Los Angeles county have been reported.[25,26] *Rhipicephalus sanguineus* was considered as a possible vector in these outbreaks. In a separate study of *B. conradae* in coyote hunting greyhounds, aggressive interactions was considered a more likely means of transmission.[27]

Considered together, these studies suggest that *I. scapularis*, *A. americanum*, and *Rh. sanguineus* have contributed to an increased prevalence of well-known pathogens in endemic and expanding geographic locales, and they are likely responsible for infection with novel species as well.

THE IMPORTANCE OF COINFECTIONS

With advances in epidemiologic and molecular diagnostic tools, the high prevalence of coinfections with tick-borne disease agents has been increasingly recognized. Coinfections or coexposures to multiple agents are common in dogs with vector-borne disease.[28–32] Coinfections may affect the nature and severity of clinical signs, complicating the diagnostic process and potentially increasing morbidity in individual patients.[32,33] Unfortunately, one drug cannot treat all vector-borne disease agents. For example, although many rickettsial organisms including *Ehrlichia*, *Anaplasma*, and *Rickettsia* species are responsive to doxycycline therapy, other organisms that commonly infect dogs, including *Babesia* and *Bartonella* species, require alternate specific therapy. Similarly, appropriate antiprotozoal therapy differs depending on the infecting agent (*B. gibsoni* is treated differently than *B. vogeli*, for example), and most antiprotozoal treatment protocols would not clear infection with most rickettsial agents. To treat coinfections appropriately, they must be diagnosed. To diagnose them, clinicians must have a high index of suspicion that they are present and use diagnostic testing protocols that maximize sensitivity.

Diagnostic evidence of infection or exposure to one vector-borne disease agent should suggest to the clinician that a coinfection may be present, particularly if an appropriate response to therapy does not occur. Infection with more than one vector-borne organism may occur due to transmission of multiple organisms from a single coinfected vector, or transmission of multiple organisms from more than one vector of the same or different species. Ticks, fleas, and other vectors commonly carry more than one agent. As mentioned above, *Rh. sanguineus* is a known or suspected vector for *E. canis*, *B. vogeli*, spotted fever group *Rickettsia*, *Bartonella* species, hemotropic *Mycoplasma*, *A. platys*, and, in some locales, *H. canis*.[12–17] Single and coinfections with these agents occur in dogs with heavy exposure to this tick species.[19,29,31,32] Considered together, it can be said that dogs with exposure to *Rh. sanguineus* are commonly infected with multiple organisms known or suspected to be transmitted by this tick species.

Other ticks in the United States are also commonly coninfected with multiple agents. For example, *I. scapularis* and *I. pacificus* are well-known to transmit both

A. phagocytophilum and *B. burgdorferi* to people and dogs. In endemic areas, dogs are commonly seropositive to both *A. phagocytophilum* and *B. burgdorferi*. In fact, this was the most commonly documented coexposure in a recent large serosurvey of dogs in the United States.[28] Similarly, coinfections with *E. chaffeensis* and *E. ewingii* seem to occur commonly in dogs exposed to *A. americanum*, which carries both of these organisms.[34,35]

Recently, coinfections with *B. gibsoni* and another small babesia called *Babesia vulpus* were commonly found in pit bulls in the United States.[30] Hemotropic *Mycoplasma* were also common coinfecting agents. *Babesia conradae* and hemotropic *Mycoplasma* coinfections were common in greyhound mixes used for hunting coyotes in California.[27] As mentioned previously, evidence suggests that blood exposure during fighting and possibly vertical transmission may play a role in the transmission of these agents.[22,27]

Coexposures with the combinations of *Bartonella* and *Ehrlichia* spp, *Bartonella* and spotted fever group *Rickettsia*, *Bartonella* and *B. burgdorferi*, *Bartonella* and *Dirofilaria immitis*, and *Rickettsia* and *Ehrlichia* species also occur in dogs in the United states.[28,36] Triple coinfections with *E. canis*, *E. ewingii*, and *E. chaffeensis* likely resulting from the exposure to multiple vectors have also been documented.[31]

Although they occur frequently, coinfections can be difficult to diagnose in an individual patient due to limitations of both clinical reasoning and diagnostic testing. However, there are strategies that can be used to diagnose and treat them. Two common forms of bias in clinical reasoning that lead to diagnostic errors are premature closure and search satisfaction. These forms of bias may lead to a failure to recognize a coinfection in an individual patient. Picture a scenario where a serologic panel that tests for antibodies to *Ehrlichia* species, *Anaplasma* species, *B. burgdorferi*, and *D. immitis* antigen is run to determine whether vector-borne disease is contributing to thrombocytopenia in a dog. The dog is seropositive for *Ehrlichia* species and negative for the other agents. Given he is thrombocytopenic, you assume the antibody represents infection rather than previous exposure. You live in the Southwest United States where *Rh. sanguineus* is commonly found. Therefore, you assume the infecting *Ehrlichia* species is *E. canis* and treat appropriately with doxycycline. You also implement tick prevention measures. The thrombocytopenia improves initially with doxycycline therapy but then recurs. You assume that *E. canis* was resistant to doxycycline therapy and persistent infection with *E. canis* is causing the thrombocytopenia. The positive test for *Ehrlichia* species led to search satisfaction in this case and a failure to consider other possible differentials (premature closure). Knowledge about the possibility of coinfection with *B. vogeli* considering the probable exposure to *Rh. sanguineus* allows for consideration of this differential as a contributing cause of thrombocytopenia.

IMPLICATIONS FOR DIAGNOSTIC TESTING

Testing for tick-borne disease is important in patients with compatible clinical signs and laboratory abnormalities. These may include (but are not limited to) fever, myalgia, arthralgia, vasculitis, central nervous system signs, anemia, thrombocytopenia, proteinuria, and neutrophilic pleocytosis in joint fluid. Importantly, tick-borne infections are also associated with immune-mediated disease in dogs. Anti-red blood cell and antiplatelet antibodies occur in dogs infected with certain vector-borne disease agents.[37-41] Antinuclear antibodies and antineutrophil cytoplasmic antibodies also occur.[42,43] Furthermore, clinical and laboratory abnormalities caused by vector-borne diseases are essentially identical to those associated with idiopathic immune-mediated diseases such as immune-mediated hemolytic anemia (IMHA), immune thrombocytopenia (ITP), immune-mediated polyarthritis, or immune complex glomerulonephritis. Therefore, acute, or chronic infection with vector-borne (and other agents) should be considered in the differential diagnosis in patients with suspected immune-mediated disease. The implications of overlooking tick and other vector borne disease in patients with immune-mediated disease include failure to respond to immunosuppressive therapy, increased morbidity, and even death.

Cytologic examination of a blood smear is very important in these patients, to characterize anemia and thrombocytopenia, and on occasion, although less sensitive than polymerase chain reaction (PCR), organisms may be detected. "Tick panels" and "vector borne disease panels" offered by diagnostic laboratories or in-house test kits give clinicians the ability to test peripheral blood for multiple agents using serology, PCR, or a combination of the two. Panel choices are available on most major diagnostic laboratory websites and have recently been compiled in a review.[44] Choosing a panel requires the clinician to consider which organisms to test for, and which methodology (PCR and/or serology) to use. Diagnostic testing is not inexpensive. Being familiar with the epidemiology, including vector and disease prevalence, the clinical findings that are most commonly associated with each organism, and other risk factors such as breed and exposure risk, helps determine which agents should be included in a diagnostic panel.

Knowing which ticks are common in each geographic locale, and which organisms are transmitted by those ticks is very helpful. Useful epidemiologic information regarding tick distributions and vector-borne disease prevalence is available at the Companion Animal Parasite Councils website capcvet.org and Companion Vector Borne Disease website CVBD.org and CDC.gov. There are also helpful citizen science projects that share data about the prevalence and distribution of various tick species in the United States such as https://web.uri.edu/tickencounter/tickspotters/submit/ and https://www.showusyourticks.org/ and others.[45]

Because the overall prevalence of tick-borne disease is expanding, and the importance of coinfections is increasingly recognized, only considering classic geographic distributions of tick-borne disease, and failing to test for them outside these well-known geographic locales, may result in overlooking infection in patients. Therefore, comprehensive testing that includes multiple organisms should be considered in patients with clinical findings consistent with tick-borne disease, especially where another cause is not found, regardless of geographic locale. For example, Babesia species are not included in some diagnostic panels for tick-borne disease.[44] However, including testing for Babesia species should be considered even in a dog without breed or occupational exposure risk presenting with hemolytic anemia, suspected, ITP, or protein losing nephropathy given the expanding distribution of Rh. sanguineus, the discovery of Babesia species in other tick species, that some Babesia species are likely transmitted vertically and by other means, and compelling evidence that Babesia species cause these abnormalities.[37,41,46]

The sensitivity of serology as compared with PCR varies with characteristics of the host, the assays, and pathophysiologic characteristics of the organism. Concepts summarizing optimal diagnostic testing for specific vector-borne diseases to maximize sensitivity and identify coinfections have recently been summarized.[44] The bottom line is, comprehensive screening for multiple agents using panels that combine serology with PCR should be used to identify coinfections and maximize sensitivity (Fig. 1).[11,44,47] In addition to combining PCR with serology initially, repeat testing on the same or additional samples using PCR (before antimicrobial administration) can increase detection of organisms such as Rickettsia, Babesia, Ehrlichia, and Bartonella species and A. platys that can circulate in low numbers or intermittently.[11,44]

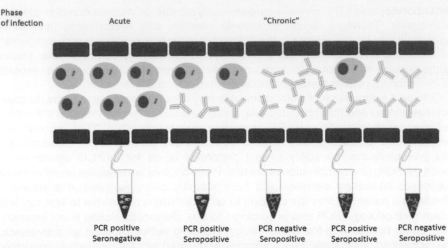

Fig. 1. Hypothetical results of PCR and serologic testing when blood is sampled at different times during infection with an organism that causes chronic infection and circulates intermittently in peripheral blood monocytes.[44] (Image copyrighted by L. Kidd. Basic shapes used in the making of this figure were purchased from and copyrighted by motifolio.com)

Convalescent serologic testing to document seroconversion can also be helpful to document acute infections, where patients may present before seroconversion and organisms are present in low numbers resulting in a negative PCR test.[44] More specialized and advanced testing for *Bartonella* species (BAPGM enrichment PCR) is often required to document infection with this organism (please see Chapter 002 of this edition).

SUMMARY

The expanding prevalence of well-known and novel tick-borne diseases necessitates an increased index of suspicion for a broad range of pathogens and the possibility of coinfection in patients with compatible clinical signs. Combined, comprehensive testing using both PCR and serology and repeat testing can help identify infection and likely improve outcomes, particularly in patients with suspected idiopathic immune-mediated disease.

CLINICS CARE POINTS

- Useful resources such as capcvet.org, cvbd.org, cdc.gov, https://web.uri.edu/tickencounter/tickspotters/submit/and https://www.showusyourticks.org/ are helpful ways to keep apprised of the distribution of ticks and tick-borne disease.

- Using comprehensive vector-borne disease diagnostic panels that combine serology and polymerase chain reaction (PCR), and repeat testing using PCR along with convalescent serologic testing increases diagnostic sensitivity for individual organisms and coinfections.

- Consider vector-borne disease in patients with suspected idiopathic immune-mediated disease.

- Consider coinfections or novel infections in dogs that do not respond to initial therapy or present with atypical clinical signs or laboratory abnormalities.

DISCLOSURE

Paid Speaker for Zoetis and IDEXX and Thought Leader for IDEXX laboratories. Currently employed by Zoetis.

REFERENCES

1. Eisen RJ, Eisen L, Beard CB. County-Scale Distribution of Ixodes scapularis and Ixodes pacificus (Acari: Ixodidae) in the Continental United States. J Med Entomol 2016;53:349–86.
2. Little SE, Beall MJ, Bowman DD, et al. Canine infection with Dirofilaria immitis, Borrelia burgdorferi, Anaplasma spp., and Ehrlichia spp. in the United States, 2010-2012. Parasit Vectors 2014;7:257.
3. Qurollo BA, Chandrashekar R, Hegarty BC, et al. A serological survey of tick-borne pathogens in dogs in North America and the Caribbean as assessed by Anaplasma phagocytophilum, A. platys, Ehrlichia canis, E. chaffeensis, E. ewingii, and Borrelia burgdorferi species-specific peptides. Infect Ecol Epidemiol 2014;4.
4. Little S, Braff J, Place J, et al. Canine infection with Dirofilaria immitis, Borrelia burgdorferi, Anaplasma spp., and Ehrlichia spp. in the United States, 2013-2019. Parasit Vectors 2021;14:10.
5. Dewage BG, Little S, Payton M, et al. Trends in canine seroprevalence to Borrelia burgdorferi and Anaplasma spp. in the eastern USA, 2010-2017. Parasit Vectors 2019;12:476.
6. Hegarty BC, Maggi RG, Koskinen P, et al. Ehrlichia muris infection in a dog from Minnesota. J Vet Intern Med 2012;26:1217–20.
7. Sagurova I, Ludwig A, Ogden NH, et al. Predicted Northward Expansion of the Geographic Range of the Tick Vector Amblyomma americanum in North America under Future Climate Conditions. Environ Health Perspect 2019;127:107014.
8. Breitschwerdt EB, Hegarty BC, Maggi RG, et al. Rickettsia rickettsii Transmission by a Lone Star Tick, North Carolina. Emerg Infect Dis 2011;17:873–5.
9. Barrett A, Little SE, Shaw E. Rickettsia amblyommii" and R. montanensis infection in dogs following natural exposure to ticks. Vector Borne Zoonotic Dis 2014; 14:20–5.
10. Grasperge BJ, Wolfson W, Macaluso KR. Rickettsia parkeri infection in domestic dogs, Southern Louisiana, USA, 2011. Emerg Infect Dis 2012;18:995–7.
11. Kidd L, Qurollo B, Lappin M, et al. Prevalence of Vector-Borne Pathogens in Southern California Dogs With Clinical and Laboratory Abnormalities Consistent With Immune-Mediated Disease. J Vet Intern Med 2017;31:1081–90.
12. Pappalardo BL, Correa MT, York CC, et al. Epidemiologic evaluation of the risk factors associated with exposure and seroreactivity to Bartonella vinsonii in dogs. Am J Vet Res 1997;58:467–71.
13. Abd Rani PA, Irwin PJ, Coleman GT, et al. A survey of canine tick-borne diseases in India. Parasit Vectors 2011;4:141.
14. Aktas M, Ozubek S. Molecular evidence for trans-stadial transmission of Anaplasma platys by Rhipicephalus sanguineus sensu lato under field conditions. Med Vet Entomol 2018;32:78–83.
15. Seneviratna P, Weerasinghe Ariyadasa S. Transmission of Haemobartonella canis by the dog tick, Rhipicephalus sanguineus. Res Vet Sci 1973;14:112–4.
16. Wikswo ME, Hu R, Metzger ME, et al. Detection of Rickettsia rickettsii and Bartonella henselae in Rhipicephalus sanguineus ticks from California. J Med Entomol 2007;44:158–62.

17. Baneth G. Perspectives on canine and feline hepatozoonosis. Vet Parasitol 2011; 181:3–11.

18. Estrada I, Balagot C, Fierro M, et al. Spotted fever group rickettsiae canine serosurveillance near the US-Mexico border in California. Zoonoses Public Health 2020;67:148–55.

19. Diniz PP, Beall MJ, Omark K, et al. High prevalence of tick-borne pathogens in dogs from an Indian reservation in northeastern Arizona. Vector Borne Zoonotic Dis 2010;10:117–23.

20. Taboada J, Harvey JW, Levy MG, et al. Seroprevalence of babesiosis in Greyhounds in Florida. J Am Vet Med Assoc 1992;200:47–50.

21. Breitschwerdt EB, Malone JB, MacWilliams P, et al. Babesiosis in the Greyhound. J Am Vet Med Assoc 1983;182:978–82.

22. Birkenheuer AJ, Correa MT, Levy MG, et al. Geographic distribution of babesiosis among dogs in the United States and association with dog bites: 150 cases (2000-2003). J Am Vet Med Assoc 2005;227:942–7.

23. Tzipory N, Crawford PC, Levy JK. Prevalence of Dirofilaria immitis, Ehrlichia canis, and Borrelia burgdorferi in pet dogs, racing greyhounds, and shelter dogs in Florida. Vet Parasitol 2010;171:136–9.

24. Kidd L, Hamilton H, Stine L, Qurollo B, Breitschwerdt EBB. Vector-borne disease and its relationship to hematologic abnormalities and microalbuminuria in retired racing and show-bred greyhounds. J Vet Intern Med 2022;36(4):1287–94.

25. Beeler E, Abramowicz KF, Zambrano ML, et al. A focus of dogs and Rickettsia massiliae-infected Rhipicephalus sanguineus in California. Am J Trop Med Hyg 2011;84:244–9.

26. Di Cicco MF, Downey ME, Beeler E, et al. Re-emergence of Babesia conradae and effective treatment of infected dogs with atovaquone and azithromycin. Vet Parasitol 2012;187:23–7.

27. Dear JD, Owens SD, Lindsay LL, et al. Babesia conradae infection in coyote hunting dogs infected with multiple blood-borne pathogens. J Vet Intern Med 2018; 32:1609–17.

28. Yancey CB, Hegarty BC, Qurollo BA, et al. Regional seroreactivity and vector-borne disease co-exposures in dogs in the United States from 2004-2010: utility of canine surveillance. Vector Borne Zoonotic Dis 2014;14:724–32.

29. Baneth G, Harrus S, Gal A, et al. Canine vector-borne co-infections: Ehrlichia canis and Hepatozoon canis in the same host monocytes. Vet Parasitol 2015; 208:30–4.

30. Barash NR, Thomas B, Birkenheuer AJ, et al. Prevalence of Babesia spp. and clinical characteristics of Babesia vulpes infections in North American dogs. J Vet Intern Med 2019;33(5):2075–81.

31. Kordick SK, Breitschwerdt EB, Hegarty BC, et al. Coinfection with multiple tick-borne pathogens in a Walker Hound kennel in North Carolina. J Clin Microbiol 1999;37:2631–8.

32. de Caprariis D, Dantas-Torres F, Capelli G, et al. Evolution of clinical, haematological and biochemical findings in young dogs naturally infected by vector-borne pathogens. Vet Microbiol 2011;149:206–12.

33. De Tommasi AS, Otranto D, Dantas-Torres F, et al. Are vector-borne pathogen co-infections complicating the clinical presentation in dogs? Parasit Vectors 2013; 6:97.

34. Starkey LA, Barrett AW, Chandrashekar R, et al. Development of antibodies to and PCR detection of Ehrlichia spp. in dogs following natural tick exposure. Vet Microbiol 2014;173:379–84.

35. Starkey LA, Barrett AW, Beall MJ, et al. Persistent Ehrlichia ewingii infection in dogs after natural tick infestation. J Vet Intern Med 2015;29:552–5.

36. Lashnits E, Correa M, Hegarty BC, et al. Bartonella Seroepidemiology in Dogs from North America, 2008-2014. J Vet Intern Med 2018;32:222–31.

37. Garden OA, Kidd L, Mexas AM, et al. ACVIM consensus statement on the diagnosis of immune-mediated hemolytic anemia in dogs and cats. J Vet Intern Med 2019;33:313–34.

38. Grindem CB, Breitschwerdt EB, Perkins PC, et al. Platelet-associated immunoglobulin (antiplatelet antibody) in canine Rocky Mountain spotted fever and ehrlichiosis. J Am Anim Hosp Assoc 1999;35:56–61.

39. Bexfield NH, Villiers EJ, Herrtage ME. Immune-mediated haemolytic anaemia and thrombocytopenia associated with Anaplasma phagocytophilum in a dog. J Small Anim Pract 2005;46:543–8.

40. Cortese L, Terrazzano G, Piantedosi D, et al. Prevalence of anti-platelet antibodies in dogs naturally co-infected by Leishmania infantum and Ehrlichia canis. Vet J 2011;188:118–21.

41. Matsuu A, Kawabe A, Koshida Y, et al. Incidence of canine Babesia gibsoni infection and subclinical infection among Tosa dogs in Aomori Prefecture, Japan. J Vet Med Sci 2004;66:893–7.

42. Smith BE, Tompkins MB, Breitschwerdt EB. Antinuclear antibodies can be detected in dog sera reactive to Bartonella vinsonii subsp. berkhoffii, Ehrlichia canis, or Leishmania infantum antigens. J Vet Intern Med 2004;18:47–51.

43. Vercellone J, Cohen L, Mansuri S, et al. Bartonella Endocarditis Mimicking Crescentic Glomerulonephritis with PR3-ANCA Positivity. Case Rep Nephrol 2018; 2018:9607582.

44. Kidd L. Optimal Vector-borne Disease Screening in Dogs Using Both Serology-based and Polymerase Chain Reaction-based Diagnostic Panels. Vet Clin North Am Small Anim Pract 2019;49:703–18.

45. Nieto NC, Porter WT, Wachara JC, et al. Using citizen science to describe the prevalence and distribution of tick bite and exposure to tick-borne diseases in the United States. PLoS One 2018;13:e0199644.

46. Ullal T, Birkenheuer A, Vaden S. Azotemia and Proteinuria in Dogs Infected with Babesia gibsoni. J Am Anim Hosp Assoc 2018;54:156–60.

47. Maggi RG, Birkenheuer AJ, Hegarty BC, et al. Comparison of serological and molecular panels for diagnosis of vector-borne diseases in dogs. Parasit Vectors 2014;7:127.

Bartonellosis in Dogs and Cats, an Update

Rachel Taber, DVM[a], Anne Pankowski, BS[b], Allison L. Ludwig, BS[c,d],
Maggie Jensen, BSE[b], Veronica Magsamen, BS[b],
Erin Lashnits, MS, DVM, PhD, DACVIM (SAIM)[e,*]

KEYWORDS

• Bartonella • Bartonellosis • Culture-negative endocarditis • Vector borne disease

KEY POINTS

• *Bartonella henselae* is transmitted by inoculation of infected flea feces into a disrupted skin barrier. Transmission routes for other zoonotic *Bartonella* spp are less clearly defined.

• Bartonellosis in dogs can manifest as culture-negative endocarditis, vascular proliferative lesions, and granulomatous or pyogranulomatous disease. Cats are often asymptomatic but can present similarly to dogs.

• Dogs and cats showing clinical signs should be treated with a combination of antibiotics for a prolonged course of 4 to 6 weeks. Monitoring for resolution of clinical signs and bacteremia/seroreactivity during and after treatment is recommended.

• Routine year-round flea and tick prevention is important to prevent *Bartonella* spp infection in dogs and cats and to prevent zoonotic transmission.

INTRODUCTION

Bartonella spp are emerging zoonotic pathogens with worldwide distribution that cause multisystemic disease in dogs, cats, and humans. The *Bartonella* genus is best known for *Bartonella henselae*, the causative agent of cat scratch disease. Members of the genus *Bartonella* are generally transmitted by arthropod vectors. There are more than 40 named species within the genus, at least 17 of which are associated with human and/or animal disease.

A. Pankowski and R. Taber contributed equally.
[a] Michigan State University Veterinary Medical Center, 736 Wilson Road, East Lansing, MI 48824, USA; [b] School of Veterinary Medicine, University of Wisconsin-Madison, 2015 Linden Drive, Madison, WI 53706, USA; [c] Department of Comparative Biomedical Sciences, School of Veterinary Medicine, University of Wisconsin-Madison, 2015 Linden Drive, Madison, WI 53706, USA; [d] Waisman Center, 1500 Highland Avenue, Madison, WI 53705, USA; [e] Department of Medical Sciences, School of Veterinary Medicine, University of Wisconsin-Madison, 2015 Linden Drive, Madison, WI 53706, USA
* Corresponding author.
E-mail address: lashnits@wisc.edu

Vet Clin Small Anim 52 (2022) 1163–1192
https://doi.org/10.1016/j.cvsm.2022.06.006
0195-5616/22/© 2022 Elsevier Inc. All rights reserved.

Chronic bartonellosis in humans is an active area of research, and veterinary species will benefit from this growing research interest. This review summarizes key advances in knowledge about transmission, clinical manifestations, diagnosis, and treatment of bartonellosis in dogs and cats. Although major funding for research is generally lacking, the number of studies of bartonellosis in dogs has increased exponentially since its discovery as a canine pathogen in 1993.[1] Despite the wealth of publications, the majority are case reports that provide limited evidence to guide clinical recommendations.[2]

The ecology and epidemiology of *Bartonella* spp—including reservoir hosts and vectors—vary geographically. Although infection with *Bartonella* spp is a global public health concern, this review focuses primarily on bartonellosis in the United States. To the extent possible, the goal of this review is to distill recent and historical research into clinically relevant recommendations for veterinarians in small animal practice.

BACTERIOLOGY AND PATHOGENESIS

Bartonella spp are gram-negative, rod-shaped alphaproteobacteria.[3] These facultative intracellular pathogens are fastidious, with a slow division time of approximately 24 hours.[4]

As with other vector-borne diseases, *Bartonella* spp are harbored in reservoir hosts but they can also infect incidental hosts. Reservoir hosts maintain the pathogen and serve as a source of infection, whereas incidental hosts do not serve as a source of infection and often show significant clinical signs when infected. Each *Bartonella* sp has coevolved with a specific mammalian reservoir host and arthropod vector, creating unique, often geographically distinct, transmission dynamics, ecology, and epidemiology (as reviewed elsewhere).[5–8] Because of this ecological diversity, for many *Bartonella* spp transmission details remain unknown; however, transmission among cats (reservoir hosts) and to humans (incidental hosts) is well understood for *B. henselae* (**Fig. 1**).[7] The typical course of bartonellosis in the reservoir host has been described in multiple animal models,[9] including *Bartonella tribocorum* in rats,[10] *Bartonella birtlesii* in mice,[11–13] and *B. henselae* in cats.[14] The pathophysiology seems similar across species, suggesting parallel coevolutionary adaptation. It has proven difficult to generate clinically relevant animal models using incidental hosts, despite attempts to induce *B. henselae* infection and disease in mice,[15,16] dogs,[17] and ferrets (Lashnits, unpublished data, 2019).

Immediately after initial inoculation into the reservoir host by the vector, *Bartonella* spp are not detectable in the bloodstream,[10] indicating that the bacteria colonize an unknown "primary niche."[18] Although no conclusive evidence yet exists to confirm the specific cellular localization of this primary niche, there are extensive data supporting the hypothesis that *Bartonella* spp infect vascular endothelial cells before their extracellular release into the bloodstream and subsequent infection of erythrocytes.[19] Within the vascular endothelial cells, *Bartonella* reside in membrane-bound intracellular compartments and are apparently released intermittently because they periodically appear within circulating erythrocytes.[18] In addition to vascular endothelial cells, other cell types are likely involved. Because the bacteria have to reach the vasculature after intradermal inoculation, it has been proposed that migratory cells such as lymphocytes or mononuclear cells that travel from the dermis through the lymphatics to the bloodstream and tissues play a role.[19] Progenitor cells within the bone marrow have also been proposed as primary niches.[19] Regardless of the cell type of the primary niche, on invasion of erythrocytes, *Bartonella* spp initially replicate. They then continue to survive without replicating for the life span of the cell, inducing only subtle membrane changes, thereby avoiding early removal.

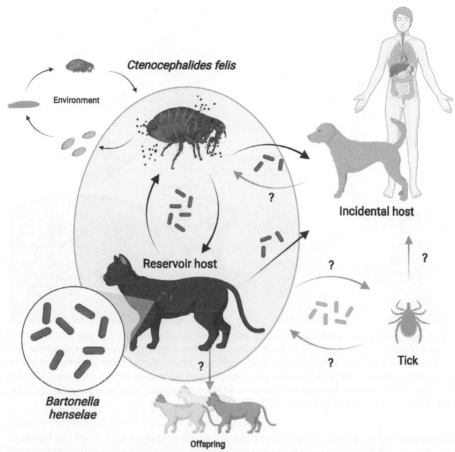

Fig. 1. *Bartonella henselae* transmission. *B. henselae* persists in cats as the primary reservoir host with transmission largely facilitated by *Ctenocephalides felis* between cats and incidental hosts. Ticks and possibly vertical transmission may contribute to spread of *B. henselae*.

Immune System Evasion and Virulence Factors

Bartonella spp have developed many well-conserved adaptations to avoid detection by the innate and adaptive arms of the immune system, as summarized in **Fig. 2**. For example, a unique lipopolysaccharide (LPS) structure antagonizes TLR4 on phagocytic cells rather than activating them, thereby disrupting inflammatory cytokine production, inflammatory cell recruitment, and the link between innate and adaptive immunity that results in B cell activation and antibody production.[3] Similarly, a unique flagellin protein may escape TLR5 recognition by phagocytes. Decreased polymorphonuclear cell activation may also contribute to the bacteria's ability to avoid phagocytosis.[20] In addition, the distinct structures of LPS and BadA, a trimeric autotransporter adhesin (TAA), may help avoid complement activation.[18,19,21,22]

The ability to survive intracellularly is also key to the ability of *Bartonella* spp to evade the immune system and to their pathogenesis. To enter cells in the reservoir host, bacteria first aggregate on cellular surfaces, and they are then internalized into cells via invasome-mediated entry (see **Fig. 2**).[23–26] Other adhesins and outer

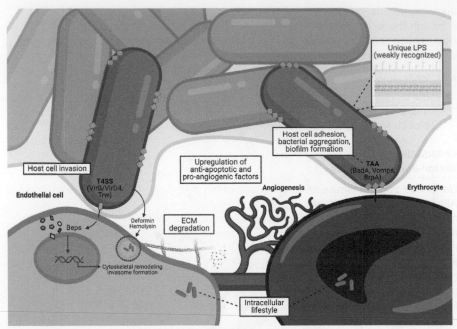

Fig. 2. *Bartonella* spp virulence factors and pathogenesis. *Bartonella* spp have evolved various virulence factors to aid in host immune system evasion, intracellular colonization, biofilm formation, and angiogenesis. Although this figure shows colonization of erythrocytes and endothelial cells, *Bartonella* spp colonize and aggregate on a multitude of diverse cell types. Beps, Bartonella effector proteins; ECM, extracellular matrix; LPS, lipopolysaccharide; TAA, Trimeric autotransporter adhesin.

membrane proteins contribute to host cell adhesion and degradation of the extracellular matrix, facilitating intracellular colonization.

Two major categories of *Bartonella* spp virulence factors that have been studied extensively in vitro include Type IV secretion systems (T4SS) and the TAAs (see **Fig. 2**).[18,19,27–31] T4SS enable translocation of *Bartonella* effector proteins within host cells to interrupt cell signaling and allow pathogen entry.[18] Although TAAs vary in size, sequence, and copy number, all *Bartonella* spp contain at least one TAA gene. BadA, the TAA of *B henselae*, was first described in the 1990s and is the most well-studied among *Bartonella* spp virulence factors; TAA variability may explain the differences in virulence among different species/strains.[18] BadA mediates bacterial autoaggregation on the surface of erythrocytes and promotes biofilm formation, which enables persistence in the host despite antibiotic therapy, and contributes to heart valve vegetations.[32–34] Thus, the degree of BadA expression may contribute to the ineffectiveness of antibiotic treatment[33,35–39] and disease pathogenesis. TAAs also partially mediate binding to erythrocytes and extracellular matrix proteins as well as invasion of, and survival within macrophages, monocytes, epithelial cells, and, perhaps most importantly in the context of pathogenesis, endothelial cells.[8,18,28,40]

In some individual hosts, invasion of endothelial cells by *Bartonella* spp results in the increasingly recognized pathologic conditions of vascular proliferation and vascular tumor formation.[41] Mechanistically, *Bartonella* spp stimulate angiogenesis through vascular endothelial growth factor (VEGF)-VEGFR2 signaling, inhibition of endothelial cell apoptosis, and reprogramming of myeloid cells.[29,41–46] Within infected cells, angiogenesis is partially controlled by BadA and HIF-1 gene expression,[38,47–50] although the exact mechanisms are not yet well characterized. It has also recently been recognized that VEGFR2-mediated angiogenesis can also be stimulated in distant, uninfected cells via a secreted factor, BafA.[40]

Key Takeaways

- *Bartonella* spp have adapted a multitude of virulence factors to aid in host immune system evasion, maintaining an intracellular lifestyle, angiogenesis, and biofilm formation.

TRANSMISSION
Vector-Borne Transmission

Bartonella spp transmission is classically associated with biting arthropod vectors. Although the specific details of transmission remain unknown for most zoonotic *Bartonella* spp, transmission of *B. henselae* is predominantly via *Ctenocephalides felis*, the cat flea (see **Fig. 1**). Experimental studies in cats show no evidence of transmission in the absence of fleas, suggesting that *B. henselae* transmission is almost exclusively flea-dependent.[51,52] Fleas ingest bacteria from infected cats during blood feeding; bacteria remain viable within the flea gastrointestinal tract, and once defecated, bacteria remain infectious for at least 9 days (longer time periods have not been studied).[53] New cats are then infected via inoculation of flea feces through a disrupted skin barrier, either from scratching, other trauma, or the flea bite itself.[53–55] Similarly, humans also become infected with *B. henselae* through inoculation of flea feces in breaks in the skin barrier, eponymously due to cat scratches, although inoculation may also occur due to any other disruptions to the dermal barrier.[53,54] Although there are no studies evaluating the role of fleas in transmission of *B. henselae* to dogs, because dogs and humans are both incidental hosts, it is assumed they can become infected in the same flea-dependent manner.[7,8]

Tick-borne transmission of *Bartonella* spp is more controversial, and reviews remain skeptical of tick transmission in humans, dogs, and cats.[56,57] However, evidence exists to support ticks as a vector for several *Bartonella* spp.[5,7,8,58] Multiple tick species found on cats and dogs in the United States, including certain *Ixodes* spp, *Rhipicephalus sanguineus*, and *Dermacentor* spp have all been shown to harbor *Bartonella* spp DNA.[7,58,59] More than 10% of *Ixodes* spp ticks collected in North Carolina and 19% of *Ixodes pacificus* ticks collected in California were found to carry *Bartonella* spp DNA.[59,60] Case reports of human bartonellosis with recent tick exposure and without cat contact further support potential tick transmission.[7,58] In addition, *R. sanguineus*[61] and *Ixodes ricinus*[62,63] have been experimentally proven to be competent vectors of *B. henselae* in artificial feeding systems, and *B. henselae* bacteremia can be induced in cats inoculated with infected *I. ricinus* salivary glands.[63] Given existing evidence, it is prudent to assume that *Ixodes* spp, *Dermacentor* spp, and *R. sanguineus* ticks may be a source of *B. henselae* in dogs and cats, although the extent that tick transmission contributes to the burden of natural infection remains unclear.

Nonvector-Borne Transmission

Although *Bartonella* spp are predominantly vector-borne, several other modes of transmission have also been proposed, including blood transfusion[64,65] and direct inoculation.[64,66,67] Indeed, 2 case reports have linked bartonellosis in veterinarians with needle stick injuries.[66,67] Although vertical transmission has been suggested in several reservoir species, including rodents[68] and cats,[69,70] as well as in incidental hosts,[71,72] horizontal and sexual transmission have not been documented to date.[51,52]

Key Takeaways

- Fleas are the main vector of *B. henselae* transmission, although evidence exists for transmission via tick vectors as well as direct inoculation and blood transfusions. Transmission for other *Bartonella* spp. affecting dogs are cats is not as well-described.

CLINICAL MANIFESTATIONS

The type and severity of bartonellosis varies widely between infected patients for reasons currently unknown but likely attributable to pathogen virulence factors and characteristics of the infected individual. Disease can range from subclinical to severe and/or fatal, the latter occurring particularly with disseminated systemic infection, endocarditis, or infections complicated by immunosuppression or coinfection.

Dogs

Bartonella henselae and *Bartonella vinsonii* subsp. *berkhoffii* are the most common pathologic species in dogs, although exposure to, and infection with these species can also be detected in dogs without clinical abnormalities.[73,74] *Bartonella rochalimae*, *Bartonella clarridgeiae*, *Bartonella koehlerae*, and *Bartonella quintana* are occasionally reported in dogs, usually as a cause of endocarditis. Risk factors associated with exposure to *Bartonella* spp in dogs seem to be mainly related to vector ecology and the potential for flea and tick exposure.[75–77]

The most common manifestations of bartonellosis in dogs include endocarditis, vascular proliferative lesions, and granulomatous or pyogranulomatous disease. A wide range of other nonspecific or less common clinical signs have also been reported, including systemic febrile illness, neurologic disease, and splenic or hepatosplenic abnormalities (**Table 1**). *Bartonella* spp infections have also been associated with immune-mediated diseases including hemolytic anemia, thrombocytopenia, polyarthritis, and immune complex glomerulonephritis.[78,82,89,124,125]

Bartonella spp are responsible for 20% to 30% of culture-negative endocarditis in dogs.[79,82,84,87,89,124–127] In one study, *Bartonella* spp would have been missed as the causative organism in more than 25% of endocarditis cases using only standard blood cultures.[89] Vegetative lesions are most commonly seen on the aortic valve but the mitral valve can also be affected.[82,124] The classic presentation of *Bartonella* spp endocarditis in dogs is a new onset of heart murmur and fever, and evidence of inflammatory disease including systemic inflammatory response syndrome or sepsis. Late stages may also have evidence of congestive heart failure.[82,87,89,124,128,129] Complications of *Bartonella* spp endocarditis include thromboembolic disease, neutrophilic polyarthritis, neurologic complications, renal injury, or immune-complex glomerulonephritis. Clinical and laboratory findings associated with these complications may indeed be presenting complaints.[82,84,89] Myocarditis has also been associated with bartonellosis, although not all endocarditis cases have concurrent myocarditis.[80,124,128]

Bartonella spp can induce vascular proliferative lesions and vasculitis, presumably due to interactions with and/or infection of vascular endothelial cells.[18,29,40] The most well-described vascular proliferative diseases in people include verruga peruana caused by *Bartonella bacilliformis* and, in immunocompromised patients, *B. henselae*-induced bacillary angiomatosis and peliosis hepatis.[130–132] *Bartonella* spp-induced vasculitis, particularly vasculitis associated with endocarditis and/or neurologic manifestations, is increasingly reported in the human literature.[133,134] Similarly, multiple case reports document amplification of *Bartonella* spp DNA from various vascular

Table 1
Clinical manifestations of bartonellosis in dogs and cats reported in the United States

Symptom	Specifics	Species	Location	Other Species
Dogs				
Endocarditis	Highly vegetative lesions with accompanying calcification, and in most cases high antibody titers[78]	B. henselae[79–81] B. vinsonii subsp. berkhoffii[78,81–83,128] B. clarridgeiae[78,84] B. washoensis[85] B. quintana[78,86] B. rochalimae[82,87] B. koehlerae[79,82,88]	CA[78,89] CO[81] WY[81] VA[87] NC[87] TX[83,87] FL[87] NY[80]	Humans, cats, cows, pumas, sea otters[32,78]
Granulomatous/ pyogranulomatous disease	Lymphadenitis, hepatosplenic, cutaneous; other multifocal/ systemic locations[90]	B. henselae[51–94,80] B. vinsonii subsp. berkhoffii[90,91]	MA[92] MN[92] PA[94] VA[91] NC[90] MT[93]	Humans, cats
Vascular proliferative lesions or vasculitis	Hemangiopericytoma,[29,95] bacillary angiomatosis,[96] peliosis hepatis,[80,135–137] vasculitis,[29] possibly hemangiosarcoma[98,99]	B. vinsonii subsp. berkhoffii[29,95,98] B. henselae[29,97–99,135,136] B. quintana[99] B. koehlerae[98,99]	NC[95,98,99] IL[97] MA, WI, CA, MI, MO, OH, TN, CO[99]	Humans,[95] cats, horses, cows, red wolves[29]
Neurologic disease	Seizures, recumbency, ataxia, paraparesis,[100–102] granulomatous meningoencephalitis,[103] meningoradiculoneuritis[104]	B. vinsonii subsp. berkhoffii[104,100,101] B. rochalimae[87]	NC[87,100,101] VA[87] TX[87] FL[87]	Humans, cats
Cats				
Asymptomatic	No obvious symptoms with chronic or recurrent bacteremia (months to years)[64,105,106]	B. henselae[64,106–108,14] B. clarridgeiae[108] B. koehlerae[111]	NC[105] IN, TX, KS, CA,[106] OK, VA,[105] (experimental)[14,64,107,111]	Humans, dogs

(continued on next page)

Table 1
(continued)

Symptom	Specifics	Species	Location	Other Species
Endocarditis/myocarditis	Blood culture-negative endocarditis, endomyocarditis with left ventricular endocardial fibrosis,[113] pyogranulomatous myocarditis[114]	B. henselae[113,114,115] B. koehlerae[113] B. vinsonii subsp. berkhoffii[113]	CA[115] NY[113] NC, FL[113,114,116]	Humans, dogs, cows, pumas, sea otters[32,78]
Fever	Can be seen with or without other clinical signs	B. henselae[117] B. clarridgeiae[110]	NC[112,117] CA[115]	Humans, dogs
Lymphadenopathy	Local or generalized (often begins near site of inoculation) necrotizing granulomas, granulomatous lymphadenitis[114,117]	B. henselae[114,117] B. clarridgeiae[117]	NC[114,117]	Humans, dogs
Neurologic disease	Various manifestations[117–119]	B. henselae[117–119] B. clarridgeiae[117]	NC[117,118] CO[119]	Humans, dogs
Ocular disease	Anterior uveitis, [120,121] chorioretinitis[118]	B. henselae[118,120,121]	AL[121] CO[120] NC[118]	Humans, dogs
Orthopedic or joint disease	Osteomyelitis, [122,123]	B. vinsonii subsp. berkhoffii[122]	NC[122]	Humans
Reproductive failure	Male and female cats[70]	B. henselae[70]	IN, TX, KS (experimental)[70]	Humans, [71] horses[72]

Bold text indicates manifestations with higher levels of evidence to support an association with *Bartonella* spp infection. Locations reported may reflect publication bias by research groups interested in investigating bartonellosis in dogs and cats.

lesions of dogs: *B. vinsonii* subsp. *berkhoffii* in cases of hemangiopericytoma[95] and bacillary angiomatosis,[96] and *B. henselae* in peliosis hepatis[97] and systemic or localized vasculitis.[100,135–137] In one case report[96] a dog that developed bacillary angiomatosis due to *B. vinsonii* subsp. *berkhoffii* was immunosuppressed, but vascular proliferative lesions have also been reported in association with *B. vinsonii* subsp. *berkhoffii* infection in an apparently immunocompetent dog.[95] In addition, bartonellosis has been documented in up to 70% of dogs with hemangiosarcoma,[98,99,138] although further research is needed to determine if a hemangiosarcoma is indeed caused by *Bartonella* spp in some patients. Vasculitis has also been reported in multiple dogs with bartonellosis,[80,135,136] and one study documented evidence of *B. henselae* infection in 15% of dogs with pleural or peritoneal effusions.[139]

As with many intracellular infections, bartonellosis is associated with granulomatous and pyogranulomatous lesions, particularly lymphadenitis and hepatosplenic disease.[90–93,140,141] In one illustrative case of bartonellosis there were granulomatous to pyogranulomatous lesions in the salivary glands, lungs, mediastinum, hilar lymph node, and heart, with multifocal histopathologic involvement of the liver, kidneys, omentum, and spleen.[91] Bartonellosis is thus an important differential diagnosis to consider in dogs with unexplained granulomatous or pyogranulomatous inflammation, particularly in cases of lymphadenitis or hepatosplenic disease.

Although only sporadically documented in canine case reports thus far, central nervous system (CNS) manifestations of bartonellosis are increasingly appreciated in people.[142–145] In dogs, bartonellosis has been diagnosed in association with meningoradiculoneuritis, meningoencephalitis, meningitis, and myelitis.[100–102,104] Interestingly, dermatitis or panniculitis have also been reported in some dogs with CNS signs presumably due to bartonellosis, and human neurobartonellosis cases also often present with cutaneous manifestations.[102,104,145] Granulomatous or vasculitic lesions in the CNS may be a more common cause of CNS disease in dogs than is currently appreciated, particularly because of the difficulty of diagnosing neurobartonellosis.[103]

In summary, clinicians should test for bartonellosis in dogs with evidence of endocarditis, lymphadenitis, or other granulomatous or pyogranulomatous lesions (particularly in the liver or spleen). Other clinical manifestations of bartonellosis have been more rarely reported in dogs but *Bartonella* spp testing should also be considered as part of a complete workup of patients with immune-mediated disease, hypercalcemia (in association with granulomatous disease), idiopathic effusions (particularly chylothorax or other vasculitides), fever of unknown origin, or other nonspecific systemic disease consistent with a vector-borne cause. Higher consideration should be given to bartonellosis in dogs with risk factors for exposure, including history of flea infestation, tick bites, and a history of exposure to or infection with other vector-borne diseases.

Cats

Bartonellosis in cats can be more difficult to study because cats are the reservoir host for multiple *Bartonella* spp including *B. henselae*, *B. clarridgeiae*, and *B. koehlerae*.[146–148] Infections with species other than *B. henselae* and *B. clarridgeiae* are rarely reported; however, *B. quintana*, *B. vinsonii* subsp. *berkhoffii*, and *Bartonella bovis* (previously *Bartonella weissii*) have been isolated from cats as incidental hosts.[108–111,149–152] This is important to consider clinically and diagnostically because cats infected with *Bartonella* spp for which they are not reservoir hosts seem to experience more severe symptoms.[8]

Bartonella henselae is most thoroughly studied in cats, where bacteremia can persist or recur for more than a year in some cases but in others it can be self-limiting.[64,105,106] The duration and recurrence of bacteremia seems to depend at least partially on reexposure to vectors but experimentally bacteremia recurs every 1 to 4.5 months.[107,108,110,111,117] The prevalence of bacteremia is variable depending on the cat population tested, ranging from less than 1% in healthy indoor owned adult cats[107] to nearly 70% in young adult cats with abundant vector exposure.[153] Although risk factors for infection have not been extensively studied, it seems that cats residing in warm, humid climates conducive to year-round flea survival are at greater risk of exposure to, and infection with, B. henselae,[110,152,154,155] particularly in cats that spend time outdoors without flea and tick preventatives.[108,149,155] Although there do seem to be geographic differences in exposure to Bartonella spp for cats (similar to those in dogs), it is estimated that 20% to 30% of cats across the United States are seroreactive to one or more of the 3 cat-adapted Bartonella spp.

It is currently unclear exactly why some cats remain asymptomatic while others develop illness related to bartonellosis, but is likely influenced by both host and pathogen factors; the range of clinical manifestations of bartonellosis is shown in **Table 1**.[156] Similar to dogs and humans, cats with bartonellosis may have cardiac manifestations. Several Bartonella spp have been associated with endocarditis and myocarditis in cats,[113,114,117,150–152,157] and bartonellosis is thought to be an underlying cause of feline endomyocarditis/left ventricular endocardial fibrosis syndrome.[113] In a recent case-control study, 50% of cats with this syndrome had evidence of bartonellosis compared with only 8% of control cats with hypertrophic cardiomyopathy.[113]

In addition to cardiovascular disease, other systemic manifestations of bartonellosis in cats have been proposed. Bartonella spp should be a differential for fever of unknown origin in cats, particularly if other common causes have been ruled out and/ or the cat has a known history of exposure to fleas.[158] Experimental studies have demonstrated acute clinical signs on inoculation of certain Bartonella spp and strains, including fever, lymphadenopathy, lethargy, and anorexia.[159,160] Laboratory abnormalities, if present, are often nonspecific, and include hyperglobulinemia, eosinophilia, neutropenia, anemia, or thrombocytopenia.[78,117,151,161] There can also be histopathologic abnormalities in cats with bartonellosis, even in the absence of clinical signs. In cats experimentally infected with B. henselae, follicular lymphoid hyperplasia of the lymph nodes with enlarged germinal centers and occasional necrotizing granulomas, as well as lymphoid hyperplasia of the spleen have been reported.[14,107,117]

Other manifestations in cats are less well-documented. A link between ocular manifestations such as chorioretinitis and uveitis and infection with B. henselae or B. clarridgeiae has been proposed.[120,121,162] Bartonella vinsonii subsp. berkhoffii has been found in cats presenting with osteomyelitis or polyarthropathy.[150–152,163] In addition, various neurologic signs have been reported in experimentally inoculated and naturally infected cats. B. henselae has been grown from brain tissue of experimentally infected cats, although attempts to prove an association between neurologic signs and bartonellosis using serology alone have been confounded by high seroprevalence in control cats.[119] There may be potential for impacts on reproduction, although further studies are needed to determine if bartonellosis is a major cause of decreased fertility or abortion in cats.[69,70] Interestingly, one study explored B. henselae infection-induced changes in human and cat endothelial cells and rapid angiogenesis was only observed in human cells,[164] potentially explaining why despite chronic bacteremia, vascular tumor formation is rarely seen as a clinical sign in cats.

Key Takeaways

- Bartonellosis in dogs most commonly presents as endocarditis, vascular lesions, or granulomatous/pyogranulomatous disease, although other systemic disease manifestations can be seen.

- Cats infected with cat-adapted species often are asymptomatic, although cats can develop disease secondary to *Bartonella* spp infection; if symptomatic, they can present with cardiac manifestations or systemic disease including lymphadenopathy, fever, or various less common manifestations.

DIAGNOSTIC TESTING
General Diagnostic Considerations

The intermittent bacteremia, low abundance, and stealth nature of *Bartonella* spp presents unique challenges—even for experienced clinicians—to definitively diagnose bartonellosis. There is currently no perfect gold standard test, so combinations of tests are often used. The major limitation for many tests is poor sensitivity, falsely negative results are common. Developing highly sensitive diagnostic assays without sacrificing specificity is an area of growing research.[8,99,156] The clinical utility of available diagnostic tests for cats and dogs has generally been extrapolated from human medicine, although a limited number of studies have investigated the accuracy of commonly used *Bartonella* spp assays in naturally infected cats[105,165] and dogs.[73,99,165–167] Thus, recommendations continue to be influenced by case series and even single case reports, as well as by expert opinion and anecdotal experience. A summary of diagnostic tests used to detect bartonellosis in dogs since the 1990s is shown in **Fig. 3**, highlighting the changes in diagnostic assays in use over time.

Currently available diagnostic tests either directly detect the pathogen or its DNA with microbiological, molecular, or histopathologic techniques, or indirectly assess *Bartonella* spp exposure via serology (**Table 2**). Because of low-level and intermittent bacteremia, and slow dividing times, *Bartonella* spp are notoriously difficult to detect

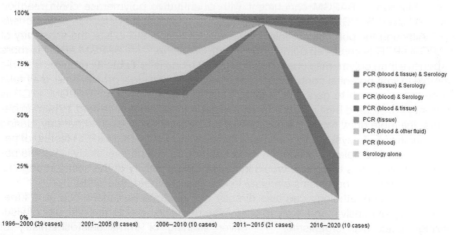

Fig. 3. Diagnostic tests reported for bartonellosis in dogs (1996–2020). Information provided based on available published case reports and case series (1996–2000, 29 cases; 2001–2005, 8 cases; 2006–2010, 10 cases; 2011–2015, 21 cases; 2016–2020, 10 cases).[29,79–81,83,84,87,88,90,91,93,95–97,100,135,136,140,141,168–179] Diagnostic assays are represented by color. Only diagnostic assays that contributed to definitive diagnosis of bartonellosis are included. Year is assigned based on the year the diagnostic test was performed, not the year the article was published. If the year of diagnosis was not given in the text of any particular case report or case series, the year was imputed using the year of paper publication and follow-up time reported. Tissues tested include biopsies from heart valve, myocardium, spleen, liver, masses, lymph nodes, and nasal epithelium. Other fluid samples tested include synovial fluid and seroma fluid.

Table 2
Sample selection guidelines and cost associated with select assays for *Bartonella* spp

Test	Sample	Estimated Cost ($)
qPCR[a]	Affected tissue: 0.5–1 g fresh frozen tissue in sterile container Effusion or other fluid: 2–3 mL in EDTA (purple top) Blood: 2–3 mL blood in EDTA (purple top)	50–100
BAPGM enrichment (ePCR)[a,b]	Affected tissue: 0.5–1 g fresh frozen tissue in sterile container Effusion or other fluid: 2–3 mL in EDTA (purple top) Blood: 2–3 mL blood in EDTA (purple top)	150–250
IFA serology (panel using multiple *Bartonella* spp antigens)	2–3 mL serum (red top or tiger top; centrifuged)	50–100

[a] Not recommended if patient is receiving an antibiotic with activity against *Bartonella* spp
[b] Triple draw may increase sensitivity (see text).
Abbreviation: EDTA, ethylenediamine tetraacetic acid

---

directly in blood samples with traditional culture methods.[8,149] A specialized insect-based liquid media,[180] *Bartonella-Alphaproteobacteria* growth medium (BAPGM),[4] has been developed to address the organism's fastidious growth requirements, and a combination of BAPGM enrichment with quantitative polymerase chain reaction (qPCR) (called BAPGM ePCR) has been used to enhance the detection of *Bartonella* spp. Although the potential for false-negative test results still exists, the sensitivity of BAPGM ePCR is improved compared with qPCR alone.[73,137] BAPGM ePCR is more expensive than polymerase chain reaction (PCR) alone (see **Table 2**), requires a sterile sample to limit potential contaminants, and, because of a slow growth time, may take more than a month to generate results. Despite these limitations, BAPGM ePCR is currently considered best practice for molecular/microbiological testing. In human patients, the triple draw method (collection of 3 blood samples, every other day, during the course of 5–7 days) further increases the sensitivity of BAPGM ePCR testing of peripheral blood samples.[181] Although there has not been a parallel study in canine patients, it is likely this technique would increase the sensitivity of the assay in dogs as well, given that the organisms circulate in low copy number, intermittently.

Although histopathology can also directly demonstrate *Bartonella* spp, it is time-consuming, expensive, and likely to yield false negatives due to the difficulty of visualizing intracellular organisms.[17,182] Silver staining or immunohistochemistry of affected tissues may help detect the intracellular bacilli if histopathologic confirmation is needed.[86,114,170,182]

Bartonella spp DNA has successfully been detected in clinical samples using conventional and quantitative PCR,[8,180] which are available through several commercial veterinary diagnostic laboratories. The accuracy of PCR will differ slightly based on numerous factors including the primers and protocols used, so it is important to confirm the sensitivity and specificity for each commercially available test. In another attempt to improve sensitivity, droplet digital PCR (ddPCR) has been adapted for the detection of rare pathogen DNA in samples with abundant inhibitors such as host DNA. A ddPCR assay originally developed for *Bartonella* spp detection in people[145,183,184] was recently validated in a retrospective study of dogs with heman-giosarcoma,[99] suggesting its potential as a highly sensitive diagnostic in veterinary patients. At the time of writing, *Bartonella* spp ddPCR is not yet commercially available to veterinarians.

As for other infectious diseases, serology is affordable but its diagnostic utility is limited to determining exposure rather than infection unless both acute and convalescent samples are tested. As such, serology seems to be most useful in acute cases in which seroconversion can be demonstrated. An immunofluorescence assay (IFA) panel detecting *B. henselae*, *B. koehlerae*, and *B. vinsonii* subsp. *berkhoffii* antibodies is most widely available. Interpretation of IFA can be subjective, and even when evaluated by experienced scientists, disagreements on the final dilution that demonstrates a positive titer occur, so small changes in IFA titer should be interpreted cautiously.[156,185] Although immunoglobulin M (IgM) and immunoglobulin G (IgG) detection is routinely used in human medicine in an attempt to distinguish acute infection from past exposure,[186–188] there is no established timeline of IgM or IgG production following infection,[185,189,190] and there is currently insufficient evidence for the diagnostic utility of reporting IgM-specific and IgG-specific titers in veterinary medicine. Although available commercially for more than 20 years, the validation of specific criteria to interpret quantitative Western blot assays for the serodiagnosis of *B. henselae* in dogs was only recently published.[191–193] Enzyme-linked immunoassay[76] is not widely used for serodiagnosis but is commercially available. Whether using IFA or another serologic test, the occurrence of seroconversion and the persistence of antibodies following exposure in incidental hosts seems highly variable.[190]

Given the challenges associated with diagnostic test selection and interpretation, it is prudent to contact the diagnostic laboratory in advance for specific guidance on sample collection and preparation and to confirm the sensitivity and specificity of diagnostic assays before sample submission.

Dogs

Molecular and microbiological tests for *Bartonella* spp are inherently insensitive due to low level, intermittent, and transient bacteremia. Peripheral blood is the most widely tested sample, and while the specificity is high, results are often negative in the face of infection for this reason.[8,76] To increase sensitivity, BAPGM ePCR is the preferred method for detecting *Bartonella* spp in canine peripheral blood samples.[73,137] It is important to remember that PCR-positive blood has been detected in apparently healthy dogs screened as potential blood donors.[74,194,195] Therefore, a positive PCR test does not always mean the organism is causing the presenting abnormalities in a given patient. In addition, because of the potential for false negatives, culture and PCR-based testing are of limited utility in patients treated with antibiotics with known efficacy against *Bartonella* spp at the time of sample collection.

Because of the challenges associated with direct detection in peripheral blood samples, a variety of other sample sources have been investigated to improve sensitivity and clarify the clinical importance of a positive PCR test. For example, effusion, if present, can be tested. BAPGM ePCR can successfully detect *Bartonella* spp in pleural and peritoneal effusions more effectively than PCR alone.[139] The utility of testing pericardial effusion with BAPGM ePCR is unknown but *Bartonella* spp DNA has not been found in pericardial effusions using PCR alone.[99,139,196] CSF does not seem to be a high-yield sample for the detection of *Bartonella* spp DNA with either PCR or BAPGM ePCR.[101,103] Aqueocentesis in cases of idiopathic anterior uveitis and/or choroiditis may prove useful;[174] *Bartonella* spp DNA and antibodies against *Bartonella* spp in aqueous humor have been linked to anterior uveitis in cats and testing of aqueous humor may be of similar utility in canine patients.[120,162,197,198]

More recent studies have suggested that *Bartonella* spp DNA is most readily detected using PCR on DNA extracted from affected tissues and that fresh/frozen specimens are better than formalin fixed because DNA degradation can occur with the latter.[98,99,138,199] In a recent study comparing ddPCR and qPCR on blood and tissue samples, ddPCR was more sensitive than qPCR (36% vs 0%) for blood samples but the assay with the highest sensitivity was qPCR performed on fresh/frozen tissue samples (estimated sensitivity 94%).[99] The specificity of this assay on tissue samples was also high (100%).

Although serology is often used to confirm a diagnosis of bartonellosis in humans, it has proven challenging to interpret in dogs. Sensitivity estimates range from less than 10% up to approximately 60% in naturally infected dogs, despite sensitivities of 100% in experimentally infected dogs.[17,73,99,166,200] In one experimental study, dogs seroconverted within approximately 1 month to the species and strain they were infected with.[200] In another report a single dog experimentally infected with *B henselae* SA2 seroconverted to *B henselae* SA2 by 2 weeks after infection and maintained seroreactivity for approximately 6 weeks, after which titers waxed and waned until finally remaining less than 1:16 after 12 weeks.[17] Despite these experimental findings, multiple studies in naturally exposed/infected dogs have suggested a poor correlation between the species/strain of *Bartonella* dogs are seroreactive to using IFA, and the species/strain found on PCR.[17,73,138,166,167,200] The specificity of IFA is difficult to estimate in naturally infected dogs but has been estimated at 85% to 88%.[99,166] The discrepancies between the sensitivity and specificity of serologic testing in laboratory studies compared with natural infections may reflect variation in immunologic clearance and the effectiveness of immune evasive strategies, differences in antibody specificity with exposure to multiple species or strains of *Bartonella*, repeated exposures due to chronic flea infestations, differences in the immune response associated with exposure to particular vectors, or individual host factors.

Collectively, current evidence for diagnostic testing in dogs suggests qPCR or BAPGM ePCR on fresh/frozen unfixed tissue samples has the highest sensitivity for detecting *Bartonella* spp in clinically affected animals.[156] When antemortem sampling of affected tissue is not feasible, BAPGM ePCR (or ddPCR once commercially available in dogs) may also be useful for identifying *Bartonella* spp in blood samples and should be combined with IFA serology to improve sensitivity.[73,99] If present, samples of peritoneal and/or pleural effusion should be submitted for BAPGM ePCR in addition to blood; aqueous humor may also be useful in cases of idiopathic anterior uveitis. Pericardial effusions and CSF are less likely to be of diagnostic value but if collected, samples should be submitted for BAPGM ePCR rather than PCR alone. If BAPGM ePCR is cost prohibitive or a sterile sample cannot be obtained, a peripheral blood sample can be submitted for qPCR alone but this approach risks a higher likelihood of false-negative results. Acute and convalescent serology should be performed for acute disease; convalescent serology alone can be performed in the case of chronic disease or in patients with a recent history of antibiotics that may interfere with reliable microbiologic or molecular testing.[141] Finally, consider repeating microbiologic/molecular testing in immunosuppressed dogs because they are more likely to become bacteremic when immunosuppressed.[141]

Cats

Similar diagnostic assay options exist for cats, and typical tests include BAPGM ePCR, qPCR, and IFA serology. Guidelines for selecting appropriate diagnostics for cats are similar to those outlined above for dogs. However, because cats serve as the primary reservoir host for *B. henselae*, *B. koehlerae*, and *B. clarridgeiae*, they are more likely to have prolonged and higher-level bacteremia when infected with these particular species, making blood samples a higher yield test.[105,106,149] It is important to remember that because of high exposure rates and their status as a reservoir host, seroreactivity or a positive microbiologic test are not always indicative of disease causation in cats.[201,202] However, cats are not reservoir hosts for all *Bartonella* spp, and they can be incidental hosts and develop pathologic condition when infected with *Bartonella* species other than *B. henselae*, *B. koehlerae* and *B. clarridgeiae*.[156] Moreover, infection with *B. henselae*, *B. koehlerae*, and *B. clarridgeiae* is not always incidental or subclinical in cats. Indeed, *Bartonella* spp with human reservoir hosts (*B. quintana* and *B. bacilliformis*) can cause serious and even fatal disease in people,[203] just as severe disease due to *B. henselae* has been reported in cats.[114]

Although not investigated independently in cats, qPCR or BAPGM ePCR on fresh/frozen unfixed tissue is thought to be useful; otherwise, for systemically ill cats with suspected bartonellosis, a peripheral blood sample for BAPGM ePCR and serum for IFA are considered the standard diagnostic tests. A negative serum IFA in cats is highly predictive for the absence of bacteremia but should be carefully considered in the context of the duration and severity of clinical signs before definitively ruling out feline bartonellosis.[106]

Key Takeaways

- Fresh/frozen unfixed tissue biopsy of affected organs (or fluids), tested with qPCR or BAPGM ePCR seems to be the most sensitive diagnostic test currently available.
- In the absence of samples from affected organs, peripheral blood should be tested with BAPGM ePCR, combined with IFA serologic testing.
- If cost is a limiting factor or sterile sample collection is not possible, qPCR testing of peripheral blood combined with IFA serologic testing can be considered.

TREATMENT AND PREVENTION
Indications for Treatment

Cats, as a natural reservoir of some *Bartonella* species, are typically only treated if they are displaying clinical signs compatible with bartonellosis and other differentials have been ruled out.[8,110,149,151] In contrast, even apparently healthy dogs with evidence of bartonellosis should be evaluated and monitored for the possibility of preclinical or subclinical abnormalities. It is likely that in certain animals, as in certain people, an appropriate immune response can clear acute bartonellosis without medical intervention. As such, the decision to treat asymptomatic *Bartonella* spp positive dogs is at the discretion of the clinician and should be considered on a case-by-case basis.

Treatment Options

Randomized controlled trials assessing optimal treatment protocols for dogs have not yet been conducted, and are limited for cats.[217,218] As with diagnostic testing guidelines, treatment recommendations are thus based on anecdotal experience and expert advice,[204] case reports, in vitro studies, and extrapolation from human treatment protocols. Antibiotic recommendations continue to evolve as clinicians gain experience with treating canine and feline bartonellosis. **Fig. 4** shows antibiotics reported as being used to treat bartonellosis in dogs since 1990, highlighting the more recent shift to the use of multiple drug combinations rather than single agents.

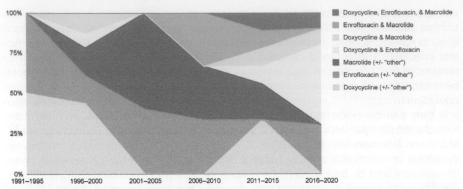

Fig. 4. Treatments reported for bartonellosis in dogs (1990–2020). Information provided based on available published case reports and case series (1991–1995, 2 cases; 1996–2000, 23 cases; 2001–2005, 5 cases; 2006–2010, 3 cases; 2011–2015, 9 cases; 2016–2020, 10 cases).[83,84,87,88,90,93,95,96,100,135,136,140,141,168,169,171–175,177,178,205] Other antibiotics used include ampicillin, clavamox, benzathine penicillin, metronidazole, cephalexin. Only antibiotic treatments with efficacy against gram negative and/or intracellular bacteria were included, and any antibiotic with potential efficacy against, or intended to treat, *Bartonella* spp given during the course of the illness was included, regardless of outcome.

Current treatment protocols generally combine antibiotics with different mechanisms of action to achieve high concentrations both in plasma and intracellularly.[8] Although in vitro studies have reported conflicting results on the need for multiple antibiotics,[206,207] case reports suggest that antibiotic monotherapy is clinically less effective than multiple agent therapy.[8] Antimicrobial susceptibility testing is not currently available to guide therapy but antimicrobial resistance is beginning to be recognized.[217,208]

Currently first-line recommendations are a fluoroquinolone (typically enrofloxacin in dogs or pradofloxacin in cats) combined with doxycycline, at standard doses.[204] Other antibiotics, including rifampin, macrolides (clarithromycin or azithromycin), or amikacin are also occasionally prescribed.[37,126,209] In vitro studies have documented resistance to single-agent macrolides, fluoroquinolones, and rifampin; therefore, different combinations may be useful if resistance is suspected.[156] A recent in vitro study found that although no single agent was effective against biofilm formation, combining a fluoroquinolone with azithromycin or rifampin rapidly eliminated *B henselae* biofilms.[37] Studies in humans with *Bartonella* spp endocarditis have established that aminoglycosides improve prognosis and decrease hospitalization time,[210] and the current standard of care in people is several weeks of doxycycline combined with a shorter (2–4 week) course of gentamicin, or rifampin when renal toxicity is a concern.[211,212] However, aminoglycosides are infrequently recommended in veterinary medicine due to potential nephrotoxicity; their use is reserved for severely ill hospitalized patients along with intensive monitoring of renal function.[126,209]

Due to antibiotic resistance, potential for biofilm formation, and ability to thrive intracellularly, a prolonged treatment course of at least 4 to 6 weeks is recommended in both dogs and cats.[8,204] If there is improvement, but not resolution of infection, antibiotic therapy should be extended, particularly in the context of chronic or severe infections such as endocarditis.[126]

Treatment Monitoring

Response to therapy should be evaluated after initiating therapy and at multiple points during treatment.[8,156] Generally, BAPGM ePCR and IFA after 2 to 4 weeks of therapy and again before discontinuing antibiotics is recommended. Because it can be difficult to clear infection, these tests should be repeated within weeks of stopping antibiotics, or if clinical signs recur once antibiotics are discontinued. In experimental studies, antibody titers in successfully treated dogs decreased over 3 to 6 months to become undetectable.[17,150] Therefore, persistence of antibody titers for longer than 3 to 6 months following treatment may indicate treatment failure, recrudescence, or reinfection.[76,141,150]

A rare systemic inflammatory reaction to bacterial die-off, similar to the Jarisch-Herxheimer reaction reported in humans,[213] has been documented in at least one cat[118] and is suspected to potentially occur in some dogs with bartonellosis after initiating treatment.[8] Based on human medical literature, reactions occur within 4 to 7 days of initiating antibiotic treatment and can appear as worsening of infection. If signs of a Jarisch-Herxheimer-like reaction are seen, antibiotics should be continued and supportive care initiated. Some patients may benefit from a short course of anti-inflammatory glucocorticoids. For dogs and cats that are stable, initiating treatment with one antibiotic for 5 to 7 days before adding the second antibiotic may prevent this reaction.[8]

Cats should also be monitored during treatment but it is possible that cats will remain bacteremic even after treatment. In cats, therefore, it is most important to monitor for resolution of clinical signs attributable to bartonellosis before discontinuing treatment.[8,156]

Prevention

Because of potentially severe complications and lengthy treatment duration of bartonellosis in dogs and cats, prevention is especially important. There is currently no vaccine for the prevention of bartonellosis in any species. The most effective preventative measure against bartonellosis in cats and dogs is year-round use of flea and tick control, which can be achieved with a variety of commercially available products.[152,154,158,160,214] Cat colonies or homes with cats known to be infected with *Bartonella* spp should be especially diligent with flea and tick preventatives. Moreover, because human bartonellosis is often linked to flea-infested cats,[8,156] eliminating fleas from pets and the environment should drastically decrease the risk for zoonotic transmission.

Due to the potential for transmission via blood transfusion, current guidelines suggest potential blood donors be screened for infection with IFA and BAPGM ePCR.[152,215,216] Based on the potential for transmission via direct inoculation, caution should also be exercised to prevent needle stick injury and exposure to potentially infectious materials.[66,67] It has been proposed that vertical transmission may also be possible,[69,70] particularly for *B. henselae* in cats, so it may also be prudent to avoid breeding infected cats or dogs and consider screening in prospective breeding animals.

Key Takeaways

- Dogs and cats that have been definitively diagnosed (or with a high degree of clinical suspicion) and are showing clinical signs should be treated with antibiotics as well as any other supportive care targeted at specific disease manifestations.
- Antimicrobial treatment should include a combination of antibiotics, typically doxycycline and enrofloxacin (dog) or doxycycline and pradofloxacin (cat); antibiotics are usually prescribed for at least 4 to 6 weeks or until resolution of clinical signs.
- Year-round flea and tick prevention is the mainstay of bartonellosis prevention in dogs and cats and to prevent zoonotic transmission.

SUMMARY

Due to the unique pathogenesis of *Bartonella* spp, bartonellosis remains difficult to diagnose and treat. Understanding how *Bartonella* spp cause disease allows clinician to better recognize cases that may warrant diagnostic testing, as well as recommend the most effective diagnostic testing and treatment plans to improve clinical outcomes.

CLINICS CARE POINTS

- Fleas are the main vector of *B. henselae* transmission, although evidence exists for transmission via tick vectors as well as direct inoculation and blood transfusions. Transmission for other Bartonella spp. affecting dogs are cats is not as well-described.

- Dogs can present with endocarditis, vascular proliferative lesions, and granulomatous or pyogranulomatous disease. Cats are often asymptomatic but can present similarly to dogs. Less common presentations include orthopedic, neurologic, ocular, or possibly reproductive abnormalities.

- Fresh/frozen unfixed tissue biopsy of affected organs (or fluids), tested with qPCR or BAPGM ePCR, seems to be the most sensitive diagnostic test currently available. In the absence of samples from specific affected organs, peripheral blood should be tested with BAPGM ePCR and combined with IFA serologic testing.

- Dogs and cats showing clinical symptoms should be treated with a combination of antibiotics, often doxycycline and a fluoroquinolone, for a prolonged course of 4 to 6 weeks. Monitoring for resolution of clinical signs and bacteremia/seroreactivity should be performed during and after treatment.

- Year-round flea and tick prevention is the mainstay of preventing *Bartonella* spp infection in dogs and cats and zoonotic transmission.

DISCLOSURE

A Ludwig was supported by fellowship NIH/NEI F30EY031230. E Lashnits has research grant support from the AKC, ASPCA, Elanco, and University of Wisconsin-Madison, and is a key opinion leader and research collaborator with IDEXX and research collaborator with Galaxy Diagnostics; none of these influenced the research or writing of this manuscript. Other authors have nothing to disclose.

REFERENCES

1. Breitschwerdt EB, Kordick DL, Malarkey DE, et al. Endocarditis in a dog due to infection with a novel Bartonella subspecies. J Clin Microbiol 1995;33(1): 154–60.
2. Breitschwerdt EB, Linder KL, Day MJ, et al. Koch's Postulates and the Pathogenesis of Comparative Infectious Disease Causation Associated with Bartonella species. J Comp Pathol 2013;148(2):115.
3. Deng H, Rhun D le, Buffet JPR, et al. Strategies of exploitation of mammalian reservoirs by Bartonella species. Vet Res 2012;43(1):15.
4. Maggi RG, Duncan AW, Breitschwerdt EB. Novel chemically modified liquid medium that will support the growth of seven bartonella species. J Clin Microbiol 2005;43(6):2651–5.
5. Regier Y, Órourke F, Kempf VAJ. Bartonella spp. - a chance to establish One Health concepts in veterinary and human medicine. Parasites Vectors 2016;9(1).

6. Chomel BB, Kasten RW. Bartonellosis, an increasingly recognized zoonosis. J Appl Microbiol 2010;109(3):743–50.
7. Billeter SA, Levy MG, Chomel BB, et al. Vector transmission of Bartonella species with emphasis on the potential for tick transmission. Med Vet Entomol 2008;22(1):1–15.
8. Álvarez-Fernández A, Breitschwerdt EB, Solano-Gallego L. Bartonella infections in cats and dogs including zoonotic aspects. 2018;11(1):1–21.
9. Seubert A, Schulein R, Dehio C. Bacterial persistence within erythrocytes: A unique pathogenic strategy of Bartonella spp. Int J Med Microbiol 2001; 291(6):555–60.
10. Schülein R, Seubert A, Gille C, et al. Invasion and Persistent Intracellular Colonization of Erythrocytes: A Unique Parasitic Strategy of the Emerging Pathogen Bartonella. J Exp Med 2001;193(9):1077.
11. Marignac G, Barrat F, Chomel B, et al. Murine model for Bartonella birtlesii infection: New aspects. Comp Immunol Microbiol Infect Dis 2010;33(2):95–107.
12. Boulouis HJ, Barrat F, Bermond D, et al. Kinetics of Bartonella birtlesii infection in experimentally infected mice and pathogenic effect on reproductive functions. Infect Immun 2001;69(9):5313–7.
13. Koesling J, Aebischer T, Falch C, et al. Cutting edge: antibody-mediated cessation of hemotropic infection by the intraerythrocytic mouse pathogen Bartonella grahamii. J Immunol 2001;167(1):11–4.
14. Guptill L, Slater L, Wu CC, et al. Experimental infection of young specific pathogen-free cats with Bartonella henselae. J Infect Dis 1997;176(1):206–16.
15. Choi E, Lee H, Lee J, et al. Ahnak-knockout mice show susceptibility to Bartonella henselae infection because of CD4+ T cell inactivation and decreased cytokine secretion. BMB Rep 2019;52(4):289–94.
16. da Silva MN, Vieira-Damiani G, Ericson ME, et al. Acute and Late Bartonella henselae Murine Model Infection. Vector-Borne Zoonotic Dis 2017;17(3):206–8.
17. Balakrishnan N, Cherry NA, Linder KE, et al. Experimental infection of dogs with Bartonella henselae and Bartonella vinsonii subsp. berkhoffii. Vet Immunol Immunopathol 2013;156(1–2):153–8.
18. Deng H, Pang Q, Zhao B, et al. Molecular Mechanisms of Bartonella and Mammalian Erythrocyte Interactions: A Review. Front Cell Infect Microbiol 2018;8:431.
19. Harms A, Dehio C. Intruders below the radar: molecular pathogenesis of Bartonella spp. Clin Microbiol Rev 2012;25(1):42–78.
20. Fumarola D, Pece S, Fumarulo R, et al. Downregulation of human polymorphonuclear cell activities exerted by microorganisms belonging to the alpha-2 subgroup of Proteobacteria (Afipia felis and Rochalimaea henselae). Immunopharmacol Immunotoxicol 1994;16(3):449–61.
21. Popa C, Abdollahi-Roodsaz S, Joosten LAB, et al. Bartonella quintana Lipopolysaccharide Is a Natural Antagonist of Toll-Like Receptor 4. Infect Immun 2007; 75(10):4831.
22. Zähringer U, Lindner B, Knirel YA, et al. Structure and biological activity of the short-chain lipopolysaccharide from Bartonella henselae ATCC 49882T. J Biol Chem 2004;279(20):21046–54.
23. Kang JG, Lee HW, Ko S, et al. Comparative proteomic analysis of outer membrane protein 43 (omp43)-deficient Bartonella henselae. J Vet Sci 2018; 19(1):59.
24. Dehio C, Meyer M, Berger J, et al. Interaction of Bartonella henselae with endothelial cells results in bacterial aggregation on the cell surface and the

subsequent engulfment and internalisation of the bacterial aggregate by a unique structure, the invasome. J Cell Sci 1997;110(18):2141–54.

25. Burgess AWO, Anderson BE. Outer membrane proteins of Bartonella henselae and their interaction with human endothelial cells. Microb Pathogenesis 1998; 25(3):157–64.

26. Burgess AWO, Paquet JY, Letesson JJ, et al. Isolation, sequencing and expression of Bartonella henselae omp43 and predicted membrane topology of the deduced protein. Microb Pathogenesis 2000;29(2):73–80.

27. Chomel BB, Boulouis HJ, Breitschwerdt EB, et al. Ecological fitness and strategies of adaptation of Bartonella species to their hosts and vectors. Vet Res 2009;40(2):29.

28. Dehio C. Molecular and Cellular Basis of Bartonella Pathogenesis. Annu Rev Microbiol 2004;58:365–90.

29. Beerlage C, Varanat M, Linder K, et al. Bartonella vinsonii subsp. berkhoffii and Bartonella henselae as potential causes of proliferative vascular diseases in animals. Med Microbiol Immunol 2012;201:319–26.

30. Osherov N, Ben-Ami R. Modulation of Host Angiogenesis as a Microbial Survival Strategy and Therapeutic Target. PLoS Pathog 2016;12(4).

31. Padmalayam I, Karem K, Baumstark B, et al. The gene encoding the 17-kDa antigen of Bartonella henselae is located within a cluster of genes homologous to the virB virulence operon. DNA Cel Biol 2000;19(6):377–82.

32. Okaro U, Addisu A, Casanas B, et al. Bartonella Species, an Emerging Cause of Blood-Culture-Negative Endocarditis. Clin Microbiol Rev 2017;30(3):709–46.

33. Okaro U, George S, Anderson B. What is in a cat scratch? Growth of bartonella henselae in a biofilm. Microorganisms 2021;9(4):1–14.

34. Bjarnsholt T. The role of bacterial biofilms in chronic infections. APMIS 2013; 121(136):1–58.

35. Kaiser PO, Linke D, Schwarz H, et al. Analysis of the BadA stalk from Bartonella henselae reveals domain-specific and domain-overlapping functions in the host cell infection process. Cell Microbiol 2012;14(2):198–209.

36. Kaiser PO, Riess T, Wagner CL, et al. The head of Bartonella adhesin A is crucial for host cell interaction of Bartonella henselae. Cell Microbiol 2008;10(11): 2223–34.

37. Zheng X, Ma X, Li T, et al. Effect of different drugs and drug combinations on killing stationary phase and biofilms recovered cells of Bartonella henselae in vitro. BMC Microbiol 2020;20(1).

38. Tu N, Carroll RK, Weiss A, et al. A family of genus-specific RNAs in tandem with DNA-binding proteins control expression of the badA major virulence factor gene in Bartonella henselae. MicrobiologyOpen 2017;6(2).

39. Okaro U, George S, Valdes S, et al. A non-coding RNA controls transcription of a gene encoding a DNA binding protein that modulates biofilm development in Bartonella henselae. Microb Pathogenesis 2020;147(May):104272.

40. Tsukamoto K, Shinzawa N, Kawai A, et al. The Bartonella autotransporter BafA activates the host VEGF pathway to drive angiogenesis. Nat Commun 2020;11(1).

41. Dehio C. Bartonella–host-cell interactions and vascular tumour formation. Nat Rev Microbiol 2005;3(8):621–31.

42. Resto-Ruiz SI, Schmiederer M, Sweger D, et al. Induction of a potential paracrine angiogenic loop between human THP-1 macrophages and human microvascular endothelial cells during Bartonella henselae infection. Infect Immun 2002;70(8):4564–70.

43. Schmid MC, Scheidegger F, Dehio M, et al. A translocated bacterial protein protects vascular endothelial cells from apoptosis. PLoS Pathog 2006;2(11): 1083–97.

44. Kirby JE, Nekorchuk DM. Bartonella-associated endothelial proliferation depends on inhibition of apoptosis. Proc Natl Acad Sci U S A 2002;99(7):4656–61.

45. Kirby JE. In vitro model of Bartonella henselae-induced angiogenesis. Infect Immun 2004;72(12):7315–7.

46. Varanat M, Maggi RG, Linder KE, et al. Infection of human brain vascular pericytes (HBVPs) by Bartonella henselae. Med Microbiol Immunol 2013;202(2): 143–51.

47. Kempf VAJ, Lebiedziejewski M, Alitalo K, et al. Activation of hypoxia-inducible factor-1 in bacillary angiomatosis: Evidence for a role of hypoxia-inducible factor-1 in bacterial infections. Circulation 2005;111(8):1054–62.

48. Kempf VAJ, Volkmann B, Schaller M, et al. Evidence of a leading role for VEGF in Bartonella henselae-induced endothelial cell proliferations. Cell Microbiol 2001; 3(9):623–32.

49. Riess T, Andersson SGE, Lupas A, et al. Bartonella adhesin a mediates a proangiogenic host cell response. J Exp Med 2004;200(10):1267–78.

50. O'Rourke F, Mändle T, Urbich C, et al. Reprogramming of myeloid angiogenic cells by Bartonella henselae leads to microenvironmental regulation of pathological angiogenesis. Cell Microbiol 2015;17(10):1447–63.

51. Zanutto MDS, Mamizuka EM, Raiz-Júnior R, et al. Experimental infection and horizontal transmission of Bartonella henselae in domestic cats. Rev Inst Med Trop Sao Paulo 2001;43(5):257–61.

52. Chomel BB, Kasten RW, Floyd-Hawkins K, et al. Experimental transmission of Bartonella henselae by the cat flea. J Clin Microbiol 1996;34(8):1952–6.

53. Higgins JA, Radulovic S, Jaworski DC, et al. Acquisition of the cat scratch disease agent Bartonella henselae by cat fleas (Siphonaptera:Pulicidae). J Med Entomol 1996;33(3):490–5.

54. Foil L, Andress E, Freeland RL, et al. Experimental infection of domestic cats with Bartonella henselae by inoculation of Ctenocephalides felis (Siphonaptera: Pulicidae) feces. J Med Entomol 1998;35(5):625–8.

55. Abbott RC, Chomel BB, Kasten RW, et al. Experimental and natural infection with Bartonella henselae in domestic cats. Comp Immunol Microbiol Infect Dis 1997;20(1):41–51.

56. Lantos PM, Wormser GP. Chronic coinfections in patients diagnosed with chronic lyme disease: a systematic review. Am J Med 2014;127(11):1105–10.

57. Wormser GP, Pritt B. Update and Commentary on Four Emerging Tick-Borne Infections: Ehrlichia muris-like Agent, Borrelia miyamotoi, Deer Tick Virus, Heartland Virus, and Whether Ticks Play a Role in Transmission of Bartonella henselae. Infect Dis Clin North Am 2015;29(2):371–81.

58. Angelakis E, Billeter SA, Breitschwerdt EB, et al. Potential for tick-borne bartonelloses. Emerg Infect Dis 2010;16(3):385–91.

59. Maggi RG, Toliver M, Richardson T, et al. Regional prevalences of Borrelia burgdorferi, Borrelia bissettiae, and Bartonella henselae in Ixodes affinis, Ixodes pacificus and Ixodes scapularis in the USA. Ticks Tick-Borne Dis 2019;10(2): 360–4.

60. Chang CC, Chomel BB, Kasten RW, et al. Molecular evidence of Bartonella spp. in questing adult Ixodes pacificus ticks in California. J Clin Microbiol 2001;39(4): 1221–6.

61. Wechtaisong W, Bonnet SI, Lien YY, et al. Transmission of Bartonella henselae within Rhipicephalus sanguineus: Data on the Potential Vector Role of the Tick. PLoS Negl Trop Dis 2020;14(10):1–14.

62. Król N, Militzer N, Stöbe E, et al. Evaluating Transmission Paths for Three Different Bartonella spp. in Ixodes ricinus Ticks Using Artificial Feeding. Microorganisms 2021;9(5).

63. Cotté V, Bonnet S, le Rhun D, et al. Transmission of Bartonella henselae by Ixodes ricinus. Emerg Infect Dis 2008;14(7):1074–80.

64. Kordick DL, Breitschwerdt EB. Relapsing bacteremia after blood transmission of Bartonella henselae to cats. Am J Vet Res 1997;58(5):492–7.

65. Magalhães RF, Pitassi LHU, Salvadego M, et al. Bartonella henselae survives after the storage period of red blood cell units: is it transmissible by transfusion? Transfus Med (Oxford, England) 2008;18(5):287–91.

66. Lin JW, Chen CM, Chang CC. Unknown fever and back pain caused by bartonella henselae in a veterinarian after a needle puncture: A case report and literature review. Vector-Borne Zoonotic Dis 2011;11(5):589–91.

67. Oliveira AM, Maggi RG, Woods CW, et al. Suspected needle stick transmission of Bartonella vinsonii subspecies berkhoffii to a veterinarian. J Vet Intern Med 2010;24(5):1229–32.

68. Kosoy MY, Regnery RL, Kosaya OI, et al. Isolation of Bartonella spp. from embryos and neonates of naturally infected rodents. J Wildl Dis 1998;34(2):305–9.

69. Manvell C, Ferris K, Maggi R, et al. Prevalence of Vector-Borne Pathogens in Reproductive and Non-Reproductive Tissue Samples from Free-Roaming Domestic Cats in the South Atlantic USA. Pathogens 2021;10(9).

70. Guptill L, Slater LN, Wu CC, et al. Evidence of reproductive failure and lack of perinatal transmission of Bartonella henselae in experimentally infected cats. Vet Immunol Immunopathol 1998;65(2–4):177–89.

71. Breitschwerdt EB, Maggi RG, Farmer P, et al. Molecular evidence of perinatal transmission of Bartonella vinsonii subsp. berkhoffii and Bartonella henselae to a child. J Clin Microbiol 2010;48(6):2289–93.

72. Johnson R, Ramos-Vara J, Vemulapalli R. Identification of Bartonella henselae in an aborted equine fetus. Vet Pathol 2009;46(2):277–81.

73. Pérez C, Maggi RG, Diniz PPVP, et al. Molecular and Serological Diagnosis of Bartonella Infection in 61 Dogs from the United States. J Vet Intern Med 2011;25(4):805–10.

74. Balakrishnan N, Musulin S, Varanat M, et al. Serological and molecular prevalence of selected canine vector borne pathogens in blood donor candidates, clinically healthy volunteers, and stray dogs in North Carolina. Parasites Vectors 2014;7(1).

75. Pappalardo BL, Correa MT, York CC, et al. Epidemiologic evaluation of the risk factors associated with exposure and seroreactivity to Bartonella vinsonii in dogs. Am J Vet Res 1997;58(5):467–71.

76. Lashnits E, Thatcher B, Carruth A, et al. Bartonella spp. seroepidemiology and associations with clinicopathologic findings in dogs in the United States. J Vet Intern Med 2021.

77. Henn JB, Liu CH, Kasten RW, et al. Seroprevalence of antibodies against Bartonella species and evaluation of risk factors and clinical signs associated with seropositivity in dogs. Am J Vet Res 2005;66(4):688–94.

78. Chomel BB, Kasten RW, Williams C, et al. Bartonella Endocarditis. Ann N Y Acad Sci 2009;1166(1):120–6.

79. Ohad DG, Morick D, Avidor B, et al. Molecular detection of Bartonella henselae and Bartonella koehlerae from aortic valves of Boxer dogs with infective endocarditis. Vet Microbiol 2010;141(1–2):182–5.

80. Donovan TA, Fox PR, Balakrishnan N, et al. Pyogranulomatous Pancarditis with Intramyocardial Bartonella henselae San Antonio 2 (BhSA2) in a Dog. J Vet Intern Med 2017;31(1):142–8.

81. Fenimore A, Varanat M, Maggi R, et al. Bartonella spp. DNA in cardiac tissues from dogs in Colorado and Wyoming. J Vet Intern Med 2011;25(3):613–6.

82. Roura X, Santamarina G, Tabar MD, et al. Polymerase chain reaction detection of Bartonella spp. in dogs from Spain with blood culture-negative infectious endocarditis. J Vet Cardiol 2018;20(4):267–75.

83. Shelnutt LM, Balakrishnan N, DeVanna J, et al. Death of Military Working Dogs Due to Bartonella vinsonii Subspecies berkhoffii Genotype III Endocarditis and Myocarditis. Mil Med 2017;182:e1864–9.

84. André MR, Canola RAM, Braz JB, et al. Aortic valve endocarditis due to Bartonella clarridgeiae in a dog in Brazil. Rev Bras Parasitol Vet 2019;28(4):661–70.

85. Chomel BB, Wey AC, Kasten RW. Isolation of Bartonella washoensis from a dog with mitral valve endocarditis. J Clin Microbiol 2003;41(11):5327–32.

86. Kelly P, Rolain JM, Maggi R, et al. Bartonella quintana endocarditis in dogs. Emerg Infect Dis 2006;12(12):1869–72.

87. Ernst E, Qurollo B, Olech C, et al. Bartonella rochalimae, a newly recognized pathogen in dogs. J Vet Intern Med 2020;34(4):1447–53.

88. Tabar MD, Altet L, Maggi RG, et al. First description of Bartonella koehlerae infection in a Spanish dog with infective endocarditis. Parasites Vectors 2017;10(1).

89. MacDonald KA, Chomel BB, Kittleson MD, et al. A Prospective Study of Canine Infective Endocarditis in Northern California (1999–2001): Emergence of Bartonella as a Prevalent Etiologic Agent. J Vet Intern Med 2004;18(1):56–64.

90. Pappalardo BL, Brown T, Gookin JL, et al. Granulomatous Disease Associated with Bartonella Infection in 2 Dogs. J Vet Intern Med 2000;14(1):37.

91. Saunders GK, Monroe WE. Systemic Granulomatous Disease and Sialometaplasia in a Dog with *Bartonella* Infection. Vet Pathol 2006;43(3):391–2.

92. Morales SC, Breitschwerdt EB, Washabau RJ, et al. Detection of *Bartonella henselae* DNA in two dogs with pyogranulomatous lymphadenitis. J Am Vet Med Assoc 2007;230(5):681–5.

93. Tucker MD, Sellon RK, Tucker RL, et al. Bilateral mandibular pyogranulomatous lymphadenitis and pulmonary nodules in a dog with Bartonella henselae bacteremia. Can Vet J 2014;55(10):970–4.

94. Gillespie TN, Washabau RJ, Goldschmidt MH, et al. Detection of Bartonella henselae and Bartonella clarridgeiae DNA in hepatic specimens from two dogs with hepatic disease. J Am Vet Med Assoc 2003;222(1):47–51.

95. Breitschwerdt EB, Maggi RG, Varanat M, et al. Isolation of *Bartonella vinsonii* subsp. *berkhoffii* Genotype II from a Boy with Epithelioid Hemangioendothelioma and a Dog with Hemangiopericytoma. J Clin Microbiol 2009;47(6):1957–60.

96. Yager JA, Best SJ, Maggi RG, et al. Bacillary angiomatosis in an immunosuppressed dog. Vet Dermatol 2010;21(4):420–8.

97. Kitchell BE, Fan TM, Kordick D, et al. Peliosis hepatis in a dog infected with Bartonella henselae. J Am Vet Med Assoc 2000;216(4):519–23.

98. Varanat M, Maggi RG, Linder KE, et al. Molecular prevalence of Bartonella, Babesia, and hemotropic Mycoplasma sp. in dogs with splenic disease. J Vet Intern Med 2011;25(6):1284–91.

99. Lashnits E, Neupane P, Bradley JM, et al. Comparison of Serological and Molecular Assays for Bartonella Species in Dogs with Hemangiosarcoma. Pathogens 2021;10(7).

100. Breitschwerdt EB, Blann KR, Stebbins ME, et al. Clinicopathological Abnormalities and Treatment Response in 24 Dogs Seroreactive to Bartonella Vinsonii (Berkhoffii) Antigens. J Am Anim Hosp Assoc 2004;40:92–101.

101. Barber RM, Li Q, Diniz PPVP, et al. Evaluation of brain tissue or cerebrospinal fluid with broadly reactive polymerase chain reaction for Ehrlichia, Anaplasma, spotted fever group Rickettsia, Bartonella, and Borrelia species in canine neurological diseases (109 cases). J Vet Intern Med 2010;24(2):372–8.

102. Mellor PJ, Fetz K, Maggi RG, et al. Alpha1-proteinase inhibitor deficiency and Bartonella infection in association with panniculitis, polyarthritis, and meningitis in a dog. J Vet Intern Med 2006;20(4):1023–8.

103. Bartner LR, McGrath S, Drury A, et al. Testing for Bartonella ssp. DNA in cerebrospinal fluid of dogs with inflammatory central nervous system disease. J Vet Intern Med 2018;32(6):1983–8.

104. Cross JR, Rossmeisl JH, Maggi RG, et al. Bartonella-associated meningoradiculoneuritis and dermatitis or panniculitis in 3 dogs. J Vet Intern Med 2008; 22(3):674–8.

105. Kordick DL, Wilson KH, Sexton DJ, et al. Prolonged Bartonella Bacteremia in Cats Associated with Cat-Scratch Disease Patients. J Clin Microbiol 1995; 33(12):3245–51.

106. Chomel BB, Abbott RC, Kasten RW, et al. Bartonella henselae prevalence in domestic cats in California: risk factors and association between bacteremia and antibody titers. J Clin Microbiol 1995;33(9):2445–50.

107. Guptill L, Slater L, Wu C-C, et al. Immune response of neonatal specific pathogen-free cats to experimental infection with Bartonella henselae. Vet Immunol Immunopathol 1999 Nov 30;71(3–4):233–43.

108. Gurfield AN, Boulouis HJ, Chomel BB, et al. Coinfection with Bartonella clarridgeiae and Bartonella henselae and with different Bartonella henselae strains in domestic cats. J Clin Microbiol 1997;35(8):2120–3.

109. Qurollo B. Feline Vector-Borne Diseases in North America. Vet Clin North Am Small Anim Pract 2019;49(4):687–702.

110. Guptill L. Feline Bartonellosis. Vet Clin North Am Small Anim Pract 2010;40(6): 1073–90.

111. Yamamoto K, Chomel BB, Kasten RW, et al. Experimental Infection of Domestic Cats with Bartonella koehlerae and Comparison of Protein and DNA Profiles with Those of Other Bartonella Species Infecting Felines. J Clin Microbiol 2002;40(2): 466–74.

112. Breitschwerdt EB, Broadhurst JJ, Cherry NA. Bartonella henselae as a cause of acute-onset febrile illness in cats. JFMS open Rep 2015;1(2). 205511691560045.

113. Donovan TA, Balakrishnan N, Carvalho Barbosa I, et al. Bartonella spp. as a Possible Cause or Cofactor of Feline Endomyocarditis-Left Ventricular Endocardial Fibrosis Complex. J Comp Pathol 2018;162:29–42.

114. Varanat M, Broadhurst J, Linder KE, et al. Identification of Bartonella henselae in 2 Cats With Pyogranulomatous Myocarditis and Diaphragmatic Myositis. Vet Pathol 2012;49(4):608–11.

115. Chomel BB, Wey AC, Kasten RW, et al. Fatal Case of Endocarditis Associated with Bartonella henselae Type I Infection in a Domestic Cat. J Clin Microbiol 2003;41(11):5337–9.

116. Palerme JS, Jones AE, Ward JL, et al. Infective endocarditis in 13 cats. J Vet Cardiol 2016;18(3):213–25.

117. Kordick DL, Brown TT, Shin K, et al. Clinical and Pathologic Evaluation of Chronic Bartonella henselae or Bartonella clarridgeiae Infection in Cats. J Clin Microbiol 1999;37(5):1536–47.

118. Castel A, Olby NJ, Breitschwerdt EB, et al. Co-infection with Bartonella henselae and Sarcocystis sp. in a 6-year-old male neutered domestic longhair cat with progressive multifocal neurological signs. Vet Q 2019;39(1):168–73.

119. Leibovitz K, Pearce L, Brewer M, et al. Bartonella species antibodies and DNA in cerebral spinal fluid of cats with central nervous system disease. J feline Med Surg 2008;10(4):332–7.

120. Lappin MR, Black JC. Bartonella spp infection as a possible cause of uveitis in a cat. J Am Vet Med Assoc 1999;214(8):1205–7.

121. Lappin MR, Kordick DL, Breitschwerdt EB. Bartonella spp antibodies and DNA in aqueous humour of cats. J Feline Med Surg 2000;2(1):61–8.

122. Varanat M, Travis A, Lee W, et al. Recurrent Osteomyelitis in a Cat due to Infection with Bartonella vinsonii subsp. berkhoffii Genotype II. J Vet Intern Med 2009; 23(6):1273–7.

123. Tomas A, Pultorak EL, Gruen ME, et al. Relationship between degenerative joint disease, pain, and Bartonella spp. seroreactivity in domesticated cats. J Vet Intern Med 2015;29(1):21–7.

124. Sykes JE, Kittleson MD, Pesavento PA, et al. Evaluation of the relationship between causative organisms and clinical characteristics of infective endocarditis in dogs: 71 cases (1992-2005). J Am Vet Med Assoc 2006;228(11):1723–34.

125. Santilli RA, Battaia S, Perego M, et al. Bartonella-associated inflammatory cardiomyopathy in a dog. J Vet Cardiol 2017;19(1):74–81.

126. MacDonald K. Infective Endocarditis in Dogs: Diagnosis and Therapy. Vet Clin North Am Small Anim Pract 2010;40(4):665–84.

127. Davis AZ, Jaffe DA, Honadel TE, et al. Prevalence of Bartonella sp. in United States military working dogs with infectious endocarditis: a retrospective case-control study. J Vet Cardiol 2020;27:1–9.

128. Breitschwerdt EB, Atkins CE, Brown TT, et al. Bartonella vinsonii subsp. berkhoffii and related members of the alpha subdivision of the Proteobacteria in dogs with cardiac arrhythmias, endocarditis, or myocarditis. J Clin Microbiol 1999; 37(11):3618–26.

129. Tabar MD, Maggi RG, Altet L, et al. Gammopathy in a Spanish dog infected with Bartonella henselae. J Small Anim Pract 2011;52(4):209–12.

130. Cheslock MA, Embers ME. Human Bartonellosis: An Underappreciated Public Health Problem? Trop Med Infect Dis 2019;4(2).

131. Relman DA, Loutit JS, Schmidt TM, et al. The agent of bacillary angiomatosis. An approach to the identification of uncultured pathogens. N Engl J Med 1990;323(23):1573–80.

132. Perkocha LA, Geaghan SM, Yen TSB, et al. Clinical and pathological features of bacillary peliosis hepatis in association with human immunodeficiency virus infection. N Engl J Med 1990;323(23):1581–6.

133. Beydon M, Rodriguez C, Karras A, et al. Bartonella and Coxiella infections presenting as systemic vasculitis: case series and review of literature. Rheumatology 2021.

134. Balakrishnan N, Ericson M, Maggi R, et al. Vasculitis, cerebral infarction and persistent Bartonella henselae infection in a child. Parasit Vectors 2016; 9(1):254.
135. Friedenberg SG, Balakrishnan N, Guillaumin J, et al. Splenic vasculitis, thrombosis, and infarction in a febrile dog infected with Bartonella henselae. J Vet Emerg Crit Care 2015;25(6):789–94.
136. Southern BL, Neupane P, Ericson ME, et al. Bartonella henselae in a dog with ear tip vasculitis. Vet Dermatol 2018;29(6):537.e180.
137. Cherry NA, Diniz PPVP, Maggi RG, et al. Isolation or Molecular Detection of Bartonella henselae and Bartonella vinsonii subsp. berkhoffii from Dogs with Idiopathic Cavitary Effusions. J Vet Intern Med 2009;23(1):186–9.
138. Lashnits E, Neupane P, Bradley JM, et al. Molecular prevalence of Bartonella, Babesia, and hemotropic Mycoplasma species in dogs with hemangiosarcoma from across the United States. PLoS One 2020;15(1):e0227234.
139. Weeden AL, Cherry NA, Breitschwerdt EB, et al. Bartonella henselae in canine cavitary effusions: prevalence, identification, and clinical associations. Vet Clin Pathol 2017;46(2):326–30.
140. Drut A, Bublot I, Breitschwerdt EB, et al. Comparative microbiological features of Bartonella henselae infection in a dog with fever of unknown origin and granulomatous lymphadenitis. Med Microbiol Immunol 2014;203(2):85–91.
141. Golly E, Breitschwerdt EB, Balakrishnan N, et al. Bartonella henselae, Bartonella koehlerae and Rickettsia rickettsii seroconversion and seroreversion in a dog with acute-onset fever, lameness, and lymphadenopathy followed by a protracted disease course. Vet Parasitol Reg Stud Rep 2017;7:19–24.
142. Zakhour R, Mancias P, Heresi G, et al. Transverse Myelitis and Guillain-Barré Syndrome Associated with Cat-Scratch Disease, Texas, USA, 2011. Emerg Infect Dis 2018;24(9):1754–5.
143. Canneti B, Cabo-López I, Puy-Núñez A, et al. Neurological presentations of Bartonella henselae infection. Neurol Sci 2019;40(2):261–8.
144. Nawrocki CC, Max RJ, Marzec NS, et al. Atypical Manifestations of Cat-Scratch Disease, United States, 2005–2014 - Volume 26, Number 7—July 2020 - Emerging Infectious Diseases journal - CDC. Emerging Infect Dis 2020;26(7): 1438–46.
145. Breitschwerdt EB, Bradley JM, Maggi RG, et al. Bartonella Associated Cutaneous Lesions (BACL) in People with Neuropsychiatric Symptoms. Pathogens (Basel, Switzerland) 2020;9(12):1–19.
146. Kordick DL, Hilyard EJ, Hadfield TL, et al. Bartonella clarridgeiae, a newly recognized zoonotic pathogen causing inoculation papules, fever, and lymphadenopathy (cat scratch disease). J Clin Microbiol 1997;35(7):1813–8.
147. Avidor B, Graidy M, Efrat G, et al. Bartonella koehlerae, a new cat-associated agent of culture-negative human endocarditis. J Clin Microbiol 2004;42(8): 3462–8.
148. Koehler JE, Glaser CA, Tappero JW. Rochalimaea henselae infection. A new zoonosis with the domestic cat as reservoir. JAMA 1994;271(7):531–5.
149. Breitschwerdt EB. Feline bartonellosis and cat scratch disease. Vet Immunol Immunopathol 2008;123(1–2):167–71.
150. Breitschwerdt EB, Maggi RG, Chomel BB, et al. Bartonellosis: An emerging infectious disease of zoonotic importance to animals and human beings. J Vet Emerg Crit Care 2010;20(1):8–30.
151. Stützer B, Hartmann K. Chronic Bartonellosis in Cats: What are the potential implications? J Feline Med Surg 2012;14(9):612–21.

152. Pennisi MG, Marsilio F, Hartmann K, et al. Bartonella Species Infection in Cats: ABCD guidelines on prevention and management. J Feline Med Surg 2013; 15(7):563–9.

153. Fleischman DA, Chomel BB, Kasten RW, et al. Bartonella Infection among Cats Adopted from a San Francisco Shelter, Revisited. Appl Environ Microbiol 2015; 81(18):6446–50.

154. Lappin MR. Update on flea and tick associated diseases of cats. Vet Parasitol 2018;254:26–9.

155. Mada PK, Zulfiqar H, Chandranesan ASJ. Bartonellosis. StatPearls. Published online January 7, 2022. Available at: https://www.ncbi.nlm.nih.gov/books/NBK430874/. Accessed January 13, 2022.

156. Breitschwerdt EB. Bartonellosis, One Health and all creatures great and small. Vet Dermatol 2017;28(1):96.e21.

157. Chomel BB, Boulouis HJ, Maruyama S, et al. Bartonella spp. in pets and effect on human health. Emerg Infect Dis 2006;12(3):389–94.

158. Lappin MR, Tasker S, Roura X. Role of vector-borne pathogens in the development of fever in cats: 1. Flea-associated diseases. J Feline Med Surg 2020; 22(1):31–9.

159. Breitschwerdt EB, Kordick DL. Bartonella Infection in Animals: Carriership, Reservoir Potential, Pathogenicity, and Zoonotic Potential for Human Infection. Clin Microbiol Rev 2000;13(3):428.

160. Bradbury CA, Lappin MR. Evaluation of topical application of 10% imidacloprid-1% moxidectin to prevent Bartonella henselae transmission from cat fleas. J Am Vet Med Assoc 2010;236(8):869–73.

161. Whittemore JC, Hawley JR, Radecki Sv, et al. Bartonella species antibodies and hyperglobulinemia in privately owned cats. J Vet Intern Med 2012;26(3):639–44.

162. Stiles J. Bartonellosis in cats: A role in uveitis? Vet Ophthalmol 2011;14(SUPPL. 1):9–14.

163. Sykes JE, Westropp JL, Kasten RW, et al. Association between Bartonella species infection and disease in pet cats as determined using serology and culture. J feline Med Surg 2010;12(8):631–6.

164. Berrich M, Kieda C, Grillon C, et al. Differential effects of bartonella henselae on human and feline macro- and micro-vascular endothelial cells. PLoS ONE 2011;6(5).

165. Maggi R, Breitschwerdt EB, Qurollo B, et al. Development of a Multiplex Droplet Digital PCR Assay for the Detection of Babesia, Bartonella, and Borrelia Species. Pathogens 2021;10(11):1462.

166. Neupane P, Hegarty BC, Marr HS, et al. Evaluation of cell culture-grown Bartonella antigens in immunofluorescent antibody assays for the serological diagnosis of bartonellosis in dogs. J Vet Intern Med 2018;32(6):1958–64.

167. Duncan AW, Maggi RG, Breitschwerdt EB. A combined approach for the enhanced detection and isolation of Bartonella species in dog blood samples: Pre-enrichment liquid culture followed by PCR and subculture onto agar plates. J Microbiol Methods 2007;69(2):273–81.

168. Randell MG, Balakrishnan N, Gunn-Christie R, et al. Bartonella henselae infection in a dog with recalcitrant ineffective erythropoiesis. Vet Clin Pathol 2018; 47(1):45–50.

169. Easley F, Taylor L, Breitschwerdt E B. Suspected Bartonella osteomyelitis in a dog. Clin Case Rep 2021;9(7):e04512.

170. Rossi MA, Balakrishnan N, Linder KE, et al. Concurrent Bartonella henselae infection in a dog with panniculitis and owner with ulcerated nodular skin lesions. Vet Dermatol 2015;26(1):60.e22.
171. de Paiva Diniz PPV, Wood M, Maggi RG, et al. Co-isolation of Bartonella henselae and Bartonella vinsonii subsp. berkhoffii from blood, joint and subcutaneous seroma fluids from two naturally infected dogs. Vet Microbiol 2009;138(3–4): 368–72.
172. Kordick SK, Breitschwerdt EB, Hegarty BC, et al. Coinfection with Multiple Tick-Borne Pathogens in a Walker Hound Kennel in North Carolina. J Clin Microbiol 1999;37(8):2631.
173. Tuttle AD, Birkenheuer AJ, Juopperi T, et al. Concurrent bartonellosis and babesiosis in a dog with persistent thrombocytopenia. J Am Vet Med Assoc 2003; 223(9):1306–10.
174. Michau TM, Breitschwerdt EB, Gilger BC, et al. Bartonella vinsonii subspecies berkhoffi as a possible cause of anterior uveitis and choroiditis in a dog. Vet Ophthalmol 2003;6(4):299–304.
175. Cockwill KR, Taylor SM, Philibert HM, et al. Bartonella vinsonii subsp. berkhoffii endocarditis in a dog from Saskatchewan. Can Vet J 2007;48(8):839.
176. Cherry NA, Maggi RG, Rossmeisl JH, et al. Ecological Diversity of Bartonella Species Infection Among Dogs and Their Owner in Virginia. Vector Borne Zoonotic Dis 2011;11(11):1425–32.
177. Breitschwerdt EB, Goldkamp C, Castleman WL, et al. Hyperinsulinemic Hypoglycemia Syndrome in 2 Dogs with Bartonellosis. J Vet Intern Med 2014;28(4): 1331.
178. Berkowitz ST, Gannon KM, Carberry CA, et al. Resolution of spontaneous hemoabdomen secondary to peliosis hepatis following surgery and azithromycin treatment in a Bartonella species infected dog. J Vet Emerg Crit Care 2016; 26(6):851–7.
179. Mexas AM, Hancock SI, Breitschwerdt EB. Bartonella henselae and Bartonella elizabethae as Potential Canine Pathogens. J Clin Microbiol 2002;40(12): 4670–4.
180. Wolf LA, Cherry NA, Maggi RG, et al. In Pursuit of a Stealth Pathogen: Laboratory Diagnosis of Bartonellosis. Clin Microbiol Newsl 2014;36(5):33–9.
181. Pultorak EL, Maggi RG, Mascarelli PE, et al. Serial Testing from a 3-Day Collection Period by Use of the Bartonella Alphaproteobacteria Growth Medium Platform May Enhance the Sensitivity of Bartonella Species Detection in Bacteremic Human Patients. J Clin Microbiol 2013;51(6):1673.
182. Caponetti GC, Pantanowitz L, Marconi S, et al. Evaluation of Immunohistochemistry in Identifying Bartonella henselae in Cat-Scratch Disease. Am J Clin Pathol 2009;131(2):250–6.
183. Lashnits E, Maggi R, Jarskog F, et al. Schizophrenia and Bartonella spp. Infection: A Pilot Case-Control Study. Vector Borne Zoonotic Dis (Larchmont, NY) 2021;21(6):413–21.
184. Maggi RG, Richardson T, Breitschwerdt EB, et al. Development and validation of a droplet digital PCR assay for the detection and quantification of Bartonella species within human clinical samples. J Microbiol Methods 2020;176.
185. Vermeulen MJ, Herremans M, Verbakel H, et al. Serological testing for Bartonella henselae infections in The Netherlands: clinical evaluation of immunofluorescence assay and ELISA. Clin Microbiol Infect 2007;13(6):627–34.
186. Theel ES, Ross T. Seasonality of Bartonella henselae IgM and IgG antibody positivity rates. J Clin Microbiol 2019;57(12):e01263.

187. Herremans M, Vermeulen MJ, van de Kassteele J, et al. The use of Bartonella henselae-specific age dependent IgG and IgM in diagnostic models to discriminate diseased from non-diseased in Cat Scratch Disease serology. J Microbiol Methods 2007;71(2):107–13.

188. Bayart JL, Gusbin C, Lardinois B, et al. Analytical and clinical evaluation of new automated chemiluminescent immunoassays for the detection of IgG and IgM anti-Bartonella henselae antibodies. Diagn Microbiol Infect Dis 2020;98(4):115203.

189. Bergmans AMC, Peeters MF, Schellekens JFP, et al. Pitfalls and fallacies of cat scratch disease serology: evaluation of Bartonella henselae-based indirect fluorescence assay and enzyme-linked immunoassay. J Clin Microbiol 1997;35(8):1931–7.

190. Metzkor-Cotter E, Kletter Y, Avidor B, et al. Long-term serological analysis and clinical follow-up of patients with cat scratch disease. Clin Infect Dis 2003;37(9):1149–54.

191. Neupane P, Sevala S, Balakrishnan N, et al. Validation of bartonella henselae western immunoblotting for serodiagnosis of bartonelloses in dogs. J Clin Microbiol 2020;58(4):e01335.

192. Breitschwerdt EB, Suksawat J, Chomel B, et al. The immunologic response of dogs to Bartonella vinsonii subspecies berkhoffii antigens: as assessed by Western immunoblot analysis. J Vet Diagn Invest 2003;15(4):349–54.

193. Michael G, Yehudith K, Avidor B, et al. Enzyme immunoassay for the diagnosis of cat-scratch disease defined by polymerase chain reaction. Clin Infect Dis 2001;33(11):1852–8.

194. Wardrop KJ, Birkenheuer A, Blais MC, et al. Update on Canine and Feline Blood Donor Screening for Blood-Borne Pathogens. J Vet Intern Med 2016;30(1):15.

195. Nury C, Blais MC, Arsenault J. Risk of transmittable blood-borne pathogens in blood units from blood donor dogs in Canada. J Vet Intern Med 2021;35(3):1316–24.

196. Tabar MD, Movilla R, Serrano L, et al. PCR evaluation of selected vector-borne pathogens in dogs with pericardial effusion. J Small Anim Pract 2018;59(4):248–52.

197. Jinks MR, English Rv, Gilger BC. Causes of endogenous uveitis in cats presented to referral clinics in North Carolina. Vet Ophthalmol 2016;19:30–7.

198. Fontenelle JP, Powell CC, Acvo D, et al. Prevalence of serum antibodies against Bartonella species in the serum of cats with or without uveitis. J Feline Med Surg 2008;10:41–6.

199. Lashnits E, Neupane P, Maggi RG, et al. Detection of Bartonella spp. in dogs after infection with Rickettsia rickettsii. J Vet Intern Med 2020;34(1):145–59.

200. Hegarty BC, Bradley JM, Lappin MR, et al. Analysis of seroreactivity against cell culture-derived Bartonella spp. antigens in dogs. J Vet Intern Med 2014;28(1):38–41.

201. Osikowicz LM, Horiuchi K, Goodrich I, et al. Exposure of Domestic Cats to Three Zoonotic Bartonella Species in the United States. Pathogens 2021;10(3):354.

202. Bergmans AMC, de Jong CMA, van Amerongen G, et al. Prevalence of Bartonella species in domestic cats in The Netherlands. J Clin Microbiol 1997;35(9):2256–61.

203. Santhanam H, Nguyen MHN, Muthukumarasamy N, et al. Bartonella endocarditis in patients with right ventricle-to-pulmonary artery conduit: 2 case reports and literature review. IDCases 2021;26.

204. Breitschwerdt DVM E. Treatment of Canine and Feline Bartonellosis. Available at: www.galaxydx.com. Accessed February 1, 2022.
205. Kordick DL, Breitschwerdt EB. Persistent infection of pets within a household with three Bartonella species. Emerg Infect Dis 1998;4(2):325.
206. Podsiadły E, Żabicka D, Demkow U, et al. Susceptibility of Polish Bartonella henselae Strains. Polish J Microbiol 2012;61(2):143–5.
207. Li T, Feng J, Xiao S, et al. Identification of FDA-Approved Drugs with Activity against Stationary Phase Bartonella henselae. Antibiotics 2019;8(2).
208. Biswas S, Rolain JM. Bartonella infection: treatment and drug resistance. Future Microbiol 2010;5(11):1719–31.
209. Gadila SKG, Embers ME. Antibiotic Susceptibility of Bartonella Grown in Different Culture Conditions. Pathogens 2021;10(6).
210. Rolain JM, Brouqui P, Koehler JE, et al. Recommendations for treatment of human infections caused by Bartonella species. Antimicrob Agents Chemother 2004;48(6):1921–33.
211. Baddour LM, Wilson WR, Bayer AS, et al. Infective endocarditis: diagnosis, antimicrobial therapy, and management of complications: a statement for healthcare professionals from the Committee on Rheumatic Fever, Endocarditis, and Kawasaki Disease, Council on Cardiovascular Disease in the Young, and the Councils on Clinical Cardiology, Stroke, and Cardiovascular Surgery and Anesthesia, American Heart Association: endorsed by the Infectious Diseases Society of America. Circulation 2005;111(23):3167–84.
212. Tattevin P, Watt G, Revest M, et al. Update on blood culture-negative endocarditis. Med Mal Infect 2015;45(1–2):1–8.
213. Butler T. The Jarisch–Herxheimer Reaction After Antibiotic Treatment of Spirochetal Infections: A Review of Recent Cases and Our Understanding of Pathogenesis. Am J Trop Med Hyg 2017;96(1):46.
214. Lappin MR, Elston T, Evans L, et al. 2019 AAFP Feline Zoonoses Guidelines. J feline Med Surg 2019;21(11):1008–21.
215. Pennisi MG, Hartmann K, Addie DD, et al. Blood transfusion in cats: ABCD guidelines for minimising risks of infectious iatrogenic complications. J feline Med Surg 2015;17(7):588–93.
216. Taylor S, Spada E, Callan MB, et al. 2021 ISFM Consensus Guidelines on the Collection and Administration of Blood and Blood Products in Cats. J feline Med Surg 2021;23(5):410–32.
217. Kordick DL, Papich MG, Breitschwerdt EB. Efficacy of enrofloxacin or doxycycline for treatment of Bartonella henselae or Bartonella clarridgeiae infection in cats. Antimicrob Agents Chemother 1997;41(11):2448–55.
218. Regnery RL, Rooney JA, Johnson AM, et al. Experimentally induced Bartonella henselae infections followed by challenge exposure and antimicrobial therapy in cats. Am J Vet Res 1996;57(12):1714–9.

Babesia in North America
An Update

Jonathan D. Dear, DVM, MAS, DACVIM (SAIM)[a],*,
Adam Birkenheuer, DVM, PhD, DACVIM (SAIM)[b]

KEYWORDS

- Babesia • Babesiosis • Canine • Tick-borne • Thrombocytopenia • Anemia

KEY POINTS

- Canine babesiosis is caused by 5 unique species of *Babesia* in North America.
- Clinical signs can vary from subclinical or mild to severe and life-threatening.
- Fever, lymph node enlargement, and splenomegaly are the most common physical examination findings. Thrombocytopenia and anemia are the most common clinicopathologic findings.
- Although tick vectors are known or suspected for several species, other routes of transmission include transplacental, blood transfusion, and direct transmission via dog bites.

INTRODUCTION
Demystifying Canine Babesia

Since their discovery, members of the genus *Babesia* have been referred to as bacteria (*Micrococcus*), parasitic fungi (*Coniothecium stilesiarum*), and various names referring to protozoa (*Piroplasma canis*, *Pyrosoma bigeminum* var *canis*, and so forth). Formal changes in eukaryotic nomenclature should be proposed through the International Commission on Zoological Nomenclature (ICZN). Unfortunately, most of the proposed name changes for canine *Babesia* species have not followed ICZN guidelines or submitted to the organization. The resulting shifting nomenclature of these organisms reflects the challenges clinician scientists have had, and continue to have, categorizing and understanding the complex biology of this genus.

The first scientific mention of the organisms was in 1888 by Victor Babes who described the cytologic appearance of a parasite in the peripheral blood of cattle as "round and bright,.......about 0.5 μm in the middle it is divided by a light line in two parts, others in 4 by a second transverse line."[1] Initially it was not clear whether the

[a] Department of Medicine and Epidemiology, School of Veterinary Medicine, University of California, One Shields Avenue, Davis, CA 95616, USA; [b] Department of Clinical Sciences, College of Veterinary Medicine, North Carolina State University, 1060 William Moore Drive, Raleigh, NC 27607, USA
* Corresponding author.
E-mail address: jddear@ucdavis.edu

Vet Clin Small Anim 52 (2022) 1193–1209
https://doi.org/10.1016/j.cvsm.2022.07.016
0195-5616/22/© 2022 Elsevier Inc. All rights reserved.

organisms he was describing caused disease. In 1893 the physician and veterinarian duo, Drs Theobald Smith and Frederick Kilbourne, identified *Pyrosoma bigeminum* as the cause of Texas fever and, in doing so, postulated that it was a tick-vectored disease (the first ever identified).[2,3] We now know that *Babesia bigeminum* and *Babesia bovis* are the organisms that cause this disease of cattle.

Around the turn of the twentieth century *Piroplasma canis* and *Pyrosoma bigeminum* var *canis* were described as a cause of anemia in dogs in Europe, Asia, and Africa. However, the genus *Babesia* was not used to describe disease in dogs until 1918. Research occurring into the 1930s highlighted differences in vector ecology of canine *Babesia* despite them having similar cytopathologic appearance. During this period canine *Babesia* tended to be identified cytologically by their relative size, with large (2.5–5 μm) *Babesia* being considered *B. canis* and small organisms (1–2.5 μm) being named *B. gibsoni*. Differences in clinical disease manifestations and geographic distributions also informed speciation efforts.

Work in the late 1980s by Uilenberg and colleagues[4] and Zahler and colleagues[5] defined characteristics of 3 "large" *Babesia* and suggested that there were 3 subspecies: *B. canis* subsp *canis*, *rossi*, and *vogeli*.

Meanwhile, things were just starting to get confusing in the world of small *Babesia*. *Babesia gibsoni* was initially described in India in 1910, and historically, until molecular identification nearly 100 years later all small babesia were called *B. gibsoni*.[6] In 1991 Conrad and colleagues[7] documented what was suspected to be *B. gibsoni* in dogs in southern California. Then in 1999, Birkenheuer and colleagues described a series of dogs in North Carolina that were infected with *B. gibsoni*. Both of these reports were beyond the suspected geographic range of that protozoa.

As time marched on and molecular techniques facilitated phylogenetics, 2 major shifts occurred: the large *Babesia* subspecies in the *B. canis* group are now considered to represent 3 distinct species: *B. canis*, *B. rossi*, and *B. vogeli*. In addition, DNA sequencing determined that the *B. gibsoni* strains from North America and Asia were genetically divergent. In addition, the North American strains are composed of 3 distinct species of small piroplasma, *B. conradae*, *B. gibsoni*, and *B. vulpes*.[8,9] *Babesia conradae* was previously referred to as *B. gibsoni* and the "California isolate" and *B. vulpes*[10] was referred to as *Babesia microti*-like, the "Spanish isolate" and *Theileria annae*.[11,12]

BABESIA BASICS

Although we continue to learn about the ecologic and molecular differences that unite and separate *Babesia* species, there are certain key characteristics that likely apply to all species. *Babesia* undergo an asexual reproductive cycle in the dog, which serves as an intermediate host. Sexual reproduction occurs in the definitive host, which is suspected to be ticks for most *Babesia* species. Using the strictest criteria for genus designation, *Babesia* are considered to be obligate erythrocyte parasites, and species capable of infecting monocytes in addition to red blood cells are typically given an alternate genus designation, such as *Theileria* or *Cytauxzoon*. Thus, because it may infect both mononuclear cells and red blood cells, *B. vulpes* may, at some point in the future, no longer be considered to be a babesial organism.

When *Babesia* organisms are transmitted to a dog, they travel through connective tissue to reach capillary beds where they are able to infect red blood cells and undergo the aforementioned asexual reproduction. During this time *Babesia* can split via binary fission appearing in pairs or as intraerythrocytic inclusions with varied morphology (**Fig. 1**).

Following infection, there is a spectrum of disease that develops in the dog that varies depending on the infecting species, the immune response, and the inoculated

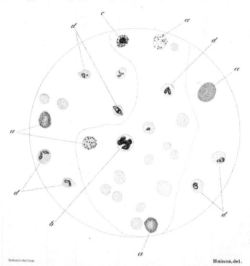

MICRO-ORGANISM WITHIN THE RED BLOOD CORPUSCLES.

Fig. 1. An illustration from the seminal publication *Investigations into the nature, causation, and prevention of Texas or southern cattle fever* demonstrating different cytologic appearances of *Babesia* organisms (d) in bovine blood. (Public domain https://collections.nlm.nih.gov/bookviewer?PID=nlm:nlmuid-62350480R-bk). The original figure legend reads: … "*a* represents modified red corpuscles, *b* a leukocyte, *c* a hematoblast, and *d* the parasites. Note the variation in the size of the red corpuscles. The parasites are mainly in pairs, they vary in size and form, and perhaps represent stages of degeneration." Modified red corpuscles refer to reticulocytes, and hematoblasts refer to rubricytes. Investigations into the nature, causation, and prevention of Texas or southern cattle fever, Washington: Government Printing Office, 1893. http://resource.nlm.nih.gov/62350480R.

parasite burden. Clinical signs can range from subclinical to mild to severe. In dogs with less severe infection, splenomegaly, lymphadenomegaly, lethargy, and anorexia may be the only clinical signs detected. Severe disease manifestations can include systemic inflammatory disease, shock, and death.

Several species of *Babesia* seem to be geographically constrained, which is likely related to the distribution of the corresponding reservoir hosts and tick vectors. As with all infectious diseases, it is important to consider travel history in patients with clinical and laboratory findings consistent with babesiosis in both endemic and non-endemic areas.[13]

TRANSMISSION

Transmission can occur through tick bite, dog fight, blood transfusion, or transplacentally.

Tick Transmission

Ticks are likely the definitive hosts for all *Babesia* species. Competent tick vectors have been identified for many (**Table 1**). In Asia, *Haemaphysalis longicornis* (the longhorn tick), *Haemaphysalis bispinosa*, and *Haemaphysalis hystricis* have been implicated as the major vectors for *B. gibsoni*.[14,15] Historically, these ticks have not been found in North America. However, *H. longicornis* was recently documented in New Jersey and subsequently reported in 9 states between 2017 and

Table 1
Species name, former names, references in which new names were proposed, and known or suspected tick vectors for Babesia species that infect dogs in North America

	Former Nomenclature	Prior References	Tick Vector
Babesia sp. 'coco'	Unnamed Large *Babesia*	Birkenheuer 2004, Sikorski 2010	*Amblyomma Americanum* (suspected)
Babesia conradae	"California isolate" "California genotype" *B. gibsoni*	Conrad 1991, Wozniak 1997, Yamane 1993, Zahler 2000, Macintire 2002 Birkenheuer 2003, 2005	Unknown
Babesia gibsoni	"Asian genotype"	Birkenheuer 2003, 2004, 2005	*Haemaphysalis longicornis*[a] *Haemaphysalis bispinosa* *Haemaphysalis hystricis* (Jongejan 2018)
Babesia vogeli	*B. canis* *B. canis vogeli*	Zahler 1998, Freeman 1994 Solano-Gallego 2008, Carli 2009, Uilenberg 1989	*Rhipicephalus sanguineus*
Babesia vulpes	*B. microti*-like "Spanish isolate" *Theileria annae*	Birkenheuer 2010, Garrett 2022 Garcia 2006, Yeagley 2009 Baneth 2015, Dixit 2010, Camacho 2003	Unknown in the United States

[a] No documented cases of tick transmission in North America.

2018. Other means of transmission are more important in the United States as detailed later.[16,17] *Rhipicephalus sanguineus* (the brown dog tick) is thought to be the major vector of *B. vogeli*, which accounts for its worldwide distribution, including North America.

The tick vectors and reservoir hosts for *B. 'coco'*, *B. conradae*, and *B. vulpes* have not been definitively determined. However, *Amblyomma americanum* is suspected to be the likely tick vector for *B. coco* based on the geographical congruence of vector and disease distribution.[18] Early studies evaluated *R. sanguineous* and *Dermacentor* spp ticks as potential vectors for *B. conradae*, but transmission did not occur in these experimental settings.[14] A recent survey of ticks in the United States detected *B. conradae* DNA in 2 *Dermacentor albipictus* ticks found on cats, but evidence for competence of transmission cannot be assumed.[19] Using polymerase chain reaction (PCR), a study of California coyotes found the overall prevalence of *B. conradae* to be 4.3%. Whether coyotes serve as reservoir or incidental hosts for this organism is not known.[20] In Spain, *Ixodes hexagonus* is thought to be the primary vector of *B. vulpes.* This tick has not been documented in North America. Other *Ixodes* spp may be involved in the transmission of this species of *Babesia.*[21]

Transfusion

Although there are only a few published reports of blood transfusion leading to transmission of *Babesia* species to naïve recipients in the literature,[22,23] experimental infections are induced by injection of infected blood.[24,25] Consequently, it seems reasonable that routine screening of donors should include PCR testing for *Babesia.*[26] Moreover, blood bank personnel should be aware that some PCR assays designed to detect *B. gibsoni* and *B. vogeli* do not detect *B. 'coco'*, *B. conradae*, and *B. vulpes.* Thus familiarity with the sensitivity and specificity of PCR assays for all relevant *Babesia* species in North America is important in developing blood donor screening protocols.

Transmission via Biting

Many *Babesia* species are suspected of being transmitted during dog fights. For instance, *B. gibsoni* lacks a competent tick vector in most of North America. It was likely introduced by imported dogs from Asia used for dog fighting. Several studies continue to document a greater prevalence in American pit bull terriers and related breeds (hereafter referred to as American pit bull terriers [APBT]) and dogs rescued from dog fighting operations in both North America and Asia.[27–30] Likewise, studies have documented *B. conradae* infections in dogs used for coyote hunting. A history of aggressive interactions with coyotes was found to be a risk factor associated with infection in one study.[31,32] *Babesia vulpes* has also been linked to a history of dog fighting.[33]

Transplacental Transmission

Transplacental transmission has been definitively documented or suspected for most canine *Babesia*. Although direct infection via a shared environmental source (ie, a tick vector or other mechanism of infection) cannot be definitely excluded, 7 of 12 dogs infected with *B. conradae* in one case series of naturally infected dogs descended from a single bitch.[34] In another study, experimental infection during pregnancy led to transmission in utero of the entire litter; 1 puppy was stillborn and the remaining 4 puppies died shortly after birth.[35]

DIAGNOSIS, TREATMENT, AND PREVENTION
General Diagnostic Principles

In general, there are 3 methods to diagnose *Babesia* infections in dogs: blood smear cytology, serology and PCR. Each method has its own strengths and limitations. Cytology is inexpensive and can be performed within the clinic; however, identification of intraerythrocytic piroplasma on a blood smear can be hampered by very low levels of parasites circulating in blood and inadequate staining. Wright stain is superior to rapid in-clinic staining but is often not available in small animal practices. PCR is sensitive; however, as cytology, a negative test can occur in actively infected patients due to low numbers of circulating organisms. In addition, some PCR assays that target certain species do not detect all species of *Babesia*. Serologic testing is available for several of the more commonly diagnosed *Babesia* species and can be less expensive than PCR testing. Unfortunately, the lag in antibody response makes serology less helpful for diagnosing acute disease. In addition, the degree of serologic cross-reactivity between species of *Babesia* is not clear. Clinicians should contact individual laboratories to determine the sensitivity and specificity of the assays used. Generally speaking, when possible, combining PCR with serology can increase overall clinical sensitivity.

General Treatment Principles

A number of antiprotozoal medications have been used to treat dogs with babesiosis. Details of treatment trials are discussed in the context of the individual species later in this article, but there are some common strategies for treatment that are discussed here. *Babesia vogeli* seems to be the parasite most responsive to treatment and is generally cleared after 2 doses of imidocarb (**Table 2**). Pretreatment with anticholinergics helps to prevent side effects. Resolution of clinical signs occurs in response to treatment with the combination therapy of atovaquone and azithromycin for infection with the small *Babesia* (*B. conradae*, *B. gibsoni*, and *B. vulpes*; **Table 2**), but there is a concern that infection with *B. gibsoni* and *B. vulpes* might persist despite clinical improvement. Persistence of *B. conradae* following treatment seems to occur less frequently. Not enough is known about *B. 'coco'* to make evidence-based recommendations for its treatment.

Table 2
Medications reported for use in the treatment of canine babesiosis in North America

Medication	Dose	Route	Frequency	Duration
Artesunate[a]	12.5 mg/kg	PO	Q 24h	10 days
Atovaquone[a]	13.3 mg/kg	PO	Q 8h	10 days
Azithromycin[a]	10 mg/kg	PO	Q 24 h	10 days
Clindamycin[b]	25 mg/kg	PO	Q 12 h	90 days
Doxycycline[b]	5 mg/kg	PO	Q 12 h	90 days
Diminazene aceturate	3.5 mg/kg	IM	Once	N/A
Imidocarb dipropionate	6.6 mg/kg	IM or SQ	Twice	14 days apart
Metronidazole[b]	10 mg/kg	PO	Q 12 h	90 days

Drug efficacy varies with infecting species, and drugs are used in specific combinations. See text for details.

[a] Atovaquone and azithromycin are always used in combination for treatment of *B. conradae*, *B. gibsoni*, *B. vulpes*, and, potentially, *Babesia* sp. 'Coco.' Artesunate was added to this combination in one study and appeared well tolerated.

[b] Clindamycin, doxycycline, and metronidazole have been used in combination for treatment of dogs with *B. gibsoni* that do not respond to atovaquone and azithromycin.

Following treatment, dogs should be retested by PCR at 60 and 90 days to help verify remission; this is recommended even in the absence of an initial negative PCR, as dogs can remain seropositive for months to years following successful treatment. Dogs respond clinically within a few days and become PCR negative very quickly with treatment (eg, as soon as 5 days) but disease can relapse after treatments. Clinicopathologic abnormalities begin to resolve within days to weeks but some, including hyperglobulinemia and proteinuria, might take several months to resolve. If a dog fails to clinically respond within 7 to 10 days, testing for coinfection or concurrent disease is recommended.

Atovaquone is a hydroxynaphthoquinone antiprotozoal medication that inhibits electron transport in parasite mitochondria. Two commercial formulations exist: Mepron (GlaxoSmithKline, Brentford, UK) and Malarone (GlaxoSmithKline, Brentford, UK). Both formulations should be administered with a fatty meal to promote absorption. In the past Mepron has been recommended because Malarone contains proguanil and may result in more frequent adverse effects including vomiting and anorexia; this has raised a concern that subtherapeutic drug levels secondary to vomiting. The resulting lack of absorption might facilitate the development of cytochrome B mutations that convey resistance to atovaquone.[36] In spite of this concern, a recent case series evaluating the combination of Malarone azithromycin and artesunate, showed promising results for the treatment of *B. gibsoni*. Gastrointestinal side effects such as vomiting and diarrhea were not reported to occur following treatment in this trial. Interestingly, artesunate is a derivative of artemisinin, which is a compound extracted from a Chinese herb with antiprotozoal properties.

Treating splenectomized dogs infected with *Babesia* poses a particular challenge, as the spleen plays a central role in disease premunition. For dogs that develop clinical disease after splenectomy, the "kitchen sink" approach, along with the use of alternating therapies, can minimize clinical disease. In splenectomized dogs that have failed to clear the infection with atovaquone and azithromycin, one author (AB) has had success using a combination of atovaquone and azithromycin, imidocarb, artemisinin, clindamycin, doxycycline, and metronidazole. Antiemetics are typically used preemptively in these cases. For dogs that have not been splenectomized, a 90-day course of clindamycin, doxycycline, and metronidazole with or without artemisinin has led to clinical improvement in dogs infected with *B. gibsoni* that fail to respond to atovaquone and azithromycin.

General principles for prevention

As transmission can occur via tick bite, dog bite, blood transfusion, or transplacentally, there is not a "one-size-fits-all" approach to disease prevention. It seems reasonable to support the use of acaricidal medications for the prevention of *B. vogeli* and *B. coco*, as tick transmission is probably the primary method of transmission of these infections. However, prevention of infection with *B. conradae*, *B. gibsoni*, and *B. vulpes* may not be accomplished using this same strategy, as infection largely occurs via dog bites or transplacentally and more rarely via blood transfusions. Given this reality, intact or pregnant APBT should be screened for *B. gibsoni* and *B. vulpes* routinely, as should all blood donor dogs in North America.

SPECIES-SPECIFIC INFORMATION
Babesia vogeli

Babesia vogeli has been described by some as being the "cosmopolitan" *Babesia* given its worldwide distribution.[37] In North America, infections in domestic dogs tend to correlate with heaviest burdens of its tick vector, *R. Sanguineus*. As one of the least virulent of the large *Babesia* species, most immunocompetent dogs infected with *B. vogeli* seem to have subclinical infections.[38] However, young dogs or dogs that are immunocompromised (eg, dogs that are splenectomized, coinfected with *Ehrlichia canis*, or receiving chemotherapy or other immunosuppressive medications) tend to develop clinical disease and are at greater risk of death from infection.[25,39–41]

Infected dogs tend to present with nonspecific clinical signs such as anorexia and lethargy. Fever is the most common physical examination finding.[25,40] When affected, moderate to marked thrombocytopenia is the most common clinicopathologic disturbance.[25] Immune-mediated hemolysis seems to be common in dogs with *B. vogeli*, as antierythrocyte immunoglobulin G has been detected in many infected dogs, although immunocompetent dogs might not develop anemia.[42]

In a small case series of 11 dogs infected with *B. vogeli*, 3 died or were euthanized, presumably from consequences related to their primary disease. In this report there was a single dog with chronic kidney disease along with severe and diffuse membranoproliferative glomerulonephritis likely resulting from babesiosis given the dog's young age (7 months).[40] Given this finding, it seems likely that chronic *B. vogeli* infection might result in protein-losing nephropathy similar to that seen in dogs with other *Babesia* infections.

Definitive diagnosis of *B. vogeli* can be achieved by a PCR assay using whole blood. PCR assays that detect *B. gibsoni* are widely available at commercial laboratories and academic centers. Although cytologic identification of erythrocyte piroplasms is specific for babesiosis, as with other babesial parasites it is impossible to speciate the organism on morphology alone. Furthermore, the sensitivity of microscopy is limited by the typically low parasitemia (often < 1% of erythrocytes) even in severely affected dogs (**Fig. 2**).[39] Serologic testing (indirect fluorescent antibody test) is available and can be used in the diagnosis of *B. vogeli*, although PCR is more specific. Combining PCR with serologic testing, using acute and convalescent serologic testing and repeat testing using PCR may increase sensitivity.

B. vogeli can be treated with imidocarb with a favorable prognosis. It is thought that the parasite is eliminated after 2 doses administered 14 days apart.[39,40] That said, controlled clinical trials using PCR for follow-up testing have not been performed. Given that they share the same tick vector, dogs with *B. vogeli* infections should also be screened for *E canis*, as concurrent infections can result in more severe clinical disease.

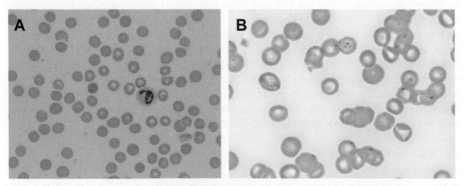

Fig. 2. Representative blood smears showing small (*A*; *B. conradae*) and large (*B*; –*B. vogeli*) *Babesia* spp in canine erythrocytes. Although blood smear can often help to differentiate between large and small *Babesia*, it is impossible to speciate further with cytology alone.

Babesia gibsoni

Babesia gibsoni is the most common *Babesia* species infecting North American dogs. In one study the organism accounted for 79% of *Babesia* positive samples submitted to a commercial laboratory.[43] *Babesia gibsoni* has been diagnosed across North America. Most of the infected dogs are APBT. American Pitbull Terrier type dogs accounted for approximately 75% of the positive cases in samples submitted to one university laboratory.[36]

Although most of the dogs diagnosed with *B. giboni* are APBT, approximately 25% of positive dogs belong to other breeds. In infected dogs from breeds other than APBT, there has been an association between infection and history of dog bite, particularly bites from APBT.[28,44] Given that most dogs in North America infected with *B. gibsoni* have a history of a dog bite, coinfections with haemotropic *Mycoplasma* spp and *B. vulpes* are relatively common.

Although not often described, transfusion-associated infections do occur and, in the investigators' opinion, are probably more common than reported.[22]

Most dogs that are infected with *B. gibsoni* have mild to moderate disease. The most common clinical and laboratory findings are pale mucous membranes, splenomegaly, thrombocytopenia, and hemolytic regenerative anemia. Splenomegaly can be occasionally detected on abdominal palpation or diagnostic imaging. The splenomegaly can be generalized or associated with benign splenic masses.[45] Therefore, *B. gibsoni* infection should be ruled out and/or treated in all APBT dogs before any nonemergent splenectomy.

Thrombocytopenia can be mild to severe. As is observed canine infection with other *Babesia* species found in North America, petechiation and ecchymosis rarely or never occur, even when thrombocytopenia is severe.[46] The anemia can also vary from mild to severe and tends to be regenerative, although nonregenerative anemia can occur early in acute disease. Hyperbilirubinemia seems to occur more frequently with *B. gibsoni* infections than other species.[46] Hemolysis can occur because of oxidative damage or antierythrocyte antibody targeting.[47] Consequently, testing for *B. gibsoni* should be considered for all dogs suspected of having immune-mediated hemolytic anemia before immunosuppressive therapy, especially in at-risk breeds.[48]

Hyperglobulinemia and protein-losing nephropathy have also been reported as a consequence of *B. gibsoni* infection. Proteinuria does not develop frequently and may resolve with treatment of the infection.[45]

Identifying characteristic intraerythrocytic organisms with cytologic examination of blood smears can confirm the clinical suspicion of babesiosis in a typical breed with compatible clinical signs. However, cytology is insensitive and cannot allow differentiation among species of small *Babesia*, as they seem morphologically identical (see **Fig. 2**). Likewise, seroreactivity supports a diagnosis but is not definitive due to serologic cross-reactivity with other species and that without documenting seroconversion, seroreactivity indicates exposure but not necessarily active infection. PCR is the only way to definitely identify the species and confirm active infection. PCR assays that target *B. gibsoni* are available through most veterinary reference laboratories. Combining PCR with serology and repeat testing of the same or additional samples using PCR increases diagnostic sensitivity.[49]

Combination therapy with atovaquone and azithromycin has been considered the optimal treatment protocol to induce clinical remission. However, as with all *Babesia* sp infections, splenectomy posttreatment followed by subinoculation of blood into naïve splenectomized dogs would be required to determine if infection is truly cleared (see **Table 2**).[50] Combination therapy with atovaquone (Malarone), azithromycin, and artesunate seems to result in remission based on long-term PCR monitoring similar to atovaquone (Mepron) and azithromycin alone.[51] Controlled studies directly comparing Mepron and azithromycin with Malarone, azithromycin, and artesunate are indicated.

In dogs with infections resistant to atovaquone, long-term therapy using a combination of clindamycin, doxycycline, and metronidazole improves clinical health and in some dogs may result in clearance of infection based on long-term PCR monitoring.[52] Unfortunately, no controlled trials have been performed, and evidence-based therapeutic protocols using these drugs are not available. Treatment with imidocarb and diminazene aceturate can reduce clinical signs and laboratory abnormalities but does not clear the parasite.[50,53] Lumefantrine has been studied in vitro for its potential synergism with artemisinin-related compounds, but there are no published reports documenting its efficacy, and limited clinical observations suggest that it, too, cannot clear infection.[54]

Babesia vulpes

As mentioned at the beginning of this article, B. vulpes has been referred to by many names (B. microti-like, Theileria annae, Babesia Spanish dog isolate and B. gibsoni in some early studies), and it will likely be renamed again. B. microti, the type species for the clade of organisms to which B. vulpes belongs, has a lifecycle that involves both an erythrocytic and a monocytic phase in vertebrate hosts, differentiating it from "true" Babesia. Babesia vulpes has been detected in dogs in Europe and the Eastern United States and was the third most frequently identified canine Babesia in one North American veterinary diagnostic laboratory.[43] In Spain Ixodes hexagonus is suspected of being its main vector, although its vector in North America has not been determined. Transmission has been reported to occur frequently in dogs used in fighting, and APBT accounted for 92% of PCR-positive dogs in one study.[33] Foxes are likely the reservoir host of this parasite. Both red and gray foxes are infected in North America with a prevalence between 25% and40%.[55] Other wildlife such as the American river otter can be infected and might also play a role in the epidemiology of this disease.[56]

Clinical disease in dogs infected with B. vulpes resembles infection with other small species of Babesia with splenomegaly, asplenia from previous splenectomy, or bite wounds reported in many dogs. Clinicopathologic evaluation often reveals moderate to marked anemia (typically regenerative), mild to marked thrombocytopenia, and hyperglobulinemia.[33] Coinfection with B. gibsoni is common. Azotemia and proteinuria have been reported in dogs infected with B. vulpes, but whether infection caused the renal abnormalities is not fully known.[33]

As is the case for other small Babesia, microscopic evaluation of a blood smear can facilitate diagnosis; however, cytologic examination cannot differentiate between related species (see **Fig. 2**). There is no serologic assay designed to detect B. vulpes-specific antibodies. The amount of serologic cross-reactivity that occurs when using assays designed to detect antibodies that target other Babesia species has not been thoroughly studied but some cross-reactivity has been documented.[33] PCR is the only way to definitively diagnose infection; however, it is important to note that not all Babesia spp PCR assays will detect this species and identify it as B. vulpes.

Combination therapy with atovaquone and azithromycin has been used to treat dogs with B. vulpes infections, but no long-term, controlled trials have been performed to explore their efficacy.[33] There are no published reports of alternative therapies for B. vulpes infections. Coinfections with B. gibsoni and haemotropic Mycoplasma are common.[33,57]

Babesia conradae

As one of the small parasites originally identified as *B. gibsoni*, much of the early work documenting the epidemiology and pathophysiology of *B. conradae* is published under its former species designation. Most of these sentinel studies originated from Dr Patricia Conrad's laboratory at University of California Davis, for whom this species was subsequently named.[7,14,24]

Most dogs diagnosed with *B. conradae* are from the Central Valley or Southern part of California.[32,34,58] There is one of coyote hunting dogs in Oklahoma that have been infected with this species.[31] It is unclear whether these dogs were infected in Oklahoma or whether they were imported from or traveled to California as a result of interstate trading.

Infected dogs tend to develop acute disease that typically presents as lethargy and anorexia. On physical examination dogs often have pale mucous membranes, an elevated body temperature, splenomegaly, and, in the case of coyote hunting dogs, evidence of wounds.[59] Complete blood count tends to reveal mild to marked regenerative hemolytic anemia and moderate thrombocytopenia along with leukopenia characterized by neutropenia.[7,32] Infected dogs also tend to have low serum albumin and high serum globulin concentrations. Although the magnitude of thrombocytopenia is typically not low enough to cause spontaneous bleeding, some dogs with untreated *B. conradae* infections have bleeding diatheses. Because the magnitude of thrombocytopenia is typically not low enough to cause spontaneous hemorrhage, additional mechanisms may contribute to disordered hemostasis (**Fig. 3**).

Diagnosing infection is best accomplished using species-specific PCR. Some assays targeting the Genus *Babesia* will not detect this organism.[32] Blood smears can reveal intraerythrocytic parasites, but as for other *Babesia* species, the sensitivity of microscopy is usually hampered by low levels of parasitemia. Typically, less than 2% to 3% of erythrocytes are infected, even with severe clinical disease (see **Fig. 2**). As with other *Babesia* infections, it is impossible to determine the infecting species by visual inspection alone. An indirect fluorescent antibody test has been developed but is not commercially available.[60]

The combination of atovaquone and azithromycin effectively clears infection, which is defined as a negative PCR test of peripheral blood 60 and 90 days posttreatment along with resolution of clinical and laboratory abnormalities.[31,34,61] Dogs infected with *B. conradae* do not seem to relapse with disease as can be observed with *B. gibsoni* infections. Although the investigator has encountered dogs effectively treated with

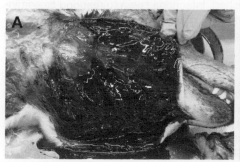
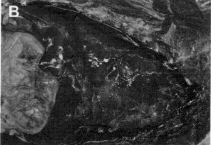

Fig. 3. Necropsy images from a 3-year-old male Greyhound mix that was diagnosed with *B conradae* but died suddenly before treatment. Postmortem findings included multisystemic (including mandibular (*A*) and cavitary (*B*) hemorrhage despite only a moderate thrombocytopenia (122,000/μL). (UC Davis VMTH Anatomic Pathology Service.)

combination therapy that test positive years later, in all cases, reinfection was suspected based on a high incidence of recurrence in dogs with continued aggressive interactions with coyotes. Imidocarb and diminazene aceturate seem to be ineffective in clearing the organism.[7] Coinfections with hemotropic *Mycoplasma* are common in dogs with wildlife contact. The combination of atovaquone and azithromycin seems to clear infection with "*Candidatus* Mycoplasma haematoparvum" but not *Mycoplasma haemocanis*.[61]

Babesia sp. 'Coco'

Babesia 'coco' was initially described in a case report of a dog ('Coco') with multicentric lymphoma who developed clinical signs of babesiosis but sequencing of the involved piroplasm was inconsistent with known species.[62] Subsequently, this species has been detected in dogs with clinical babesiosis from the mid-Atlantic, Southeastern, and Southcentral United States. It seems that immunocompromised dogs are more susceptible to this disease, as all 7 dogs in a small case series had identifiable cause of immunocompromise (splenectomy in 6 dogs).[63]

The prevalence of *B. 'coco'* is unknown although a review of *Babesia* positive samples submitted to the North Carolina State University Vector Borne Disease Diagnostic Laboratory documented approximately the same prevalence as *B. vogeli* (0.17% of dogs tested).[33]

When clinical signs are present, fever may be the only abnormal physical examination finding. Petechiation and ecchymosis are absent, even when severe thrombocytopenia is present. Thrombocytopenia and mild anemia, which can be regenerative or nonregenerative, are the most common hematologic findings.[63]

Although published reports of ill dogs infected with *B. 'coco'* have identifiable exogenous or endogenous causes of immunocompromise (splenectomy or chemotherapy), recent information suggests that approximately 25% of positive cases do not. (Birkenheuer unpublished data, 2021) *B. 'coco'* has been suspected as the cause of fever of unknown origin in some unpublished observations, but further study is needed to characterize the role of the protozoa in these cases.

As with other species of *Babesia*, microscopic evaluation of blood smears can facilitate the diagnosis of *B. 'coco'*, but visual evaluation cannot determine species (see **Fig. 2**). Serologic testing is not currently commercially available, and cross-reactivity with other species is inconsistent. PCR is the only method of establishing definitive diagnosis, although negative PCR does not rule out infection in cases of low parasitemia or if an appropriate species-specific assay is not used.

Optimal treatment has not been established. Infections seem to respond to administration of either imidocarb or combination atovaquone and azithromycin (see **Table 2**).[63] Anecdotally, it seems that dogs are more likely to become PCR negative with the latter approach.

Prevention

Although there is evidence that many *Babesia* spp are transmitted through tick bites, there is a paucity of data evaluating acaricide use as a strategy in the prevention of canine babesiosis in North America. Most of the studies evaluating the ability of acaracides to reduce the risk of transmission have used a European *Babesia* species, *Babesia canis (canis)*, as the pathogen. Studies evaluating the natural tick-vectors of the canine *Babesia* species in North America and whether acaracides reduce the risk of their transmission are needed. Although acaracide use is important, the reality is that many North American dogs are infected via alternate routes such as vertical transmission and biting.

Human Health Implications

Canine babesiosis is not a zoonotic disease. Although several *Babesia* species that infect humans such as *Babesia microti* and *Babesia duncani* have wildlife reservoirs, transmission of these protozoa likely requires a tick vector. In addition, infection with the organisms that infect people has not been documented in canine patients.

SUMMARY

Canine babesiosis in North America is caused by 1 of 5 identified *Babesia* species and results in multisystemic disease. *Babesia* are intracellular parasites of erythrocytes and can be transmitted transplacentally, via tick bite, blood transfusion, or aggressive interactions. Clinical signs include lethargy, anorexia, and depression, whereas physical examination findings include pallor and splenomegaly. Clinicopathologic findings associated with babesiosis include hemolytic anemia, thrombocytopenia, hyperglobulinemia, and proteinuria. Diagnosis can be achieved by evaluation of blood smear, serology, or PCR, but only PCR allows for speciation. Treatment can be challenging and dogs might relapse following cessation of therapy (especially those undergoing immunosuppression such as chemotherapy or splenectomy). More randomized, controlled studies are needed to assess best practices for treatment.

CLINICS CARE POINTS

- Babesiosis should be considered in dogs with thrombocytopenia, anemia, hyperglobulinemia, splenomegaly, proteinuria, or azotemia.

- Diagnostics should include blood smear examination and PCR assays that can detect all relevant *Babesia* spp and serology.

- In high-risk breeds (APBT or Greyhounds) or dogs with high risk of infection (tick exposure, dog bites, or blood transfusions from high-risk breeds) consider empirical treatment.

- To determine if therapy has been successful, monitoring for resolution of laboratory abnormalities, and performing PCR to document at least 2 consecutive negative tests approximately 60 and 90 days posttreatment is recommended.

- Antibody titers can remain positive for months to years after treatment and are therefore less useful for determining whether infection has been cleared.

DISCLOSURE

J.D. Dear: no financial or conflicts of interest to disclose. A. Birkenheuer: Co-Director of the Vector Borne Disease Diagnostic Laboratory at North Carolina State University (no financial compensation) and consulting and continuing education provided for Idexx Laboratories Inc, Boehringer-Ingelheim and Merck.

REFERENCES

1. Babes V. Sur l'hemoglobinurie bacterienne du boeuf. CR Acad Sci 1888;107: 692–4.
2. Assadian O, Stanek G. Theobald Smith — the discoverer of ticks as vectors of disease. Wien Klin Wochenschr 2002;114:479–81.

3. Smith T, Kilborne FL. Investigations into the nature, causation, and prevention of Texas or southern cattle fever. Washington, DC.: Government Printing Office; 1893.

4. Uilenberg G, Franssen FF, Perie NM, et al. Three groups of *Babesia canis* distinguished and a proposal for nomenclature. Vet Q 1989;11:33–40.

5. Zahler M, Schein E, Rinder H, et al. Characteristic genotypes discriminate between *Babesia canis* isolates of differing vector specificity and pathogenicity to dogs. Parasitol Res 1998;84:544–8.

6. Patton WS. Preliminary report on a new piroplasm (*Piroplasma gibsoni* sp. nov.) found in the blood of the hounds of the Madras Hunt and subsequently discovered in the blood of the jackal *Canis aureus*. Bull de la Société de pathologie exotique 1910;3:274–80.

7. Conrad P, Thomford J, Yamane I, et al. Hemolytic anemia caused by *Babesia gibsoni* infection in dogs. J Am Vet Med Assoc 1991;199:601–5.

8. Kjemtrup AM, Kocan AA, Whitworth L, et al. There are at least three genetically distinct small piroplasms from dogs. Int J Parasitol 2000;30:1501–5.

9. Zahler M, Rinder H, Zweygarth E, et al. *Babesia gibsoni'* of dogs from North America and Asia belong to different species. Parasitology 2000;120(Pt 4):365–9.

10. Baneth G, Florin-Christensen M, Cardoso L, et al. Reclassification of *Theileria annae* as *Babesia vulpes* sp. nov. Parasit Vectors 2015;8:207.

11. Garcia AT. Piroplasma infection in dogs in northern Spain. Vet Parasitol 2006;138: 97–102.

12. Dixit P, Dixit AK, Varshney JP. Evidence of new pathogenic *Theileria* species in dogs. J Parasit Dis 2010;34:29–32.

13. Allison RW, Yeagley TJ, Levis K, et al. *Babesia canis rossi* infection in a Texas dog. Vet Clin Pathol/Am Soc Vet Clin Pathol 2011;40:345–50.

14. Yamane I, Gardner IA, Telford SR, et al. Vector Competence of *Rhipicephalus sanguineus* and *Dermacentor variabilis* for American Isolates of *Babesia gibsoni*. Exp Appl Acarol 1993;17:913–9.

15. Jongejan F, Su BL, Yang HJ, et al. Molecular evidence for the transovarial passage of *Babesia gibsoni* in *Haemaphysalis hystricis* (Acari: Ixodidae) ticks from Taiwan: a novel vector for canine babesiosis. Parasit Vectors 2018;11:134.

16. Rainey T, Occi JL, Robbins RG, et al. Discovery of *Haemaphysalis longicornis* (Ixodida: Ixodidae) Parasitizing a Sheep in New Jersey, United States. J Med Entomol 2018;55:757–9.

17. Beard CB, Occi J, Bonilla DL, et al. Multistate Infestation with the Exotic Disease-Vector Tick *Haemaphysalis longicornis* - United States, August 2017-September 2018. MMWR Morb Mortal Wkly Rep 2018;67:1310–3.

18. Shock BC, Moncayo A, Cohen S, et al. Diversity of piroplasms detected in blood-fed and questing ticks from several states in the United States. Ticks Tick Borne Dis 2014;5:373–80.

19. Duncan KT, Grant A, Johnson B, et al. Identification of *Rickettsia* spp. and *Babesia conradae* in *Dermacentor* spp. Collected from Dogs and Cats Across the United States. Vector Borne Zoonotic Dis 2021;21:911–20.

20. Javeed N, Foley JE, Quinn N, et al. Prevalence and geographic distribution of Babesia conradae in California coyotes (Canis latrans). In: International Babesiosis Meeting III, New Haven, CT, April 24-25, 2021.

21. Camacho AT, Pallas E, Gestal JJ, et al. *Ixodes hexagonus* is the main candidate as vector of *Theileria annae* in northwest Spain. Vet Parasitol 2003;112:157–63.

22. Stegeman JR, Birkenheuer AJ, Kruger JM, et al. Transfusion-associated *Babesia gibsoni* infection in a dog. J Am Vet Med Assoc 2003;222:959–63, 952.

23. Freeman MJ, Kirby BM, Panciera DL, et al. Hypotensive shock syndrome associated with acute *Babesia canis* infection in a dog. J Am Vet Med Assoc 1994; 204:94–6.

24. Wozniak EJ, Barr BC, Thomford JW, et al. Clinical, anatomic, and immunopathologic characterization of *Babesia gibsoni* infection in the domestic dog (Canis familiaris). J Parasitol 1997;83:692–9.

25. Wang J, Zhang J, Kelly P, et al. First description of the pathogenicity of *Babesia vogeli* in experimentally infected dogs. Vet Parasitol 2018;253:1–7.

26. Nury C, Blais MC, Arsenault J. Risk of transmittable blood-borne pathogens in blood units from blood donor dogs in Canada. J Vet Intern Med 2021;35:1316–24.

27. Macintire DK, Boudreaux MK, West GD, et al. *Babesia gibsoni* infection among dogs in the southeastern United States. J Am Vet Med Assoc 2002;220:325–9.

28. Yeagley TJ, Reichard MV, Hempstead JE, et al. Detection of *Babesia gibsoni* and the canine small *Babesia* 'Spanish isolate' in blood samples obtained from dogs confiscated from dogfighting operations. J Am Vet Med A 2009;235:535–9.

29. Miyama T, Sakata Y, Shimada Y, et al. Epidemiological survey of *Babesia gibsoni* infection in dogs in eastern Japan. J Vet Med Sci 2005;67:467–71.

30. Jefferies R, Ryan UM, Jardine J, et al. Blood, Bull Terriers and Babesiosis: further evidence for direct transmission of *Babesia gibsoni* in dogs. Aust Vet J 2007;85: 459–63.

31. Stayton E, Lineberry M, Thomas J, et al. Emergence of *Babesia conradae* infection in coyote-hunting Greyhounds in Oklahoma, USA. Parasit Vectors 2021; 14:402.

32. Dear JD, Owens SD, Lindsay LL, et al. *Babesia conradae* infection in coyote hunting dogs infected with multiple blood-borne pathogens. J Vet Intern Med 2018; 32:1609–17.

33. Barash NR, Thomas B, Birkenheuer AJ, et al. Prevalence of *Babesia* spp. and clinical characteristics of *Babesia vulpes* infections in North American dogs. J Vet Intern Med 2019;33:2075–81.

34. Di Cicco MF, Downey ME, Beeler E, et al. Re-emergence of *Babesia conradae* and effective treatment of infected dogs with atovaquone and azithromycin. Vet Parasitol 2012;187:23–7.

35. Fukumoto S, Suzuki H, Igarashi I, et al. Fatal experimental transplacental *Babesia gibsoni* infections in dogs. Int J Parasitol 2005;35:1031–5.

36. Birkenheuer AJ, Marr HS, Wilson JM, et al. *Babesia gibsoni* cytochrome b mutations in canine blood samples submitted to a US veterinary diagnostic laboratory. J Vet Intern Med 2018;32:1965–9.

37. Penzhorn BL. Don't let sleeping dogs lie: unravelling the identity and taxonomy of *Babesia canis, Babesia rossi* and *Babesia vogeli*. Parasit Vectors 2020;13:184.

38. Di Cataldo S, Ulloa-Contreras C, Cevidanes A, et al. *Babesia vogeli* in dogs in Chile. Transbound Emerg Dis 2020;67:2296–9.

39. Irwin PJ. Canine babesiosis. Vet Clin North Am Small Anim Pract 2010;40: 1141–56.

40. Solano-Gallego L, Trotta M, Carli E, et al. *Babesia canis canis* and *Babesia canis vogeli* clinicopathological findings and DNA detection by means of PCR-RFLP in blood from Italian dogs suspected of tick-borne disease. Vet Parasitol 2008;157: 211–21.

41. Rawangchue T, Sungpradit S. Clinicopathological and molecular profiles of *Babesia vogeli* infection and Ehrlichia canis coinfection. Vet World 2020;13: 1294–302.

42. Carli E, Tasca S, Trotta M, et al. Detection of erythrocyte binding IgM and IgG by flow cytometry in sick dogs with *Babesia canis canis* or *Babesia canis vogeli* infection. Vet Parasitol 2009;162:51–7.

43. Birkenheuer AJ, Buch J, Beall MJ, et al. Global distribution of canine *Babesia* species identified by a commercial diagnostic laboratory. Vet Parasitol Reg Stud Rep 2020;22:100471.

44. Birkenheuer AJ, Correa MT, Levy MG, et al. Geographic distribution of babesiosis among dogs in the United States and association with dog bites: 150 cases (2000-2003). J Am Vet Med A 2005;227:942–7.

45. Ullal T, Birkenheuer A, Vaden S. Azotemia and Proteinuria in Dogs Infected with *Babesia gibsoni*. J Am Anim Hosp Assoc 2018;54:156–60.

46. Liu PC, Lin CN, Su BL. Clinical characteristics of naturally *Babesia gibsoni* infected dogs: a study of 60 dogs. Vet Parasitol Reg Stud Rep 2022;28:100675.

47. Otsuka Y, Yamasaki M, Yamato O, et al. The effect of macrophages on the erythrocyte oxidative damage and the pathogenesis of anemia in *Babesia gibsoni*-infected dogs with low parasitemia. J Vet Med Sci 2002;64:221–6.

48. Garden OA, Kidd L, Mexas AM, et al. ACVIM consensus statement on the diagnosis of immune-mediated hemolytic anemia in dogs and cats. J Vet Intern Med/Am Coll Vet Intern Med 2019;33:313–34.

49. Kidd L. Optimal Vector-borne Disease Screening in Dogs Using Both Serology-based and Polymerase Chain Reaction-based Diagnostic Panels. Vet Clin North Am Small Anim Pract 2019;49:703–18.

50. Birkenheuer AJ, Levy MG, Breitschwerdt EB. Efficacy of combined atovaquone and azithromycin for therapy of chronic *Babesia gibsoni* (Asian genotype) infections in dogs. J Vet Intern Med 2004;18:494–8.

51. Karasova M, Tothova C, Vichova B, et al. Clinical Efficacy and Safety of Malarone((R)), Azithromycin and Artesunate Combination for Treatment of *Babesia gibsoni* in Naturally Infected Dogs. Animals (Basel) 2022;12:708–20.

52. Almendros A, Burchell R, Wierenga J. An alternative combination therapy with metronidazole, clindamycin and doxycycline for *Babesia gibsoni* (Asian genotype) in dogs in Hong Kong. J Vet Med Sci 2020;82:1334–40.

53. Lin EC, Chueh LL, Lin CN, et al. The therapeutic efficacy of two antibabesial strategies against *Babesia gibsoni*. Vet Parasitol 2012;186:159–64.

54. Iguchi A, Matsuu A, Matsuyama K, et al. The efficacy of artemisinin, artemether, and lumefantrine against *Babesia gibsoni* in vitro. Parasitol Int 2015;64:190–3.

55. Birkenheuer AJ, Horney B, Bailey M, et al. *Babesia microti*-like infections are prevalent in North American foxes. Vet Parasitol 2010;172:179–82.

56. Garrett K, Halseth A, Ruder MG, et al. Prevalence and genetic characterization of a *Babesia microti*-like species in the North American river otter (*Lontra canadensis*). Vet Parasitol Reg Stud Rep 2022;29:100696.

57. Tuska-Szalay B, Vizi Z, Hofmann-Lehmann R, et al. *Babesia gibsoni* emerging with high prevalence and co-infections in "fighting dogs" in Hungary. Curr Res Parasitol Vector Borne Dis 2021;1:100048.

58. Kjemtrup AM, Conrad PA. A review of the small canine piroplasms from California: *Babesia conradae* in the literature. Vet Parasitol 2006;138:112–7.

59. Macur J. Bred to Seek Blood. New York Times 2010. New York, NY.

60. Yamane I, Thomford JW, Gardner IA, et al. Evaluation of the indirect fluorescent antibody test for diagnosis of *Babesia gibsoni* infections in dogs. Am J Vet Res 1993;54:1579–84.

61. Dear JD, Owens SD, Biondo AW, et al. Efficacy of azithromycin and atovaquone for treatment of Babesia conradae and hemoplasma infections in coyote hunting

dogs infected with multiple blood-borne pathogens. In: 2012 ISCAID Symposium, San Francisco, CA 2012.

62. Birkenheuer AJ, Neel J, Ruslander D, et al. Detection and molecular characterization of a novel large *Babesia* species in a dog. Vet Parasitol 2004;124:151–60.

63. Sikorski LE, Birkenheuer AJ, Holowaychuk MK, et al. Babesiosis caused by a large *Babesia* species in 7 immunocompromised dogs. J Vet Intern Med 2010; 24:127–31.

Cytauxzoonosis

Leah A. Cohn, DVM, PhD

KEYWORDS

- Hematoprotozoan • Blood parasite • Bobcat fever • Vector-borne disease • Tick

KEY POINTS

- Cytauxzoonosis is a tick-transmitted illness that results in severe morbidity and mortality in many domestic cats but infection does not always lead to illness.
- For a cat with clinical signs of cytauxzoonosis (eg, acute fever, lethargy, and icterus), blood smear is often confirmatory. When infection is suspected despite a negative smear, options include polymerase chain reaction testing, tissue aspirate for cytology, or repeat blood smear.
- Treatment includes minimization of stress, supportive care, and antiprotozoal therapy but prognosis remains guarded (60% survival).
- Rigorous tick prophylaxis is far preferred over disease treatment.

INTRODUCTION

Cytauxzoonosis is a severe, even frequently fatal illness of cats caused by infection with the tick-transmitted hematoprotozoan parasite, *Cytauxzoon felis*. The parasite has a complex life cycle involving a tick vector as well as a mammalian host. The colloquial name of the disease, "bobcat fever," is derived from the mammalian reservoir host and the most consistent clinical finding. *C. felis* was first recognized as a cause of illness in domestic cats in Missouri and surrounding states in the 1970s.[1]

Because the apicomplexan organism is a member of the family Theleridae, there was initial concern that it might be capable of causing disease in domestic livestock. This sparked intensive investigation of the pathogen including infection studies in cats and transmission studies across animal species (including livestock). Literally hundreds of cats were experimentally infected, providing important information on the course of disease and the pathologic condition associated with the illness.[2–4] When it was determined that the organism did not result in infection or illness in any studied nonfelidae host, the intense investigation largely came to a halt.[5] The rate of progress in understanding the pathogen was hampered both by an inability to culture the organism in vitro and by a perceived small geographic niche for infection around Missouri/

There are no relevant disclosures or conflicts of interest.
Small Animal Medicine, Department of Veterinary Medicine and Surgery, University of Missouri – College of Veterinary Medicine, 900 East Campus Drive, Columbia, MO 65211, USA
E-mail address: Cohnl@missouri.edu

Arkansas/Kansas. Despite many valiant attempts, the organism remains noncultivatable in vitro.[6] However, the geographic range of the pathogen has expanded dramatically (**Fig. 1**) along with the expansion in geographic range of the primary vector tick, *Amblyomma americanum* (Lone Star Tick).[7-10] Additionally, reports of cats surviving infection were made at the turn of the century, sparking renewed interest in study of the pathogen and disease.[11-13] New discoveries have been facilitated by improved molecular techniques and tick transmission studies as well as collaborative efforts between multiple institutions.[14-22]

PARASITE AND LIFE CYCLE

Cytauxzoon felis is one of a growing number of recognized *Cytauxzoon* parasites, many of which have been recognized in wild cats in Europe and Asia.[23-27] Infection in wild and domestic cats with *Cytauxzoon* parasites is also widely recognized in South America but it is not certain the parasite is identical to the *C. felis* recognized in North America.[28-31] To date, only *C. felis* has been recognized as an important pathogen of domestic cats.

Transmission of the pathogen in a natural setting requires that a competent vector tick (usually *A. americanum* but potentially *Dermacentor variabilis*) feed on a felid with piroplasms in the red blood cells (RBC; **Fig. 2**). Although Lone Star ticks can be found in all warm months, peak activity in early spring and late summer corresponds to peak incidence of disease in spring with a smaller peak in early autumn.[32] Any cat, wild or domestic, that survives the disease-causing schizogenous phase of acute infection and progresses to the chronic carrier phase of infection can transmit the pathogen to a naïve tick in as little as 36 hours of tick feeding.[15,16,33] Because bobcats (*Lynx rufus rufus*) have a limited disease-causing schizogenous phase of infection compared with domestic cats, bobcats are more likely than domestic cats to survive acute

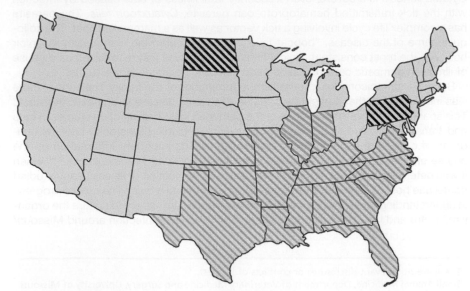

Fig. 1. Geographic distribution of *C. felis* and the vector tick, *A. americanum*. Yellow shading represents states where *A. americanum* is considered endemic. Blue diagonal stripes represent states where cytauxzoonosis has been recognized in domestic cats. Black diagonal stripes represent states where *C. felis* infection has been recognized in wild cats but not in domestic cats.[70-72]

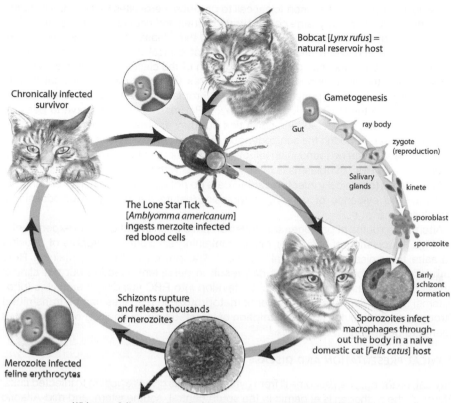

Fig. 2. Life cycle of *C. felis*. The acute tissue stage of disease (the schizogenous phase) is characterized by wide spread dissemination of schizonts that form parasitic thrombi throughout the body resulting in a disease course that is typically fatal. Hosts that survive this acute tissue phase develop a chronic yet fairly innocuous erythroparasitemia with merozoite-infected red cells. (Figure from Tarigo et al, A Novel Candidate Vaccine for Cytauxzoonosis Inferred from Comparative Apicomplexan Genomics, PLOS One, 2013. https://doi.org/10.1371/journal.pone.0071233.)

infection and go on to serve as a reservoir for the pathogen.[34] In endemic areas, the prevalence of subclinical infection in bobcats may be 70% or more.[8,35] Interestingly, parasite levels in the reservoir hosts increase when vector activity is increased by rising ambient temperature, increasing the odds of passing the parasite on to feeding ticks.[36] In recent years, it has been appreciated that some domestic cats act similarly to bobcats and survive infection with no apparent disease state having ever been recognized; because domestic cats are likely to live in close proximity to other domestic cats, even small numbers of chronically infected pet cats may serve as an important pathogen reservoir.[37–41]

The sexual phase of reproduction for *C. felis* is believed to occur in the tick gut, with ookinetes leaving the gut and migrating to the salivary glands where they further replicate as infective sporozoites. When the tick feeds during its next life-stage, sporozoites are inoculated into the felid host and penetrate mononuclear phagocytes. There they develop into large, nucleated schizonts that continue to multiply (**Fig. 3**). Schizonts undergo fission within the mononuclear cell to produce merozoites that eventually fill the entire host cell. These very large cells infiltrate tissues and occlude small vessels.[42,43] A combination of vascular obstruction, anoxia, and the release of substances secondary to cell rupture and death are the likely cause of clinical disease. This is important because clinical disease can precede recognition of the classic RBC piroplasms.

Eventually, the host mononuclear cell ruptures releasing merozoites that invade erythrocytes to become piroplasms (**Fig. 4**). Piroplasms are believed to reproduce asexually within the RBC through merogony.[44] Piroplasms not only serve to pass on the pathogen when ingested by a naïve tick but they are the usual diagnostic feature on blood smear. Although the schizogenous phase of acute infection is limited in duration, piroplasms can be found in an infected cat for months to years.[13,38,45,46] The first appearance of RBC piroplasms is often associated with presumed hemolytic anemia but recovered (chronically infected carrier) cats do not demonstrate persistent anemia and have no evidence of ongoing hemolysis despite the presence of occasional piroplasms.

Alternative routes of pathogen transmission have been investigated in experimental settings. Inoculation of tissues or blood containing schizonts is capable of causing parasite transmission and clinical illness.[2,3] Transfusion of blood containing RBC with piroplasms but not schizonts can result in persistent infection but not clinical illness since disease-causing schizonts develop into RBC invading merozoites (piroplasms) but not vice versa.[33,47] Other hematoprotozoan parasites can be transmitted through perinatal routes and consumption of infected ticks but neither of these routes seems to be important for *C. felis*.[16,48]

CLINICAL PRESENTATION AND DISEASE COURSE

Any cat, of any age, can become ill from cytauxzoonosis given exposure to infected ticks. Although the pathogen is endemic in the south central, southeastern, and mid-Atlantic United States, there are geographic pockets where it seems to occur more commonly than in nearby areas. As example, although infection is very common in Springfield, MO, it is far less commonly identified only 150 miles away in Columbia, MO. On a smaller scale, geographic pocketing is also reflected by the common phenomenon of multiple

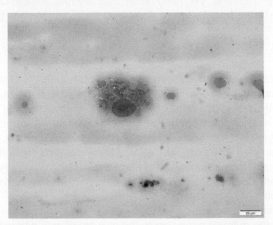

Fig. 3. Schizont, blood film: Blood film with a single schizont-laden macrophage along the feathered edge. The nucleus is peripheralized with a single macronucleus. The deep blue cytoplasm contains C. felis merozoites. Modified Wright Giemsa, 200× magnification. (Image courtesy of Dr. Erin Burton, University of Minnesota.)

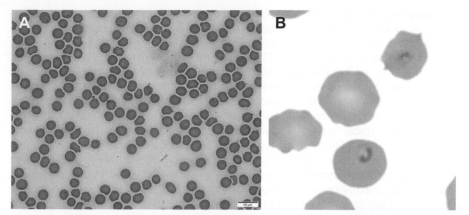

Fig. 4. (*A*) Piroplasm, blood film with several intra-erythrocytic C. felis piroplasms present. Modified Wrights Giemsa, 1000x magnification. (Image courtesy of Dr. Erin Burton, University of Minne-sota.) (*B*) Magnification of red blood cells demonstrating signet ring shaped piroplasms.

cats from a single household or neighborhood becoming sick within weeks of each other. The wider geographic range of the pathogen is expanding along with the range of the tick vector, meaning that each year disease is recognized where it had not been recognized previously (see **Fig. 1**). As mentioned, illness is most likely during the early spring and early autumn with sporadic infections throughout the summer. Most infected cats have spent time outdoors, even if this is an episode of "escape" by an otherwise indoor cat. Illness does not seem to be any more likely in immunosuppressed or retroviral positive cats. In fact, infection is most common in otherwise healthy young adult cats, more male than female, who spend time roaming outdoors.[45]

Typically, owners note that their previously healthy cat suddenly has a reduced appetite and quiet affect. Soon severe lethargy and anorexia ensues.[45] The clinical signs and examination findings will differ depending on how early in the disease process cat owners seek veterinary care. With the progression of disease, clinical signs may include respiratory effort/distress, icterus, or even neurologic signs such as seizure. Gastrointestinal signs are rare. The most consistent finding on physical examination is fever, which is often quite high.[20] However, the temperature will come down, even progressing to hypothermia, in moribund cats. Besides the aforementioned findings, examination may demonstrate pallor, systolic murmur due to anemia, and hepatosplenomegaly with or without lymphadenomegaly. Petechia and ecchymosis are occasionally seen. Lung sounds may be loud or muffled because infiltrative pneumonia, noncardiogenic edema, and pleural effusion are all possible. Tachycardia and tachypnea are commonplace. Cats often have raised third eyelids and may react as if in pain on abdominal palpation.[20]

Clinical signs associated with schizogeny typically begin between 11 to 15 days following inoculation from tick feeding.[15,18] Illness progresses very rapidly during the course of only a few days. It is common for cats to die within 2 to 4 days of the owners' first awareness that the cat was ill, or within 24 to 36 hours of presentation for veterinary care. For cats that survive the illness, fever often continues for 5 days or more.[20,45]

DIAGNOSIS

Cytologic diagnosis is often straightforward. A simple blood smear will demonstrate intraerythrocytic piroplasms (see **Fig. 4**) in many cats. Because illness begins during the schizogenous stage of infection, cats can become ill when piroplasms are absent or rare. In such cases, a repeat blood smear even 12 hours later might demonstrate the signet-ring (or less commonly, coccoid or safety-pin) shaped piroplasms singly, as pairs, or in tetrads (see **Fig. 4**). These piriforms often measure 0.3 to 0.7 μm up to 1.0 to 2.2 μm in diameter. Because cats that survive illness remain infected, on occasion rare piroplasms will be noted incidentally on the blood smear of a cat presented for reasons other than cytauxzoonosis. Therefore, identification of a rare piroplasm is not pathognomonic for the illness but finding many piroplasms in a cat demonstrating typical findings is considered confirmatory for diagnosis. Cytologic identification of any number of schizont-laden distended mononuclear cells is pathognomonic for cytauxzoonosis (see **Fig. 3**).[49] It is uncommon to see these very large cells in peripheral circulation because they become entrapped in the small vessels. However, they are often readily apparent on fine needle aspiration of infected tissues. In a recent study of cats with acute cytauxzoonosis, schizont-laden macrophages were seen in 33% of blood smears, 56% of lymph node aspirates, and 77% of splenic aspirates.[50] Early in the disease course, schizonts are smaller but later on, they may measure up to 250 μm in diameter.

The most sensitive method of diagnosis is polymerase chain reaction (PCR) testing of peripheral blood, which can become positive days before the demonstration of clinical signs of illness.[14] Multiple genetic targets for PCR are available currently for use in blood or other tissues. There remain 2 problems with PCR as a diagnostic test. First, there is currently no in-clinic PCR option, meaning that there will be some delay in sending samples for testing. Because many cats will succumb to the disease within a day to two of diagnosis, this delay in confirmation is problematic. The second problem with PCR testing is that as with cytologic recognition of rare piroplasms, cats that survived acute infection are expected to remain PCR positive potentially for life; this could lead to a mistaken diagnosis in an incidentally (chronically) infected cat.

Diagnosis is easily confirmed after death via recognition of schizont-laden macrophages within tissues. Grossly, venous distention may be seen, and the liver and spleen are often enlarged and mottled; lymphadenomegaly is commonly recognized. Tissues may be icteric and pale. The lungs may seem to have edema/pneumonia, and pleural effusion may be present. Petechial and ecchymotic hemorrhage are frequent findings. On histopathologic examination, infiltration of any or all tissues with schizont-laden macrophages is possible but spleen, liver, lung, lymph node, bone marrow, and brain are often most heavily parasitized.[42,51–54] In situ hybridization can also be used to confirm the presence of pathogen in formalin-fixed tissues.[53]

Currently, there are no commercial serologic tests for cytauxzoonosis. An important difficulty to overcome for any antibody-based test is that the illness is very acute in nature. It is entirely possible that a newly infected cat could die of the disease before mounting a detectable antibody response.[55]

There are a myriad of other potential abnormalities on routine diagnostic testing but none of them are pathognomonic. Common abnormalities found on serum biochemistry and complete blood count tests are listed in **Box 1**.[20,45] Anemia may not be present at the onset of illness related to the schizogenous phase of infection but hemolysis can occur as merozoites are released and first taken up by the RBCs. Initial anemia is nonregenerative but in surviving cats, the anemia becomes regenerative. Interestingly, although acute infection is associated with an apparent hemolytic anemia, the chronic carrier state is not despite continued presence of piroplasms (in low number) in RBC. Also, the degree of infiltration of kidneys is less than that of other tissues and most cats retain good urine concentrating ability; azotemia, if present, is generally prerenal. Disseminated intravascular coagulation (DIC) is a frequent

---

Box 1
Common abnormalities on routine laboratory testing

- Anemia (often nonregenerative due to acuity)
- RBC inclusions (piroplasms)
- Thrombocytopenia
- Lymphopenia
- Neutropenia OR neutrophilia—Neutropenia may be associated with worse prognosis
- Hyperglycemia
- Hyperbilirubinemia
- Hypoalbuminemia (mild)
- Hypocalcemia (mild)

---

complication of cytauxzoonosis, leading to thrombocytopenia as well as prolonged activated partial thromboplastin time and prothrombin time.[56] Imaging studies may be useful for identification of treatable complications of infection (eg, pleural effusion). Although imaging changes related to tissue infiltration by schizonts are present, these changes are not specific (eg, splenomegaly, pulmonary interstitial or alveolar patterns).

TREATMENT

Left untreated, most cats with clinical signs of cytauxzoonosis will die. That said, there are domestic cats that develop an inapparent or self-limiting infection similar to what is considered the norm for bobcats.[13,37,57] However, for most cats prompt institution of supportive and therapeutic measures is key to survival. Moreover, although infection is thought to be self-limiting in most bobcats, infection can be fatal in this species too (**Box 2**).[34,58]

Although specific antiprotozoal drug therapies have been investigated, there are no studies that evaluate other aspects of care for cats with cytauxzoonosis. Below are general impressions of the author based on personal experience, as well as experience in treating experimentally infected cats. Stress should be minimized for these very ill cats. If hospitalization is required (and it often is initially), they should be handled minimally and given a place to hide (box, cage covering) with efforts to reduce exposure to barking dogs or other environmental stressors. Because

---

Box 2
Comparison of what are believed to be typical for infection of bobcats versus domestic cats with C. felis

Bobcats	Domestic Cats
Primary reservoir host	Incidental host (but potential reservoir)
Limited schizogeny typical	Profound schizogeny typical
Illness (ie, cytauxzoonosis) believed to be rare	Illness (ie, cytauxzoonosis) believed to be common
Chronic carrier infection common in endemic regions (up to 79% in MO, for instance)[8]	Chronic carrier infection less common in endemic regions (up to 12.9% in MO, for instance)[41]

administration of oral drugs can be stressful in itself, the author prefers to place a nasoesophageal tube or an esophagostomy tube early in the course of treatment. This allows a simplified means of drug delivery, a route for supportive enteral nutrition, and esophagostomy tube allows enteric maintenance of hydration in a home setting. Usually, judicious intravenous crystalloid fluids are indicated at least initially but sending cats home as soon as possible may improve outcome. Because DIC is a common complication, the author administers heparin (200 U/Kg subcutaneously q 8 hours) until there is evidence of clinical improvement but the utility of this treatment is unknown. Despite a high fever, the author's impression is that cats receiving NSAID drugs to reduce fever (eg, meloxicam) do not fare as well. In fact, I consider the continued presence of fever through the first several days of treatment as a favorable prognostic sign. Nonetheless, cats often seem to be in some pain/discomfort at presentation, making analgesia important. My preference is buprenorphine (0.01 mg/kg IV or buccal application q 8 hours). Specific complications require specific supportive therapy. For instance, anemia may require transfusion of packed RBCs or whole blood, respiratory distress may be relieved by thoracocentesis if pleural effusion is present, or cats with seizure may benefit from anticonvulsants. If no feeding tube is placed, appetite stimulants may be useful. Further study of supportive therapies is needed.

Specific antimicrobial treatments have been investigated both in experimental and naturally infected cats. For now, the standard of care is a combination of the antiprotozoal (antimalarial) drug atovaquone (Mepron, GlaxoSmithKline, 15 mg/kg PO q 8 hour) with azithromycin (10 mg/kg PO q 24 hour) for 10 days. Because malaria is not endemic to the United States, atovaquone is not immediately available at local pharmacies. Therefore, veterinarians practicing in endemic areas often stock at least a limited supply in their clinic for prompt initiation of treatment. The drug is very expensive and difficult to administer. The liquid is quite viscus; it is common to think that you have loaded the appropriate volume in the syringe while in reality the sides of the syringe are coated with the substance. The author suggests letting the filled syringe sit/settle for several minutes before administration to be sure the actual desired volume is loaded. Cats do not like the taste of atovaquone so administration through a feeding tube flushed with water afterward is less stressful than oral drug administration. In a prospective randomized clinical trial, survival of cats treated with this drug combination was only 60%.[20] There are 2 likely reasons that atovaquone and azithromycin may not prove lifesaving. First, the disease course is extremely brief. Many cats do not present for veterinary care until days into the course of the illness, and these cats often die within 24 to 36 hours of presentation. The damage may already be done by the time these cats are evaluated such that no antiprotozoal treatment would prevent death. Second, atovaquone targets C. felis cytochrome b (cytb), of which there are many unique genotypes and in which mutations may occur. Some of these genotypes may be associated with resistance or susceptibility to atovaquone.[19,59] Clearly, better therapies are desired.

Other specific antimicrobial therapies have been investigated or are undergoing further investigation. Antitheilerial drugs parvaquone and buparvaquone were not effective in treating experimental infection.[60] Diminazene aceturate was given to a small number of naturally infected cats that survived illness but is not approved for use in the United States (and is therefore difficult to acquire in a timely manner).[12] The antiprotozoal drug imidocarb dipropionate (2 doses injected intramuscularly several days apart, preceded by atropine or glycopyrrolate to minimize cholinergic effects) was used for years as the default treatment option with some limited success but was inferior to atovaquone and azithromycin in a prospective clinical trial (26% survival for imidocarb-treated cats compared with 60% survival for atovaquone-treated cats).[20,61] A multiple antimicrobial combination can be used for the treatment of the related protozoal pathogen *Babesia gibsoni* in dogs but a similar combination (metronidazole, clindamycin, pradofloxacin) was not effective in experimentally infected cats[62] (Leah Cohn, 2015, personal knowledge). In an as-yet unpublished study, the author found that the combination artemether and lumefantrine (Coartem, Novartis, East Hanover, NJ) administered orally for 3 days demonstrated efficacy very similar to atovaquone and azithromycin. Study is currently underway to investigate the potential utility of the antiprotozoal drug ponazuril in the treatment of cytauxzoonosis.

Because cats that survive infection may still carry the parasite for many months or even years, the question arises as to the need to treat these survivors with antiprotozoal drugs. Survivors may live for many years after infection without experiencing ill effects, and the author has personally followed many such cats throughout their lifetime. However, these cats might serve as a reservoir to infect ticks that could then infect other cats.[16,18] Atovaquone and azithromycin will reduced parasite number dramatically but cannot eliminate the parasites with certainty.[63] Surviving cats should ideally be housed indoors and should be kept on stringent tick prophylaxis to protect neighboring cats.

PREVENTION

Although treatment of this illness is difficult, expensive, and often futile, prevention is relatively straightforward. Simply keeping cats indoors goes a long way to prevent infection but even indoor cats can be bitten by ticks after a brief escape outdoors or if ticks are carried into the home. Acaricides that act to prevent the tick bite or kill the tick very rapidly can also be effective at preventing illness. Both a tick prevention collar containing imidacloprid 10% and flumethrin 4.5% (Seresto, Elanco) and a topical formulation of selamectin plus sarolaner (Revolution Plus/Stronghold Plus, Zoetis) were extremely effective at preventing infection and illness in cats infested with infected ticks under experimental conditions.[64,65]

Efforts have been made to develop a vaccine.[66,67] Based on experimental attempts at reinfection, it was long believed that recovered cats were immune to subsequent infection.[2,60,67,68] There is now evidence that bobcats can become infected with multiple different strains of the pathogen.[69] And quite recently, for the first time, a clinically apparent second infection was confirmed in a domestic cat that survived illness after treatment with atovaquone and azithromycin only to succumb to the subsequent infection 7 years later.[49] For vaccine development, complete sequencing of the *C. felis* genome allowed for the development of a microarray of proteins that were then probed with sera from infected and naïve cats to identify differentially reactive antigens.[67] These were incorporated into polyvalent or monovalent expression library vaccines administered to naïve cats. These cats were infested with infected ticks in an experimental setting but unfortunately neither vaccine prevented infection or illness.[67] Nonetheless, vaccination offers an extremely attractive future option for prevention of this life-threatening illness.

SUMMARY

Cytauxzoonosis is the clinical illness that occurs in many domestic cats after tick-transmitted infection with the hematoprotozoan parasite *C. felis*. The initial schizogenous phase of parasite proliferation in mononuclear cells results in vascular occlusion and tissue infiltration that causes the characteristic clinical signs. Fever, anorexia, depression, icterus, anemia, neurologic or respiratory signs, and coagulopathy are common presentations. The clinical course of disease is quite brief, with death often occurring in days of the first signs of illness. Treatment with supportive care and a combination of atovaquone and azithromycin offers a guarded prognosis for recovery as of now. Despite the high morbidity and mortality of the disease in domestic cats, some cats experience a self-limiting or even inapparent illness and respond as is typical of the bobcat reservoir, leading to life-long parasitemia but no long-term illness. For cats in endemic regions, stringent tick prevention offers an excellent means of disease prevention.

CLINICS CARE POINTS

- Cats can become ill before piroplasms are seen on blood smear.
- Visualization of rare piroplasms on blood smear of a cat without clinical signs is compatible with incidental infection.
- Atovaquone is a viscous liquid that coats the syringe; care should be used in dosing.
- Minimization of stress is a key to survival of treated cats.
- Strict tick prophylaxis can prevent infection

REFERENCES

1. Wagner JE. A fatal cytauxzoonosis-like disease in cats. J Am Vet Med Assoc 1976;168(7):585–8.
2. Ferris DH. A progress report on the status of a new disease of American cats: cytauxzoonosis. Comp Immunol Microbiol Infect Dis 1979;1(4):269–76.
3. Wagner JE, Ferris DH, Kier AB, et al. Experimentally induced cytauxzoonosis-like disease in domestic cats. Vet Parasit 1980;6:305–11.
4. Kier AB, Wagner JE, Morehouse LG. Experimental transmission of *Cytauxzoon felis* from bobcats (*Lynx rufus*) to domestic cats (*Felis domesticus*). Am J Vet Res 1982;43(1):97–101.
5. Kier AB, Wightman SR, Wagner JE. Interspecies transmission of *Cytauxzoon felis*. Am J Vet Res 1982;43(1):102–5.
6. Yang TS, Reichard MV, Marr HS, et al. Direct injection of *Amblyomma americanum* ticks with *Cytauxzoon felis*. Ticks Tick Borne Dis 2022;13(1):101847.
7. Birkenheuer AJ, Marr HS, Warren C, et al. *Cytauxzoon felis* infections are present in bobcats (*lynx rufus*) in a region where cytauxzoonosis is not recognized in domestic cats. Vet Parasit 2008;153:126–30.
8. Shock BC, Murphy SM, Patton LL, et al. Distribution and prevalence of *Cytauxzoon felis* in bobcats (*Lynx rufus*), the natural reservoir, and other wild felids in thirteen states. Vet Parasitol 2011;175:325–30.
9. Birkenheuer AJ, Le JA, Valenzisi AM, et al. *Cytauxzoon felis* infection in cats in the mid-Atlantic states: 34 cases (1998-2004). J Am Vet Med Assoc 2006;228(4):568–71.
10. Raghavan RK, Peterson AT, Cobos ME, et al. Current and future distribution of the Lone Star Tick, *Amblyomma americanum* (L.) (Acari: Ixodidae) in North America. PLoS One 2019;14(1):e0209082.
11. Walker DB, Cowell RL. Survival of a domestic cat with naturally acquired cytauxzoonosis. J Am Vet Med Assoc 1995;206(9):1363–5.

12. Greene CE, Latimer K, Hopper E, et al. Administration of diminazene aceturate or imidocarb dipropionate for treatment of cytauxzoonosis in cats. J Am Vet Med Assoc 1999;215(4):497–500.

13. Meinkoth J, Kocan AA, Whitworth L, et al. Cats surviving natural infection with *Cytauxzoon felis*: 18 cases (1997-1998). J Vet Intern Med 2000;14(5):521–5.

14. Kao YF, Peake B, Madden R, et al. A probe-based droplet digital polymerase chain reaction assay for early detection of feline acute cytauxzoonosis. Vet Parasitol 2021;292:109413.

15. Allen KE, Thomas JE, Wohltjen ML, et al. Transmission of *Cytauxzoon felis* to domestic cats by *Amblyomma americanum* nymphs. Parasites Vectors 2019; 12:28.

16. Thomas JE, Ohmes CM, Payton ME, et al. Minimum transmission time of Cytauxzoon felis by Amblyomma americanum to domestic cats in relation to duration of infestation, and investigation of ingestion of infected ticks as a potential route of transmission. J Feline Med Surg 2018;20(2):67–72.

17. Schreeg ME, Marr HS, Griffith EH, et al. PCR amplification of a multi-copy mitochondrial gene (cox3) improves detection of *Cytauxzoon felis* infection as compared to a ribosomal gene (18S). Vet Parasitol 2016;225:123–30.

18. Reichard MV, Edwards AC, Meinkoth JH, et al. Confirmation of *Amblyomma americanum* (Acari: Ixodidae) as a vector for *Cytauxzoon felis* (Piroplasmorida: Theileriidae) to domestic cats. J Med Entomol 2010;47(5):890–6.

19. Schreeg ME, Marr HS, Tarigo J, et al. Pharmacogenomics of *Cytauxzoon felis* cytochrome b: implications for atovaquone and azithromycin therapy in domestic cats with cytauxzoonosis. J Clin Microbiol 2013;51(9):3066–9.

20. Cohn LA, Birkenheuer AJ, Brunker JD, et al. Efficacy of atovaquone and azithromycin or imidocarb dipropionate in cats with acute cytauxzoonosis. J Vet Intern Med 2011;25(1):55–60.

21. Birkenheuer AJ, Marr H, Alleman AR, et al. Development and evaluation of a PCR assay for the detection of *Cytauxzoon felis* DNA in feline blood samples. Vet Parasitol 2006;137(1–2):144–9.

22. Birkenheuer AJ, Levy MG, Breitschwerdt EB. Development and evaluation of a seminested PCR for detection and differentiation of *Babesia gibsoni* (Asian genotype) and *B. canis* DNA in canine blood samples. J Clin Microbiol 2003;41(9): 4172–7.

23. Panait LC, Mihalca AD, Modry D, et al. Three new species of *Cytauxzoon* in European wild felids. Vet Parasitol 2021;290:109344.

24. Willi B, Meli ML, Cafarelli C, et al. *Cytauxzoon europaeus* infections in domestic cats in Switzerland and in European wildcats in France: a tale that started more than two decades ago. Parasites Vectors 2022;15(1):1–17.

25. Naidenko SV, Erofeeva MN, Sorokin PA, et al. The first case of *Cytauxzoon* spp. in Russia: The parasite conquers Eurasia. Animals 2022;12(5):593.

26. Gallusova M, Jirsova D, Mihalca AD, et al. *Cytauxzoon* infections in wild felids from Carpathian-Danubian-Pontic space: Further evidence for a different *Cytauxzoon* species in European felids. J Parasitol 2016;102(3): 377–80.

27. Reichard MV, Van Den Bussche RA, Meinkoth JH, et al. A new species of *Cytauxzoon* from Pallas' cats caught in Mongolia and comments on the systematics and taxonomy of piroplasmids. J Parasit 2005;91(2):420–6.

28. Braga IA, de Souza Ramos DG, Marcili A, et al. Molecular detection of tick-borne protozoan parasites in a population of domestic cats in midwestern Brazil. Ticks Tick Borne Dis 2016;7(5):1004–9.

29. Andre MR, Calchi AC, Furquim MEC, et al. Molecular Detection of Tick-Borne Agents in Cats from Southeastern and Northern Brazil. Pathogens 2022; 11(1):106.

30. Furtado MM, Taniwaki SA, Metzger B, et al. Is the free-ranging jaguar (*Panthera onca*) a reservoir for *Cytauxzoon felis* in Brazil? Ticks Tick Borne Dis 2017;8(4): 470–6.

31. Andre MR, Adania CH, Machado RZ, et al. Molecular detection of Cytauxzoon spp. in asymptomatic Brazilian wild captive felids. J Wildl Dis 2009; 45(1):234–7.

32. Reichard MV, Baum KA, Cadenhead SC, et al. Temporal occurrence and environmental risk factors associated with cytauxzoonosis in domestic cats. Vet Parasit 2008;152(3–4):314–20.

33. Blouin EF, Kocan AA, Glenn BL, et al. Transmission of *Cytauxzoon felis* Kier, 1979 from bobcats, *Felis rufus* (Schreber), to domestic cats by *Dermacentor variabilis* (Say). J Wildl Dis 1984;20(3):241–2.

34. Blouin EF, Kocan AA, Kocan KM, et al. Evidence of a limited schizogonous cycle for *Cytauxzoon felis* in bobcats following exposure to infected ticks. J Wildl Dis 1987;23(3):499–501.

35. Zieman EA, Jimenez FA, Nielsen CK. Concurrent examination of bobcats and ticks reveals high prevalence of *Cytauxzoon felis* in southern Illinois. J Parasitol 2017;103(4):343–8.

36. Zieman EA, Lawson T, Nielsen CK, et al. Within-season changes in *Cytauxzoon felis* parasitemia in bobcats. J Parasitol 2020;106(2):308–11.

37. Wikander YM, Anantatat T, Kang Q, et al. Prevalence of *Cytauxzoon felis* Infection-Carriers in Eastern Kansas Domestic Cats. Pathogens 2020;9(1). Accession Number: 33092245.

38. Brown HM, Lockhart JM, Latimer KS, et al. Identification and genetic characterization of *Cytauxzoon felis* in asymptomatic domestic cats and bobcats. Vet Parasitol 2010;172(3–4):311–6.

39. Jacobs CH. Prevalence of *Cytauxzoon felis* in Feral Cats AR. J Ark Acad Sci 2018;72:123–8.

40. Nagamori Y, Slovak JE, Reichard MV. Prevalence of *Cytauxzoon felis* infection in healthy free-roaming cats in north-central Oklahoma and central Iowa. J Feline Med Surg Open Rep 2016;2(1). 2055116916655174.

41. Rizzi TE, Reichard MV, Cohn LA, et al. Prevalence of *Cytauxzoon felis* infection in healthy cats from enzootic areas in Arkansas, Missouri, and Oklahoma. Parasit Vectors 2015;8:13.

42. Kier AB, Wagner JE, Kinden DA. The pathology of experimental cytauxzoonosis. J Comp Pathol 1987;97(4):415–32.

43. Kocan AA, Kocan KM, Blouin EF, et al. A redescription of schizogony of *Cytauxzoon felis* in the domestic cat. Ann N Y Acad Sci 1992;653:161–7.

44. Jalovecka M, Hajdusek O, Sojka D, et al. The complexity of piroplasms life cycles. Front Cell Infect Microbiol 2018;8:248.

45. Sherrill MK, Cohn LA. Cytauxzoonosis: Diagnosis and treatment of an emerging disease. J Feline Med Surg 2015;17(11):940–8.

46. Schnittger L, Ganzinelli S, Bhoora R, et al. The Piroplasmida Babesia, Cytauxzoon, and Theileria in farm and companion animals: species compilation, molecular phylogeny, and evolutionary insights. Parasitol Res 2022;1–39. Accession Number: 35098377.

47. Glenn BL, Kocan AA, Blouin EF. Cytauxzoonosis in bobcats. J Am Vet Med Assoc 1983;183(11):1155–8.

48. Lewis KM, Cohn LA, Birkenheuer AJ. Lack of evidence for perinatal transmission of *Cytauxzoon felis* in domestic cats. Vet Parasitol 2012;188(1–2):172–4.

49. Cohn LA, Shaw D, Shoemake C, et al. Second illness due to subsequent *Cytauxzoon felis* infection in a domestic cat. J Feline Med Surg Open Rep 2020;6. 2055116920908963.

50. Sleznikow CR, Granick JL, Cohn LA, et al. Evaluation of various sample sources for the cytologic diagnosis of *Cytauxzoon felis*. J Vet Intern Med 2022;36(1): 126–32.

51. Snider TA, Confer AW, Payton ME. Pulmonary histopathology of *Cytauxzoon felis* infections in the cat. Vet Pathol 2010;47(4):698–702.

52. Clarke LL, Rissi DR. Neuropathology of natural *Cytauxzoon felis* infection in domestic cats. Vet Pathol 2015;52(6):1167–71.

53. Susta L, Torres-Velez F, Zhang J, et al. An in situ hybridization and immunohistochemical study of cytauxzoonosis in domestic cats. Vet Pathol 2009;46(6): 1197–204.

54. Aschenbroich SA, Rech RR, Sousa RS, et al. Pathology in practice. *Cytauxzoon felis* infection. J Am Vet Med Assoc 2012;240(2):159–61.

55. Cowell RL, Fox JC, Panciera RJ, et al. Detection of anticytauxzoon antibodies in cats infected with a *Cytauxzoon* organism from bobcats. Vet Parasitol 1988; 28(1–2):43–52.

56. Conner BJ, Hanel RM, Brooks MB, et al. Coagulation abnormalities in 5 cats with naturally occurring cytauxzoonosis. J Vet Emerg Crit Care (San Antonio) 2015; 25(4):538–45.

57. Brown HM, Latimer KS, Erikson LE, et al. Detection of persistent *Cytauxzoon felis* infection by polymerase chain reaction in three asymptomatic domestic cats. J Vet Diagn Invest 2008;20(4):485–8.

58. Nietfeld JC, Pollock C. Fatal cytauxzoonosis in a free-ranging bobcat (Lynx rufus). J Wildl Dis 2002;38(3):607–10.

59. Hartley AN, Marr HS, Birkenheuer AJ. *Cytauxzoon felis* cytochrome b gene mutation associated with atovaquone and azithromycin treatment. J Vet Intern Med 2020;34(6):2432–7.

60. Motzel SL, Wagner JE. Treatment of experimentally induced cytauxzoonosis in cats with parvaquone and buparvaquone. Vet Parasit 1990;35(1–2):131–8.

61. Greene CE, Meinkoth J, Kocan AA. Cytauxzoonosis. In: Greene GE, editor. Infectious disease of the dog and cat. 3rd edition. St Louis (MO): Saunders Elsevier; 2006. p. 716–22.

62. Lin M-Y, Huang H-P. Use of a doxycycline-enrofloxacin-metronidazole combination with/without diminazene diaceturate to treat naturally occurring canine babesiosis caused by *Babesia gibsoni*. Acta Vet Scand 2010;52(1):1.

63. Cohn LA, Birkenheuer AJ, Ratcliff E. Comparison of two drug protocols for clearance of *Cytauxzoon felis* infections. J Vet Intern Med 2008;22:704 (abstract).

64. Reichard MV, Thomas JE, Arther RG, et al. Efficacy of an Imidacloprid 10 %/Flumethrin 4.5 % Collar (Seresto((R)), Bayer) for Preventing the Transmission of *Cytauxzoon felis* to Domestic Cats by *Amblyomma americanum*. Parasitol Res 2013; 112(Suppl 1):11–20.

65. Reichard MV, Rugg JJ, Thomas JE, et al. Efficacy of a topical formulation of selamectin plus sarolaner against induced infestations of *Amblyomma americanum* on cats and prevention of *Cytauxzoon felis* transmission. Vet Parasitol 2019; 270(Suppl 1):S31–7.

66. Tarigo JL, Scholl EH, Bird DM, et al. A novel candidate vaccine for Cytauxzoonosis inferred from comparative Apicomplexan genomics. PloS one 2013;8(8): e71233.
67. Schreeg ME, Marr HS, Tarigo JL, et al. Identification of *Cytauxzoon felis* antigens via protein microarray and assessment of expression library immunization against cytauxzoonosis. Clin Proteomics 2018;15:44.
68. Uilenberg G, Franssen FF, Perie NM. Relationships between *Cytauxzoon felis* and African piroplasmids. Vet Parasitol 1987;26(1–2):21–8.
69. Zieman EA, Nielsen CK, Jimenez FA. Chronic *Cytauxzoon felis* infections in wild-caught bobcats (*Lynx rufus*). Vet Parasitol 2018;252:67–9.
70. Shock BC, Moncayo A, Cohen S, et al. Diversity of piroplasms detected in blood-fed and questing ticks from several states in the United States. Ticks Tick Borne Dis 2014;5(4):373–80.
71. Jackson CB, Fisher T. Fatal cytauxzoonosis in a Kentucky cat (*Felis domesticus*). Vet Parasit 2006;139(1–3):192–5.
72. MacNeill AL, Barger AM, Skowronski MC, et al. Identification of *Cytauxzoon felis* infection in domestic cats from southern Illinois. J Feline Med Surg 2015;17(12): 1069–72.

Ehrlichiosis and Anaplasmosis: An Update

Pedro Paulo V.P. Diniz, DVM, PhD[a],*,
Daniel Moura de Aguiar, DVM, PhD[b]

KEYWORDS

- Anaplasma • Ehrlichia • Dog • Cat • PCR • Serology • Doxycycline • Zoonosis

KEY POINTS

- A growing number of *Ehrlichia* and *Anaplasma* species have been detected in dogs and cats.
- The incidence of these diseases is expanding into new geographic areas.
- Broader availability of in-clinic diagnostic tests targeting multiple pathogens has supported better and more timely medical decision-making.
- Doxycycline remains the best therapeutic option; however, proper protocols should be used to optimize outcomes and help avoid antimicrobial resistance.
- Tick prevention is key to avoiding infection, even in urban areas.

CANINE EHRLICHIOSIS
Etiology

Ehrlichia spp are tick-borne intracellular gram-negative α-proteobacteria that multiply in microcolonies known as morulae.[1,2] They mainly infect leukocytes (monocytes, macrophages, and neutrophils) of mammals and cells of the intestine, hemocoel, and salivary glands of ticks.[3–5] Currently, the genus *Ehrlichia* is composed of six species: *Ehrlichia canis*, *Ehrlichia chaffeensis*, *Ehrlichia ewingii*, *Ehrlichia muris euauclarensis*, *Ehrlichia ruminantium*, and *Ehrlichia minasensis* (**Fig. 1**).[2,6] *Ehrlichia canis* is the most frequently documented species infecting dogs worldwide. It is transmitted by the brown dog tick *Rhipicephalus sanguineus*, and causes a syndrome called canine monocytotropic ehrlichiosis (CME, also known as canine monocytic ehrlichiosis).[4,7] In North America, other species of *Ehrlichia* have been documented in geographic regions that follow the distribution of their confirmed or suspected tick vectors. *Ehrlichia chaffeensis* and *E. ewingii* are frequently identified in the southeastern and south-

---

[a] Western University of Health Sciences, College of Veterinary Medicine, 309 East 2nd Street, Pomona, CA 91766, USA; [b] Laboratory of Virology and Rickettsiosis, Federal University of Mato Grosso State - UFMT, Avenida Fernando Correa da Costa, 2367, Cuiabá, Mato Grosso, Brazil
* Corresponding author.
E-mail address: pdiniz@westernu.edu

Vet Clin Small Anim 52 (2022) 1225–1266
https://doi.org/10.1016/j.cvsm.2022.07.002
0195-5616/22/© 2022 Elsevier Inc. All rights reserved.

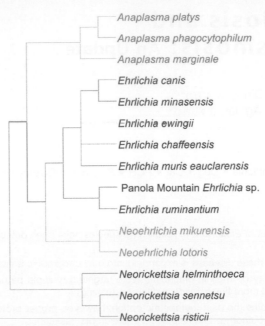

Anaplasma platys
Anaplasma phagocytophilum
Anaplasma marginale
Ehrlichia canis
Ehrlichia minasensis
Ehrlichia ewingii
Ehrlichia chaffeensis
Ehrlichia muris eauclarensis
Panola Mountain Ehrlichia sp.
Ehrlichia ruminantium
Neoehrlichia mikurensis
Neoehrlichia lotoris
Neorickettsia helminthoeca
Neorickettsia sennetsu
Neorickettsia risticii

Fig. 1. Phylogenetic tree of *Anaplasma* and *Ehrlichia* spp and closely related bacteria from the Alphaproteobacteria family based on the 16S rRNA gene. (*Courtesy of* Pedro Diniz, USA.)

central United States, from the East Coast extending westward to Texas, areas where their vector *Amblyomma americanum* (the Lone Star tick) and their main reservoir host, the white-tailed deer, are frequently present.[8,9] *Ehrlichia chaffeensis* causes monocytotropic ehrlichiosis, whereas *E. ewingii* causes granulocytotropic ehrlichiosis in dogs and people. A large survey showed that *E. ewingii* is the most seroprevalent *Ehrlichia* species in dogs in the United States.[10] Dogs may serve as reservoir hosts for this species, because chronic infection for more than 1 year has been documented experimentally.[11] Sporadic infections with *E. muris eauclarensis*, which is most likely transmitted by the black-legged tick *Ixodes scapularis*, have also been reported in dogs and people in the Upper Midwestern United States.[12,13] Similarly, a species phylogenetically close to *E. ruminantium* named Panola Mountain *Ehrlichia* sp, which was found in *A. americanum* and *Amblyomma maculatum* (the Gulf Coast tick), was documented in a sick goat, a dog, and a person in the Southeastern United States.[14–17] Recent serologic evidence indicates that dogs in the Central-West region of Brazil are also exposed to *E. minasensis*, a species originally detected from cattle, horses, and cervids, and transmitted by several ticks.[6,18–20]

Epidemiology

CME has been documented in all continents, mainly in tropical and subtropical regions where environmental conditions are favorable for the survival of *R. sanguineus* ticks (**Fig. 2**). Because no transovarial transmission of *E. canis* occurs, *R. sanguineus* larvae do not transmit the infection but they can become infected after feeding. Transstadial transmission does occur, with nymphs and adult ticks capable of transmitting *E. canis* to dogs for up to 155 days postmolting.[21] The prevalence of *E. canis* infection in *R. sanguineus* ticks ranges from 2.5% to 6% in tropical areas.[22] The existence of two distinct

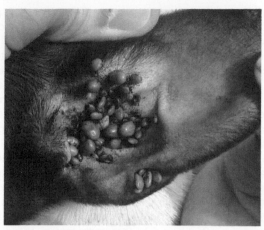

Fig. 2. Severe *Rhipicephalus sanguineus* infestation in a dog. (*Courtesy of* Daniel Moura de Aguiar, Brazil.)

lineages of *R. sanguineus* (temperate and tropical) impacts the distribution of CME because the tropical lineage is a more competent vector for *E. canis*.[23,24] The geographic distribution of the tropical lineage ranges from Brazil to Mexico and Southern parts of the United States including Florida and Southern Texas, where high *E. canis* seroprevalence is reported.[25–28] *Dermacentor variabilis* (the American dog tick) may also be a vector for *E. canis* and *E. chaffeensis*, but with a less significant role.[29] Dogs are considered the main reservoir for *E. canis* because prolonged bacteremia occurs, which facilitates the acquisition of this pathogen by ticks.[25,26] *Amblyomma* sp and *Ixodes* sp ticks are more active during the spring and summer months. In contrast, *R. sanguineus* ticks can survive indoors in homes or kennels, and be active year-round, especially in subtropical areas, such as the coastal Southern United States.[30]

In the United States, *E. canis* exposure in dogs is estimated to be 1.8%, whereas the seroprevalence of *E. chaffeensis* and *E. ewingii* ranges between 3.1% and 3.8%. *Ehrlichia canis* exposure is more frequent in the South and Western regions of the United States, whereas exposure to *E. chaffeensis* and *E. ewingii* is more frequent in the South and Mid-Atlantic regions.[27] In Central and South America, reported molecular prevalence ranges from 18% in Colombia,[31] 29% in Mexico,[32] and 64% in Panama,[33] to 88% in Brazil.[34] In Europe, Asia, and Africa reported molecular prevalence ranges from less than 3.0% to 23%.[35]

Ehrlichia sp can survive and remain infectious in preserved and refrigerated whole blood for up to 11 days.[36,37] Therefore, they are transmitted by transfusion of blood or blood components or contaminated needles especially in endemic areas, potentially causing disease in transfusion recipients.[38] Conversely, perinatal transmission has not been documented in dogs.[39,40] Dogs of all breeds and ages are susceptible to CME, with German shepherd dogs and Siberian huskies predisposed to developing more severe clinical manifestations.[41] In some endemic regions, *E. canis* infection is more frequently observed among young dogs,[42,43] whereas seroreactivity is more frequent in adult dogs.[44] This observation may be caused by a higher probability of exposure to *E. canis* over time, rather than an increase in susceptibility with age.

Infection, Clinical Presentation, and Relevance

CME caused by *E. canis* is a multisystemic disease with variable severity depending on the clinical stage. The pathogenesis involves an incubation period of 8 to

20 days followed by acute, subclinical (asymptomatic), and chronic phases. The definition of each clinical phase in naturally infected dogs is difficult because clinical and laboratory findings are similar, with variable duration and severity.[45] The most common clinical signs during acute or chronic phases in naturally infected dogs are lethargy, inappetence, anorexia, weight loss, fever, epistaxis, petechiation, lymphadenopathy, and splenomegaly (**Fig. 3**, **Table 1**). Clinical manifestations vary depending on the strain of *E. canis,* host susceptibility, and the immune response, with acute disease in some dogs manifesting with moderate to severe signs and even death, whereas other dogs tolerate the infection with limited signs of illness.[46–48] In general, *Ehrlichia* sp subvert the host innate immune system, allowing the pathogens to perpetuate within macrophages (in the case of monocytic ehrlichiosis) or granulocytes (in the case of granulocytic ehrlichiosis) causing lymphadenomegaly and lymphoreticular hyperplasia in the spleen and liver. These immunologic and inflammatory changes result in leukocyte infiltration of parenchymal organs and perivascular cuffs in several locations, such as kidneys, spleen, meninges, lungs, eyes, and spleen.[45,49] Hypergammaglobulinemia is frequently documented in severe cases, including polyclonal or monoclonal (in the case of *E. canis*) expansion. This antibody production does not confer adequate protective immunity.[50] Thrombocytopenia is the most common finding during all three phases of CME because of increased consumption, immune-mediated destruction, sequestration of platelets in the spleen, and decreased production from hypoplastic bone marrow. Cytokine-mediated thrombocytopathia also occurs.[51,52] Once the acute phase subsides, there is an apparent

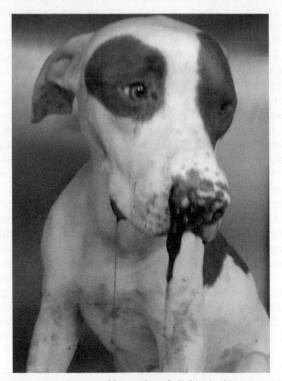

Fig. 3. Dog with severe epistaxis caused by canine ehrlichiosis. (*Courtesy of* Daniel Moura de Aguiar, Brazil.)

Table 1
Common clinical presentations and laboratory abnormalities in canine ehrlichiosis or anaplasmosis

Organism	Anaplasma phagocytophilum[a]	Anaplasma platys[b]	Ehrlichia canis[c]	Ehrlichia chaffeensis[d]	Ehrlichia ewingii[e]
Syndrome	Granulocytotropic anaplasmosis	Infectious cyclic thrombocytopenia	Monocytotropic ehrlichiosis	Monocytotropic ehrlichiosis	Granulocytotropic ehrlichiosis
Disease course	Acute or subclinical	Acute or subclinical	Acute, subclinical, or chronic	Acute or subclinical	Acute or subclinical
Clinical severity	Generally mild to moderate	Generally mild to moderate	From mild to life-threatening	Asymptomatic to mild	Asymptomatic to moderate
Main historical finding	Lethargy, inappetence, anorexia, lameness, weakness, stiffness, weight loss, rarely vomiting or diarrhea	No clinical abnormalities in most cases in the United States When present, lethargy, inappetence, anorexia, weight loss, epistaxis can occur	Lethargy, inappetence, anorexia, vomiting, diarrhea, weight loss, epistaxis, melena	No manifestations in most cases	Lameness, join pain, reluctance to move, stiffness, rarely vomiting or diarrhea It can be asymptomatic
Main signs	Fever, lymphadenopathy, splenomegaly, joint swelling, rarely epistaxis, and CNS signs	Fever, lymphadenopathy, petechiae, ecchymosis, pale mucous membranes	Fever, lymphadenopathy, splenomegaly, petechiae, ecchymosis, pale mucous membranes, melena, ocular and nasal discharge, scleral congestion, hyphema, uveitis, retinal detachment, CNS signs, cardiac arrhythmias	Fever, lymphadenopathy, petechiae	Fever, painful or swollen joints, ataxia, paresis, lymphadenopathy, splenomegaly, CNS signs

(continued on next page)

Table 1
(continued)

Organism	Anaplasma phagocytophilum[a]	Anaplasma platys[b]	Ehrlichia canis[c]	Ehrlichia chaffeensis[d]	Ehrlichia ewingii[e]
Main laboratory findings	Thrombocytopenia, neutrophilic polyarthritis, leukocytosis, neutrophilia, lymphopenia, eosinopenia, mild to moderate nonregenerative anemia, hypoalbuminemia, hyperglobulinemia, elevated ALP and ALT activities, hyperbilirubinemia, proteinuria	Thrombocytopenia, leukocytosis with neutrophilia, lymphocytosis, and monocytosis	Thrombocytopenia, neutropenia, monocytosis, eosinophilia, nonregenerative anemia, pancytopenia, polyclonal or monoclonal hyperglobulinemia, increased ALT and ALP activities, proteinuria, increased SDMA	Mild thrombocytopenia, anemia, and/or leukopenia	Thrombocytopenia, neutrophilic polyarthritis, leukocytosis, neutrophilia, monocytosis, anemia, elevated ALP and ALT activities, increased SDMA
Differential diagnoses	Other vector-borne diseases (Lyme disease, ehrlichiosis, among others), immune-mediated polyarthritis, immune-mediated hemolytic anemia, systemic lupus erythematosus	Other vector-borne diseases (anaplasmosis, ehrlichiosis, among others), immune thrombocytopenia	Other vector-borne diseases (anaplasmosis, Rocky Mountain spotted fever, leishmaniasis, among others), coccidioidomycosis, immune-mediated polyarthritis, immune-mediated hemolytic anemia, immune thrombocytopenia, systemic lupus erythematosus	Other vector-borne diseases (anaplasmosis, ehrlichiosis by E. canis or E. ewingii among others), idiopathic immune thrombocytopenia	Lyme disease, idiopathic immune-mediated polyarthritis, immune-mediated hemolytic anemia, immune thrombocytopenia, systemic lupus erythematosus

Abbreviations: ALP, alkaline phosphatase; AST, aspartate aminotransferase; CNS, central nervous system; SDMA, symmetric dimethylarginine.
[a] Refs. 46,58–65
[b] Refs. 46,47,66–70
[c] Refs. 46,58,71–74
[d] Refs. 46,58,71,72,75–77
[e] Refs. 55–58,72,78,79

clinical recovery with the disease becoming subclinical or asymptomatic for 6 to 9 weeks or persisting for years.[53] These dogs may have mild thrombocytopenia but without clinical signs of disease.[54] Chronic CME may develop in some dogs, with weight loss, myalgia, bleeding tendencies, ocular lesions, neurologic signs, cardiac arrhythmias, and a grave prognosis (**Figs. 3–7**). Complications from chronic infection include glomerulonephritis and nephrotic syndrome because of the deposition of immune complexes, and bone marrow suppression resulting in pancytopenia and secondary infections. At this stage, *E. canis* is hardly detected in circulation but may be detected in the spleen, lymph nodes, and bone marrow.[53]

Clinical manifestations of *E. ewingii* include fever and lameness associated with neutrophilic polyarthritis, but infected dogs may be asymptomatic.[55,56] Rarely, more severe neurologic signs, such as paresis, proprioceptive deficits, anisocoria, intention tremor, and head tilt, may be present.[57] Renal disease, immune-mediated hemolytic anemia, proteinuria, neutrophilia, abnormal lymphocytes, and increased liver enzyme activities were the most frequent abnormalities reported in dogs naturally infected with *E. ewingii*, although cause and effect was not established.[56] In contrast, *E. chaffeensis* infection in dogs is generally asymptomatic, or only mild signs are reported (see **Table 1**). A dog infected with *E. muris* was presented with fever, lethargy, and lameness,[13] whereas Panola Mountain *Ehrlichia* spp was reported as asymptomatic in a dog.[15]

CANINE ANAPLASMOSIS
Etiology

Canine anaplasmosis is caused by two distinct pathogens. *Anaplasma phagocytophilum* is the causative agent of granulocytotropic (also called granulocytic) anaplasmosis in domestic animals and people because it mainly targets peripheral neutrophils and eosinophils. This pathogen was previously named *Ehrlichia equi*, *Ehrlichia phagocytophila*, and in humans, the human granulocytotropic ehrlichiosis agent, but based on DNA sequencing these organisms were subsequently grouped under the genus *Anaplasma*.[2] This organism was first described in 1932 in a Scottish sheep as "a granulocytotropic ehrlichial disease."[80] In the United States, it was first identified in horses from California in 1969[81] and subsequently in dogs from California in 1982.[82] In Europe, cases were likely seen in dogs and horses in Sweden in 1989.[83] In people,

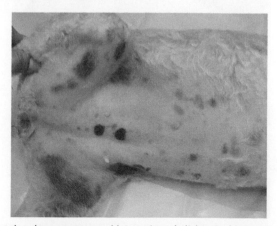

Fig. 4. Petechiae and ecchymoses caused by canine ehrlichiosis. (*Courtesy of* Ana Silvia Dagnone, Brazil.)

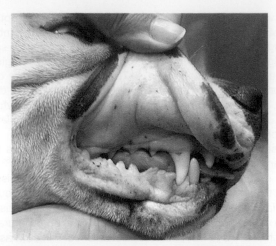

Fig. 5. Pale mucous membranes and petechiae in a dog with chronic ehrlichiosis. (*Courtesy of* Ana Silvia Dagnone, Brazil.)

A. phagocytophilum infection was first detected in Minnesota and Wisconsin between 1990 and 1993,[84,85] with canine cases identified simultaneously from those states.[86] Human anaplasmosis is an emerging disease, with more than 5000 human cases reported annually in the United States.[87]

Anaplasma platys is the causative agent of thrombocytotropic anaplasmosis (also called infectious cyclic thrombocytopenia). This pathogen was first described as basophilic inclusion bodies in platelets of thrombocytopenic dogs in the United States in 1978.[88] Since then, this organism has been detected in other domestic animals, such as cats, horses, cattle, goats, and people.[89–91] This pathogen was previously

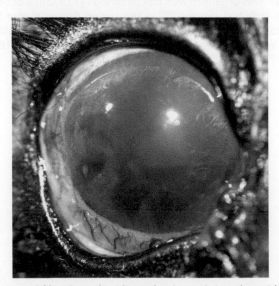

Fig. 6. Hyphema, corneal fibrosis, and evident scleral vessels in a dog with uveitis caused by ehrlichiosis. (*Courtesy of* Nathalie M. B. Dower, Brazil.)

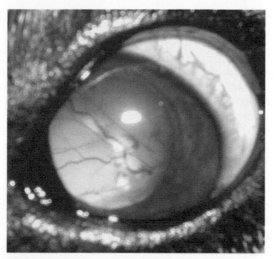

Fig. 7. Retinal detachment in a dog caused by ehrlichiosis. (*Courtesy of* José L. Laus and Ivan R. Martinez Padua, Brazil.)

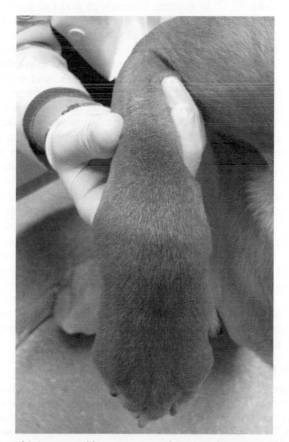

Fig. 8. Swollen carpal joint caused by canine anaplasmosis. (*Courtesy of* Matt Eberts, USA.)

named *Ehrlichia platys* but was subsequently found to belong to the genus *Anaplasma* based on DNA sequencing.[2]

Epidemiology

Anaplasma phagocytophilum has a worldwide distribution. Endemic areas follow the distribution of the *Ixodes* sp ticks.[92] *Ixodes scapularis* (black-legged tick) is the main vector in Eastern regions of United States and Canada,[93,94] where a 213% increase in the number of counties with established tick populations was documented between 1996 and 2015.[95] *Ixodes pacificus* (the Western black-legged tick) is the vector in the west coast of the United States.[96] This tick has expanded its geographic distribution to include southwest Canada and Alaska in recent years.[97,98] In Europe, *Ixodes ricinus* (the castor bean tick) is the main vector for *A. phagocytophilum*[99]; its geographic distribution is also expanding, and now includes northwestern areas of Europe.[100–102] *Ixodes persulcatus* (the taiga tick) is the main vector in eastern Europe and southeast Asia (China, Mongolia, Korea, and Russia), although several other *Ixodes* species have been implicated in carrying and transmitting *A. phagocytophilum*.[103–105] Several genetic variants of *A. phagocytophilum* from a large number of domestic and wild animals have been described worldwide.[64,106] In the United States, the white-footed mouse, the redwood chipmunk, and woodrats are the main reservoir for an *A. phagocytophilum* variant capable of causing disease in people, dogs, and horses.[107–110] In Europe, hedgehogs and red squirrels may be the main reservoir of *A. phagocytophilum* variants commonly detected in dogs and people.[111] It is estimated that 1 in every 30 dogs in the United States and 1 in every 240 dogs in Canada screened have been exposed to *Anaplasma* sp (presumably *A. phagocytophilum* for the most part), with higher frequencies in the Northeastern, upper Midwestern, and Pacific Northwestern United States, and southern regions of Canada, especially Alberta, British Columbia, and Nova Scotia provinces.[112,113] In Europe, *A. phagocytophilum* is more frequently detected in northern and central regions, especially in Hungary, Romania, and Poland, whereas in Asia it was more frequently reported in China and Malaysia. A molecular prevalence of 40% to 57% was reported from Jordan and Iran, respectively, but estimates were based on testing of a limited number of dogs. This pathogen is rarely reported from dogs in South America or Africa.[64]

Anaplasma platys also has a worldwide distribution, with infections frequently found in the same geographic regions as *E. canis*, because they share the same vector *R. sanguineus*.[114,115] *Anaplasma platys* has also been less frequently detected in other ticks, such as *Rhipicephalus turanicus*,[116] *I. persulcatus*,[117] *I. ricinus*,[118] and *Dermacentor nuttalli*.[117] Canine infections with *A. platys* are more frequently detected in southern parts of the United States, especially in Arizona and New Mexico.[119] In Europe, it is more frequently diagnosed in dogs from countries in the Mediterranean basin, including Italy, Spain, Portugal, France, Turkey, Greece, Croatia, and Romania.[41,66] This pathogen is also frequently detected in dogs from Central and South America (Brazil, Colombia, Paraguay, Uruguay, among others),[114,120–123] the Caribbean,[68,124] Africa,[125–127] Middle East,[128,129] and Asia.[130–132]

Infection, Clinical Presentation, and Relevance

Dogs with granulocytotropic anaplasmosis are generally present with lethargy, fever, inappetence or anorexia, musculoskeletal pain, reluctance to walk, and lameness (see **Table 1**), although asymptomatic dogs have been documented after natural or experimental infection.[46,62,64] Lameness, weakness, or stiffness (**Fig. 8**) are frequently reported as a consequence of monoarthropathy or polyarthropathy, secondary to the immune response triggered by the infection.[63,64] Exactly how *A. phagocytophilum* causes disease remains unknown, but proposed mechanisms include cytokine-mediated myelosuppression; the development of autoantibodies; infection of hemato-poietic precursors; and consumption of blood cells, especially platelets.[133] Thrombo-cytopenia is the most common laboratory abnormality detected, followed by anemia, increased liver enzymes, and hyperbilirubinemia.[46,58-65] Joint aspirates may reveal turbid synovial fluid with a high neutrophil count, where intracellular inclusions may be visualized. However, *A. phagocytophilum* morulae are morphologically indistin-guishable from *E. ewingii* inclusions, so molecular methods such as polymerase chain reaction (PCR) and/or DNA sequencing are required to distinguish these organisms.[133] The morulae may also be confused with stain artifacts or basophilic precipitates. Although granulocytotropic anaplasmosis is considered an acute disease (generally with 1–2 weeks of duration),[63] persistent infections in dogs from several months to a year have been documented experimentally.[46,134-136] Therefore, if antimicrobial treatment is not administered, subclinical infection with acute flare-ups could possibly develop.[136,137] Dogs may develop secondary immune-mediated diseases, such as immune-mediated hemolytic anemia, immune-mediated thrombocytopenia (ITP), and polyarthritis.[65] Fatal cases have been reported, with immune-mediated hemolytic anemia and disseminated intravascular coagulation being the most frequent cause of death.[64]

Infection with *A. platys* in the dog is characterized by recurrent thrombocytopenia that waxes and wanes on approximately a 10- to 14-day cycle during acute infec-tion.[47,88] Thrombocytopenia is believed to be a consequence of platelet phagocy-tosis by macrophages, either because of injury to platelets by the organism or opsonization by platelet-antibody.[138] Dogs can remain asymptomatic during the acute phase, although clinical manifestations, such as lethargy, inappetence, anorexia, weight loss, and epistaxis, have been reported (see **Table 1**). When pre-sent, the physical examination may reveal fever, lymphadenopathy, and petechiae. Apparently, clinical manifestations from strains in the United States are generally mild or asymptomatic,[46,47,70] whereas strains in Europe and South America are associated with more severe manifestations.[67,69,139,140] Nonetheless, subclinical carriers have been frequently reported from the United States and abroad.[124,141-143] Infectious cyclic thrombocytopenia is life-threatening especially if the patient is sub-jected to surgery or blunt trauma.

FELINE EHRLICHIOSIS AND ANAPLASMOSIS
Etiology

Infections of cats with *Ehrlichia* or *Anaplasma* species are much less frequent than in dogs. Worldwide, the most frequently reported species are *E. canis* and *A. phagocy-tophilum,* with *A. platys*, *Anaplasma bovis*, *E. chaffeensis*, *E. ewingii*, and others rarely reported.[144-148] The same vectors responsible for infections in dogs are suspected to transmit them to cats.[149,150]

Epidemiology, Clinical Presentation, and Relevance

The frequency of cats infected with or exposed to *E. canis* or *A. phagocytophilum* also varies according to the geographic region, population tested, and diagnostic method used. The seroprevalence of *E. canis* exposure in cats was reported to be 0.14% in the United States,[148] from 6% to 18% in Europe,[151] and 33% in Brazil.[152] For *A. phago-cytophilum*, reported seroprevalences ranged from 1.8% to 38% in the United States and 2% to 33% in Europe.[148,151,153] Molecular prevalence for *A. phagocytophilum* in peripheral blood varied from 0% to 23% in Europe and 0% to 7% in the United States.[154]

Not all infected cats present with clinical disease, which is characterized by nonspecific signs, such as intermittent fever, anorexia, lethargy, dehydration, joint pain, and epistaxis. Similarly, hematologic findings are variable and may include nonregenerative anemia, thrombocytopenia, lymphopenia, monocytosis, or hyperglobulinemia. In contrast to dogs infected with *A. phagocytophilum*, polyarthropathy is infrequently documented in infected cats.[155,156]

DIAGNOSIS OF EHRLICHIOSIS AND ANAPLASMOSIS

The combination of more than one diagnostic assay, especially one serology-based and one molecular-based assay, is recommended to optimize the diagnosis of ehrlichiosis and anaplasmosis across the different stages of infection.[157,158] Because every assay has strengths and limitations, a negative result from cytology, serology, or PCR does not necessarily rule out infection. A summary of the most frequently used diagnostic assays is provided in **Table 2**, but no in-clinic serology or molecular-based test for these diseases in cats is currently available. Clinical and laboratory abnormalities must be taken into consideration when evaluating a suspected case (see **Table 1**), because no single diagnostic test is capable of accurately detecting *Anaplasma* or *Ehrlichia* infection in all cases.[159]

Microscopic Examination

Microscopic examination of peripheral blood is always indicated in patients with thrombocytopenia or anemia to verify cell counts and review red blood cell and platelet morphology. However, microscopic evaluation of peripheral blood, buffy coat, or aspirates from lymph nodes or bone marrow is time consuming and have overall limited sensitivity and specificity for detecting *E. canis*, *E. chaffeensis*, *E. ewingii*, and *A. platys* when compared with other diagnostic assays.[160] For the diagnosis of *A. phagocytophilum*, review of peripheral blood smears yields moderate to high sensitivity, probably caused by the acute nature of the infection.[63,161] Morphologic features of the morulae do not allow species identification and the cell type infected (monocyte or granulocyte) does not always correlate directly with the species of *Ehrlichia* or *Anaplasma* involved (eg, *E. canis* can infect granulocytes or lymphocytes, **Figs. 9–11**).[3,162] The exception is when morulae are detected in platelets, which suggests *A. platys* infection (**Fig. 12**).[88] In summary, cytologic examination of peripheral blood and other samples may be most sensitive in cases with acute illness, when circulating numbers of organisms are highest, but not visualizing an organism does not rule out infection. More sensitive diagnostic tools should be used when ehrlichiosis and anaplasmosis is suspected.

Serology

Several assays are available for the detection of antibodies against *Anaplasma* and *Ehrlichia* species. Most in-clinic tests are based on enzyme-linked immunosorbent assays, whereas laboratory-based assays are either based on enzyme-linked immunosorbent assays or microimmunofluorescence (immunofluorescence assay [IFA]). These rely on the patient's ability to mount a detectable antibody response; consequently, most serologic assays yield negative results during early phases, generally 1 to 2 weeks postinfection.[157,163,164] Of note, after the infection is managed with antimicrobials, antibodies can remain elevated for several months to years, especially for *E. canis*.[165] In-clinic serologic assays are a valuable tool to clinicians to quickly

Table 2
Most common diagnostic assays for anaplasmosis and ehrlichiosis in dogs and cats

Assay	Specimen	Setting	Organism Detected	Advantage	Limitation
Cytology	Peripheral blood Buffy coat Lymph node Bone marrow	Point of care	*Anaplasma phagocytophilum* *Anaplasma platys* *Ehrlichia canis* *Ehrlichia chaffeensis* *Ehrlichia ewingii*	Cost-effective The assay is performed on-site or at a diagnostic laboratory Feline samples can be tested	Cannot determine bacterial species (except for *A platys*) Time-consuming when scanning a large number of oil immersion fields (500–1000) needed to increase sensitivity[160] Low to moderate specificity, depending on the operator's training level (lymphocytic azurophilic granules, lymphoglandular bodies, and phagocytosed material may resemble ehrlichial inclusions)[175] *E. canis, E. ewingii*, and *A. platys*: Low sensitivity when compared with other methods (from 0% to 10% in peripheral blood of infected dogs, but moderate sensitivity for buffy coat, bone marrow, or lymph node with *E. canis*)[63,160,176–178] *A. phagocytophilum*: moderate to high sensitivity (40%–94%), but cannot be differentiated from *E. ewingii*[63,161]

(continued on next page)

Table 2
(continued)

Assay	Specimen	Setting	Organism Detected	Advantage	Limitation
Serology: SNAP 4Dx Plus (IDEXX)	Serum, plasma, or anticoagulated whole blood	Point of care	*A. phagocytophilum* *A. platys* *Borrelia burgdorferi* *E. canis* *E. chaffeensis* *E. ewingii* *Dirofilaria immitis* (antigen)	Results in 8 min Cost-effective and easy to perform at the clinic Stored at room temperature for 90 d Reported sensitivity of 97% for *E. canis*, 98% for *E. ewingii*, 85% for *A. phagocytophilum*, and 83% for *A. platys* when compared with IFA, Western immunoblot, and/or species-specific ELISA[179] The manufacturer claims better performance than other lateral-flow ELISA assays[180] Available worldwide	Does not quantify antibody levels, therefore cannot detect a 4-fold increase between paired samples Cannot differentiate between antibodies against *A. phagocytophilum* and *A. platys*, or between *E. canis* and *E. ewingii*[181] Limited sensitivity for *E. chaffeensis*[181] Not approved for cats
Serology: VetScan Flex4 (Zoetis)	Serum, plasma, or anticoagulated whole blood	Point of care	*A. phagocytophilum* *A. platys* *B. burgdorferi* *E. canis* *E. chaffeensis* *E. ewingii* *D. immitis* (antigen)	Results in 8 min Cost-effective and easy to perform at the clinic Stored at room temperature Available in the United States and several countries across Europe and Asia	Does not quantify antibody levels, therefore cannot detect a 4-fold increase between paired samples Cannot differentiate between antibodies against *A. phagocytophilum* and *A. platys*, or among *E. canis*, *E. chaffeensis*, or *E. ewingii*

Test	Sample	Type	Target	Features	Availability/Limitations
					Reported sensitivity of 61% for *E. canis*, 59% for *E. ewingii*, 13% for *A. phagocytophilum*, and 33% for *A. platys* when compared with IFA, Western immunoblot, and/or species-specific ELISA[179] Limited peer-reviewed literature Not approved for cats
Serology: ImmunoComb (Biogal)	Serum	Point of care	*E. canis*	Results in 20 min Cost-effective and easy to perform at the clinic Results provide semiquantification of antibodies, based on the color tone of the test spot Reported sensitivity of 86% for *E. canis* when compared with IFA[182]	Not available in the United States or Canada but available in several countries in Europe, the Americas, and Asia Requires refrigeration Limited peer-reviewed literature Not approved for cats
PCRun (Biogal)	Anticoagulated whole blood	Point of care	*A. platys* *E. canis*	Based on PCR assay, so can detect active infection Results within 1 h One study reported 100% sensitivity and specificity[183] Marketed for *A. platys* and *E. canis* detection, but reported to detect *A. phagocytophilum*, *E. chaffeensis*, and *E. ewingii*	Not available in the United States, Canada, and most of Europe, but available in several countries in the Americas, Middle East, and Asia Requires specific equipment (heat block) Time-consuming when compared with other point-of-care assays One study reported sensitivity of 75%[184]

(continued on next page)

Table 2
(continued)

Assay	Specimen	Setting	Organism Detected	Advantage	Limitation
Serology: Immunofluorescent assay	Serum	Diagnostic laboratory (many private or university-based laboratories)	*A. phagocytophilum* *E. canis*	Provides quantification of antibody response (titer) A 4-fold increase in titers confirmed active infection Continuous decrease in titers may indicate treatment success Feline samples can be tested	Limited peer-reviewed literature Not approved for cats Tests must be performed at a diagnostic laboratory Results may take days to be available Acute infection may yield negative results Dogs with chronic infection may not seroconvert Not yet available for *A. platys, E. chaffeensis,* or *E. ewingii* Cannot determine species involved in the infection because cross reactivity may occur Lack of standardization among laboratories
Serology: Accuplex4 (Antech)	Serum	Diagnostic laboratory	*A. phagocytophilum* *E. canis* *B. burgdorferi* *D. immitis* (antigen)	In one experimental study, antibodies against *E. canis* were detected earlier than IFA or SNAP[185] Reported sensitivity of 100% for *E. canis* when compared with IFA[186]	Only available in the United States and Canada Tests must be performed at a diagnostic laboratory Reported sensitivity of 75% for *A. phagocytophilum* when compared with IFA[187] Limited peer-reviewed literature Not approved for cats

| PCR: Single test or tick-borne panel | Diagnostic laboratory (many private or university-based laboratories) | Anticoagulated whole blood Buffy coat Lymph node Bone marrow Other tissues | A. phagocytophilum A. platys E. canis E. chaffeensis E. ewingii Other organisms (panels vary among laboratories) | Can detect active infection High analytical sensitivity and specificity Species/strain present is identified with specific PCR assays and/or DNA sequencing Panels can detect coinfections with other vector-borne pathogens Feline samples can be tested | Tests must be performed at a diagnostic laboratory Results may take days to be available Limited sensitivity in case of subclinical or chronic infection Prone to false-positive because of cross-contamination if laboratory best practices are not properly followed Lack of standardization among laboratories |

Abbreviations: ELISA, enzyme-linked immunosorbent assay; IFA, immunofluorescence assay.

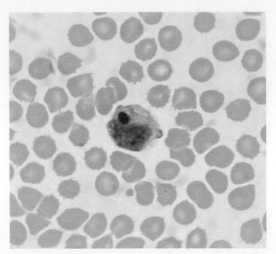

Fig. 9. Morulae of *Ehrlichia canis* in a monocyte (note that it cannot be distinguished from morulae of *Ehrlichia chaffeensis*). (*Courtesy of* Arnon Falcão Calábria, Brazil.)

document exposure to vector-borne pathogens. However, the presence of specific antibodies against *Anaplasma* and/or *Ehrlichia* spp only indicates exposure to the organisms, and should not be used alone to make a diagnosis without taking into consideration clinical and laboratory abnormalities and other case context.[166] In general, a seroreactive dog with no signs or laboratory abnormalities and negative PCR testing does not require antibiotic therapy but should be monitored to rule out subclinical infection (**Table 2**). The presence of long-lasting antibodies levels is particularly relevant in areas endemic for vector-borne pathogens, where a positive serologic test may be caused by past exposure and not necessarily associated with the current

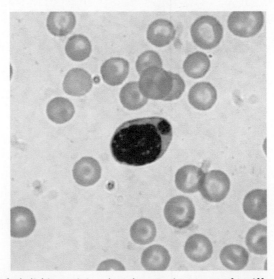

Fig. 10. Morulae of *Ehrlichia canis* in a lymphocyte. (*Courtesy of* Jeniffer Ariane de Morais, Brazil.)

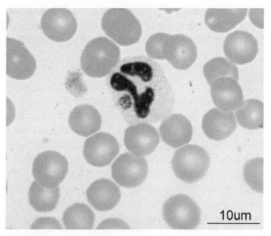

Fig. 11. Morulae of *Anaplasma phagocytophilum* on a neutrophil (note that it cannot be distinguished from morulae of *Ehrlichia ewingii*). (*Courtesy of* Kristin Nunez, USA.)

disease.[166] Chronically infected dogs generally have high titers, although some dogs may be seronegative because of the ability of the pathogen to evade the immune system.[47,56,62,89,167]

Most in-clinic serologic assays do not provide quantification of antibodies (titers), whereas laboratory-based assays can quantify specific antibody concentration and support the detection of a four-fold increase in titers between acute and convalescent samples, which confirms active infection. Therefore, clinicians should establish a routine of banking frozen specimens at the initial presentation to allow such analysis during follow-up visits.[157] The sensitivity and specificity are high for most available serology assays, but vary across reports, with no peer-reviewed studies for some tests (see **Table 2**). Serologic cross reactivity among *Anaplasma* and *Ehrlichia* species within their respective genus in some assays prevent the determination of the bacterial species involved, but it does not prevent the clinician from reaching a diagnosis and establishing appropriate antimicrobial therapy, because these infections generally

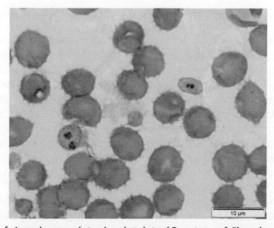

Fig. 12. Morulae of *Anaplasma platys* in platelets. (*Courtesy of* Charalampos Attipa, UK.)

respond well to doxycycline therapy.[41,168] The presence of other vector-borne agents should always be considered, given that the same vector may be capable of transmitting more than one pathogen (eg, *A. phagocytophilum* and *Borrelia burgdorferi* by *Ixodes* ticks).[169,170]

Polymerase Chain Reaction

In recent decades, PCR assays have become widely available for the diagnosis of anaplasmosis and ehrlichiosis because of a significant reduction in the cost of reagents and equipment. PCR assays have several advantages over serology, including the detection of acute infection with high levels of analytical sensitivity and specificity, the opportunity to test different specimens (eg, fine-needle aspirate or biopsy samples),[171] the ability to determine the bacterial species involved, and to screen for multiple pathogens by the use of PCR panels.[158] Tissue samples, such as the spleen, lymph nodes, or bone marrow aspirates, are more sensitive for the molecular detection of *Anaplasma* and *Ehrlichia* spp than peripheral blood, especially during subclinical/chronic phases of infection or after antibiotic therapy.[171–173] However, anticoagulated whole-blood samples are more practical to obtain and if collected during the acute phase, achieve good clinical sensitivity using PCR. Well-designed and validated PCR assays can detect few organisms in clinical specimens, at concentrations that cannot be visualized by microscopic examination.[160] In addition, these assays are paired with DNA sequencing, for the further identification of species, strains, or variants, providing valuable epidemiologic data about animal and human health.[89] However, despite advances in chemistry and equipment, PCR assays are not widely available at the point of care (see **Table 2**). In addition, results may take days to become available, limiting the clinician's ability to reach quick medical decisions. Most importantly, a negative PCR result never rules out infection, because low levels of bacteremia (seen in subclinical or chronic infections) may be lower than the level of detection of the assay or not be present in the specimen tested.[171,174] Because the phase of infection is generally unknown, PCR-based results should be interpreted in combination with serologic testing (**Table 3**).[157,158] Similar to serologic assays, clinicians should routinely bank frozen EDTA-blood samples of patients suspected of a tick-borne disease during the initial consultation and before antibiotic therapy. These samples are later used for repeat PCR testing in a highrisk patient with a negative initial result, and analyzed for additional known pathogens or novel organisms if needed.[157]

TREATMENT AND PREVENTION OF EHRLICHIOSIS AND ANAPLASMOSIS

The decision to start antimicrobial therapy depends on several factors including clinical manifestations, the results of specific diagnostic testing, and predictive values for positive and negative tests in the region. Clinicians should also consider other noninfectious differentials, and veterinary antibiotic stewardship guidelines. **Table 3** summarizes the most common clinical scenarios and treatment recommendations. Among all etiologic pathogens of anaplasmosis and ehrlichiosis, *E. canis* infection in dogs is more frequently associated with severe to life-threatening manifestations, requiring more comprehensive therapy. Conversely, *A. phagocytohilum* infection generally responds quickly to proper antimicrobial therapy. Tetracyclines remain the antibiotic class of choice to control ehrlichial infections in companion animals but their indiscriminate use increases the risk of antimicrobial resistance.[188,189] Doxycycline remains the recommended antibiotic, with other tetracyclines also being effective for dogs and cats (**Table 4**). Doxycycline treatment in dogs during the acute phase of *E. canis* infection reduces oxidative stress and promotes resolution of clinical and

Table 3
Potential clinical scenarios of suspected anaplasmosis or ehrlichiosis and treatment recommendations[a]

Compatible Clinical and/or Laboratory Findings	In-Clinic Serology	IFA[b]	PCR	Diagnosis	Treatment	Recommendations, Treatment Response, and Other Considerations
No	Positive for *Ehrlichia canis*	Negative to low titer for *E. canis*	Negative	Possible subclinical ehrlichiosis	No	Low titers may indicate past exposure with resolution of infection Repeat serologic testing after 2–3 wk because increasing titers indicate active infection Repeat CBC in 2–3 wk; consider monitoring chemistry and urinalysis Consider repeating PCR assay after a few days, because bacteria levels vary in circulation
		High titer for *E. canis*	Negative	Possible subclinical ehrlichiosis	No	High titers may indicate active infection but can persist following previous exposure Follow the recommendations above for CBC, chemistry, urinalysis, and PCR testing
	Positive for *Anaplasma*	Negative or positive for *Anaplasma*	Negative	Suspected chronic anaplasmosis	No	*Anaplasma platys* frequently cause chronic infection, whereas *Anaplasma phagocytophilum* is generally acute

(continued on next page)

Table 3
(continued)

Compatible Clinical and/or Laboratory Findings	In-Clinic Serology	IFA[b]	PCR	Diagnosis	Treatment	Recommendations, Treatment Response, and Other Considerations
						Repeat CBC for cyclic thrombocytopenia, which supports *A. platys* infection Consider repeating PCR assay after a few days, because bacteria levels vary in circulation
Yes	Negative	Negative for *E. canis*	Positive for *E. canis*	Acute ehrlichiosis	Yes	An increase in antibody titers after 2–3 wk confirms acute infection Expected rapid clinical response to treatment in 2–3 d, with improvement of laboratory abnormalities in 1–3 wk
		Negative for *Anaplasma*	Positive for *Anaplasma*	Acute anaplasmosis	Yes	Same as above
	Positive for *Anaplasma*	Negative or low titers for *Anaplasma*	Negative	Possible acute anaplasmosis	Yes	Detected antibodies may be caused by past exposure An increase in antibody titers after 2–3 wk confirms acute infection If acute presentation, consider repeating PCR after a few days

Positive for E canis	Negative to low titer for E canis	Negative	Possible acute ehrlichiosis	Yes	A. platys frequently cause chronic infection and more difficult to treat, whereas A. phagocytophilum is generally acute and responds quickly to antibiotic therapy Consider repeating PCR assay after a few days, because bacteria levels vary in circulation Consider infection with other vector-borne pathogens and other underlying diseases
	High titer for E canis	Negative or positive	Suspected chronic ehrlichiosis	Yes	Same as above If blood PCR is negative, consider PCR of lymph node aspirates (especially if enlarged) Antibody titers may remain elevated for several months after therapy Variable response to treatment, with poor prognosis in dogs with bone marrow suppression

Abbreviations: CBC, complete blood count; IFA, immunofluorescence assay.

[a] Not meant to be a comprehensive list of all possible diagnostic scenarios.

[b] IFA assays for A. platys, E. chaffeensis, or E. ewingii are not currently available in veterinary medicine.

Table 4
Recommended antimicrobial drugs for the treatment of anaplasmosis and ehrlichiosis in dogs and cats

Drug	Dose and Interval	Route	Minimum duration[a]	Considerations
Doxycycline	5 mg/kg every 12 h or 10 mg/kg every 24 h	PO[b], IV	28 d [166,168,202]	Consider liquid formulation for cats or small dogs to avoid esophageal damage
Minocycline	Dogs: 5–10 mg/kg every 12 h Cats: 5–12.5 mg/kg every 12 h	PO[b]	28 d	Recommended if doxycycline is not available
Oxytetracycline	7.5–10 mg/kg every 12 h	IV	Until the patient can tolerate oral doxycycline	Used if oral antibiotics are not tolerated because of gastrointestinal signs

Abbreviation: IV, intravenous.
[a] Extended duration may be necessary in chronic cases.
[b] If available, IV preparations of doxycycline or minocycline are preferred when the patient cannot tolerate oral medication; however, it should be diluted in 100 to 1000 mL of lactated Ringer solution or 5% dextrose and be administered over 1 to 2 hours.

hematologic abnormalities.[74,190] In these authors' experience, a dose of 5 mg/kg orally every 12 hours is associated with fewer gastrointestinal adverse effects, such as vomiting and anorexia, while remaining as effective as the dose of 10 mg/kg orally every 24 hours. Esophageal strictures caused by tablet-induced focal esophagitis have been well described in cats and may also happen in small dogs.[191–193] Thus, at least 6 mL of liquid should be given orally after each tablet,[194] or liquid formulations could be considered. Of note, if liquid doxycycline is compounded from tablets, the preparation should be used within 7 days, because a 14% to 18% decrease in doxycycline concentration has been documented in liquid formulations stored from 14 to 28 days.[195] In addition, the pharmacokinetics of tetracyclines in the gastrointestinal tract is affected by chelation by calcium (from foods, such as dairy products, or certain oral antacids), causing a decrease in absorption, bioavailability, and efficacy. Among all tetracyclines, doxycycline is the least affected by the ingestion of calcium-rich foods.[196] However, in humans, simultaneous ingestion of milk diminished the peak plasma concentration of doxycycline by 24% and absorption by 9% to 53% (mean, 30%).[197] Anecdotal evidence supports a potentially similar effect in dogs who received doxycycline with milk or cheese, where the rate of clinical improvement was delayed. Therefore, it is prudent to avoid calcium-rich foods when administering oral tetracyclines, if possible.

Minocycline may be used if doxycycline is not available (see **Table 4**).[198] If the patient cannot tolerate oral antibiotics because of gastrointestinal signs, intravenous doxycycline or oxytetracycline is used until the patient can receive oral doxycycline.[159,166,199] One study also reported clinical and hematologic recovery of dogs with CME treated with rifampicin (10 mg/kg PO, once daily for 21 days), but three out of five infected dogs remained PCR positive from blood samples.[200] Given the limited clinical experience in conjunction with a few experimental studies and drug safety profile, rifampicin may be an alternative antibiotic for CME[168] but should not be used as monotherapy or as the first line of treatment until more data are reviewed. Clinical improvement to doxycycline therapy for acute and subclinical cases of ehrlichiosis or anaplasmosis is generally rapid in dogs and cats (within 24–48 hours), with platelet count and other laboratory abnormalities returning to normal within 2 weeks.[168,201–203] However, because of this rapid improvement, some clients may consider early termination of antibiotics. In one study of *A. phagocytophilum*–infected cats without comorbidities, three out of seven did not recover clinically after 3 weeks of doxycycline treatment.[204] Clinicians should highlight the importance of the minimum recommended duration of antibiotics to avoid potential chronic infection and the development of microbial antibiotic resistance. Antibody titers decline and generally become negative within 6 to 9 months after the introduction of antibiotics, but may remain elevated for years in some cases.[166] In acute cases presented with mild to moderate manifestation, if clinical improvement is absent after 3 days of adequate antimicrobial therapy, clinicians should investigate the presence of other vector-borne diseases (babesiosis, bartonellosis, and leishmaniasis in endemic areas or for patients with a travel history), other infectious causes (coccidioidomycosis), or noninfectious underlying disease.

Because tetracyclines and rifampicin are bacteriostatic,[205] the duration of therapy necessary to control the infection remains unknown. Several studies were unable to detect *E. canis*, *A. phagocytophilum*, or *A. platys* in canine blood or tissues after 4 weeks of doxycycline treatment of acute or subclinical disease, even after immunosuppression.[47,74,202,206] However, elimination of the *E. canis* infection is not achieved in all cases, especially during chronic infection. In one study, persistent infection with *E. canis* was detected after 28 days of doxycycline when naive ticks fed on chronically infected dogs.[201] In cats, *A. phagocytophilum* PCR-positive results were also reported from 8 days, 37 days, 120 days, 150 days, to 2 years after doxycycline treatment of varying duration.[154,204] These differences in susceptibility to treatment may be caused by distinct strains of organisms, differences in host immunity, variations in dosing regimens, or reinfection.[168] Chronic CME cases with severe manifestation are challenging and have a poor prognosis because of myelosuppression and consequent pancytopenia and bleeding disorders.

The use of glucocorticoid therapy in canine ehrlichiosis and anaplasmosis remains controversial. Despite being advocated for CME by some clinicians, studies have not documented significant clinical or prognostic benefits of glucocorticoids as an adjunct to doxycycline.[207,208] Therefore, glucocorticoids are not recommended in the first line of treatment because resolution of clinical and hematologic abnormalities after administration of doxycycline is usually rapid, and they may theoretically predispose to secondary infections and the inability to clear the infection, even with antibiotic therapy.[41,168,199] Doxycycline and minocycline also have anti-inflammatory and immunomodulatory properties,[209] which may be associated with the rapid response during the first days of treatment. In cases where improvement of clinical and/or hematologic abnormalities are not documented after the first week of antibiotic therapy, anti-inflammatory doses of glucocorticoids may be considered. For uveitis, topical anti-inflammatory medications (glucocorticoids or nonsteroidal anti-inflammatory drugs) and mydriatic drugs to improve comfort and prevent pupil adhesions are also frequently used in combination with oral prednisolone at 1 mg/kg every 24 hours for 1 to 2 weeks.[210] For antibody-mediated syndromes, such as ITP, the use of higher immunosuppressive doses of glucocorticoids has been suggested for up to 7 days in addition to ongoing therapy with doxycycline if no response is documented with doxycycline alone. Glucocorticoids are not recommended in the case of *E canis*–

induced myelosuppression because the pancytopenia is not believed to be immune-mediated.[168] A few case reports have described the use of erythropoietin (100 IU/kg subcutaneously every 3 days), ferrous sulfate (100 mg/kg orally every 24 hours), and folate (5 mg/kg orally every 24 hours) for anemia; filgrastim (50 μg/kg subcutaneously every 48 hours for up to three doses) for neutropenia; and desmopressin (1 μg/kg subcutaneously every 24 hours for 3 days) for bleeding disorders.[168,211,212]

In addition to antibiotics, supportive therapy is essential for survival and may include fluid therapy with electrolyte management, appropriate blood products in the presence of severe anemia or thrombocytopenia or life-threatening hemorrhage, control of vomiting with antiemetics (maropitant, ondansetron), and prevention or treatment of gastroduodenal ulceration and erosion (proton-pump inhibitors such as omeprazole).[213] Appetite stimulants and nutritional support should be implemented in patients who are persistently anorexic. Dogs with severe thrombocytopenia with acute infection may benefit from a single intravenous injection of 0.02 mg/kg of vincristine, which is hypothesized to stimulate thrombopoiesis, accelerate fragmentation of megakaryocytes, reduce phagocytosis of platelets by macrophages, and interfere with antiplatelet antibody formation and binding.[214] The use of a single dose of levamisole at 0.5 to 2 mg/kg subcutaneously as immunostimulant in dogs receiving doxycycline therapy for E canis infection was evaluated in one study where a significant increase in leukocyte, lymphocyte, and monocyte counts was documented within a 5-day period without adverse effects.[215] Imidocarb dipropionate is no longer recommended for the treatment of E. canis infection because of a lack of documented efficacy,[216] but its use is recommended when coinfection with Babesia canis or Babesia vogeli is suspected or confirmed.[168] Enrofloxacin is not effective against Ehrlichia spp and therefore should not be used.

ZOONOTIC IMPLICATIONS

All Ehrlichia and Anaplasma species listed in this review have been reported to infect people. Direct transmission of ehrlichial species from dogs or cats to humans has not been documented. However, infection in companion animals suggests the presence of the vector in the same environment to which human companions may also be exposed. Therefore, avoiding tick bites is the most effective measure to prevent disease in humans. Ixodes and Amblyomma ticks aggressively feed on people. R. sanguineus has also been documented to attach and feed on humans, especially when exposed to high temperatures.[217] For example, this tick species was responsible for an outbreak of Rocky Mountain spotted fever in people in Arizona.[218] Although not confirmed for Ehrlichia or Anaplasma spp, accidental needle sticks or tick removal using bare hands are important modes of transmission for other tick-borne pathogens, especially to veterinarians, veterinary technicians, and animal caretakers.[219–221] The case fatality rate (ie, the proportion of anaplasmosis or ehrlichiosis patients that reportedly died as a result of infection) in people is roughly 1% to 3% of ehrlichiosis cases and 0.3% of anaplasmosis cases in the United States.[222–224] Fatalities have been rarely reported in Europe.[225,226]

PREVENTION STRATEGIES

Exposure to Ehrlichia or Anaplasma species does not confer full protective immunity. Dogs and cats remain susceptible to reinfection and subsequent clinical disease if reexposed to vectors. Protective vaccines for dogs or cats are not commercially available. Therefore, vector control is the most effective prophylactic measure, and should be based on decreasing exposure to vectors by restricting access to tick-infested areas, year-round use of acaricides, and prompt removal of ticks with forceps or gloves. Ticks spend a significant amount of their life cycle not attached to their host, with approximately 5% on dogs and the remainder (~95%) in the environment.[227] Thus successful strategies incorporate tick control for the host and the environment, especially for *R. sanguineus*, which can thrive in urban settings.[217,227] In addition, landscaping the areas where dogs and cats have access can also decrease the risk of tick infestations, by clearing tall grasses and brushes, creating a 3-foot wide barrier of wood chips or gravel between play areas and surrounding wooded areas, frequently mowing the lawn, and maintaining the area clutter free.[228,229] For dog and cat breeders, where animals travel to shows or competitions, periodic antibody screening, PCR testing, and adequate treatment of positive animals should also be considered beyond vector control.

SUMMARY

In the last decade, the understanding of the epidemiology of vector-borne diseases has significantly expanded. These diseases continue to expand in geographic distribution because of enhanced vector activity from climate change. Broader use of accurate diagnostic tests provides clinicians with timely information to support better medical decision making. Doxycycline remains the therapy of choice for *Ehrlichia* or *Anaplasma* infections, and clinical resolution is achieved in most acute and subclinical cases. Clearance of infection may not be achieved in all cases, especially in chronic presentations. With the absence of effective vaccines for ehrlichiosis or anaplasmosis in dogs or cats, continuous tick prevention is the only effective strategy to avoid these diseases.

CLINICS CARE POINTS

- PCR testing of blood or tissue samples (spleen, lymph node, and bone marrow) is a sensitive and specific diagnostic tool, but a negative PCR result never rules out infection.
- For organisms where serologic testing is possible, combining PCR with serology increases overall diagnostic sensitivity. Acute and convalescent serologic testing and repeat testing using PCR can facilitate diagnosis.
- Doxycycline or minocycline for at least 4 weeks is the treatment of choice for dogs and cats but longer treatment durations may be necessary in complex cases.
- In acute cases, rapid clinical improvement and an increase in platelet count is observed within the first week of treatment, but antibiotic therapy should not be discontinued.
- Supportive therapy not only accelerates recovery but also is essential in complicated cases, when clinical response may take more than 4 weeks.
- Decreasing antibody titers and normalization of platelet counts after antibiotic therapy supports resolution of infection, but titers can remain elevated for several months in some cases.
- No vaccine is yet available, so a robust tick control program must be implemented to avoid infection or reinfection after antibiotic treatment.

DISCLOSURE

The authors have nothing to disclose.

REFERENCES

1. Popov VL, Han VC, Chen SM, et al. Ultrastructural differentiation of the genogroups in the genus *Ehrlichia*. J Med Microbiol 1998;47(3):235–51. https://doi.org/10.1099/00222615-47-3-235.

2. Dumler JS, Barbet AF, Bekker CP, et al. Reorganization of genera in the families Rickettsiaceae and Anaplasmataceae in the order Rickettsiales: unification of some species of *Ehrlichia* with *Anaplasma, Cowdria* with *Ehrlichia* and *Ehrlichia* with *Neorickettsia*, descriptions of six new species combinations and designation of *Ehrlichia equi* and 'HGE agent' as subjective synonyms of *Ehrlichia phagocytophila*. Int J Syst Evol Microbiol 2001;51(Pt 6):2145–65.

3. Aguiar DM, Rodrigues FP, Ribeiro MG, et al. Uncommon *Ehrlichia canis* infection associated with morulae in neutrophils from naturally infected dogs in Brazil. Transbound Emerg Dis 2020;67(Suppl 2):135–41. https://doi.org/10.1111/tbed.13390.

4. Groves MG, Dennis GL, Amyx HL, et al. Transmission of *Ehrlichia canis* to dogs by ticks (*Rhipicephalus sanguineus*). Am J Vet Res 1975;36(7):937–40.

5. Seamer J, Snape T. Tropical canine pancytopaenia and *Ehrlichia canis* infection. Vet Rec 1970;86(13):375. https://doi.org/10.1136/vr.86.13.375-a.

6. Cabezas-Cruz A, Zweygarth E, Vancova M, et al. *Ehrlichia minasensis* sp. nov., isolated from the tick *Rhipicephalus microplus*. Int J Syst Evol Microbiol 2016;66(3):1426–30. https://doi.org/10.1099/ijsem.0.000895.

7. Fourie JJ, Stanneck D, Luus HG, et al. Transmission of *Ehrlichia canis* by *Rhipicephalus sanguineus* ticks feeding on dogs and on artificial membranes. Vet Parasitol 2013;197(3–4):595–603. https://doi.org/10.1016/j.vetpar.2013.07.026.

8. Dumler JS, Bakken JS. Human ehrlichioses: newly recognized infections transmitted by ticks. Annu Rev Med 1998;49:201–13. https://doi.org/10.1146/annurev.med.49.1.201.

9. Olano JP, Walker DH. Human ehrlichioses. Med Clin North Am 2002;86(2):375–92. https://doi.org/10.1016/s0025-7125(03)00093-2.

10. Beall MJ, Alleman AR, Breitschwerdt EB, et al. Seroprevalence of *Ehrlichia canis, Ehrlichia chaffeensis* and *Ehrlichia ewingii* in dogs in North America. *Parasit Vectors* 2012;5:29. https://doi.org/10.1186/1756-3305-5-29.

11. Starkey LA, Barrett AW, Beall MJ, et al. Persistent *Ehrlichia ewingii* infection in dogs after natural tick infestation. *J Vet Intern Med* Mar-apr 2015;29(2):552–5. https://doi.org/10.1111/jvim.12567.

12. Pritt BS, Sloan LM, Johnson DK, et al. Emergence of a new pathogenic *Ehrlichia* species, Wisconsin and Minnesota, 2009. N Engl J Med 2011;365(5):422–9. https://doi.org/10.1056/NEJMoa1010493.

13. Hegarty BC, Maggi RG, Koskinen P, et al. *Ehrlichia muris* infection in a dog from Minnesota. J Vet Intern Med 2012;26(5):1217–20. https://doi.org/10.1111/j.1939-1676.2012.00968.x.

14. Loftis AD, Kelly PJ, Paddock CD, et al. Panola Mountain *Ehrlichia* in *Amblyomma maculatum* from the United States and *Amblyomma variegatum* (Acari: Ixodidae) from the Caribbean and Africa. J Med Entomol 2016;53(3):696–8. https://doi.org/10.1093/jme/tjv240.

15. Qurollo BA, Davenport AC, Sherbert BM, et al. Infection with Panola Mountain *Ehrlichia* sp. in a dog with atypical lymphocytes and clonal T-cell expansion. J Vet Intern Med 2013;27(5):1251–5. https://doi.org/10.1111/jvim.12148.

16. Reeves WK, Loftis AD, Nicholson WL, et al. The first report of human illness associated with the Panola Mountain *Ehrlichia* species: a case report. J Med Case Rep 2008;2:139. https://doi.org/10.1186/1752-1947-2-139.

17. Loftis AD, Reeves WK, Spurlock JP, et al. Infection of a goat with a tick-transmitted *Ehrlichia* from Georgia, U.S.A., that is closely related to *Ehrlichia ruminantium*. J Vector Ecol 2006;31(2):213–23.

18. Aguiar DM, Araujo JP Jr, Nakazato L, et al. Complete genome sequence of an *Ehrlichia minasensis* strain isolated from cattle. Microbiol Resour Announc 2019; 8(15). https://doi.org/10.1128/MRA.00161-19.

19. Melo ALT, Luo T, Zhang X, et al. Serological evidence of *Ehrlichia minasensis* infection in Brazilian dogs. Acta Trop 2021;219:105931. https://doi.org/10. 1016/j.actatropica.2021.105931.

20. Muraro LS, Souza AO, Leite TNS, et al. First evidence of *Ehrlichia minasensis* infection in horses from Brazil. Pathogens 2021;(3):10. https://doi.org/10.3390/ pathogens10030265.

21. Lewis GE Jr, Ristic M, Smith R, et al. The brown dog tick *Rhipicephalus sanguineus* and the dog as experimental hosts of *Ehrlichia canis*. Am J Vet Res 1977; 38(12):1953–5.

22. Aguiar DM, Cavalcante GT, Pinter A, et al. Prevalence of *Ehrlichia canis* (Rickettsiales: Anaplasmataceae) in dogs and *Rhipicephalus sanguineus* (Acari: Ixodidae) ticks from Brazil. J Med Entomol 2007;44(1):126–32.

23. Moraes-Filho J, Krawczak FS, Costa FB, et al. Comparative evaluation of the vector competence of four South American populations of the *Rhipicephalus sanguineus* group for the bacterium *Ehrlichia canis*, the agent of canine monocytic ehrlichiosis. PLoS One 2015;10(9):e0139386. https://doi.org/10.1371/ journal.pone.0139386.

24. Sanches GS, Villar M, Couto J, et al. Comparative proteomic analysis of *Rhipicephalus sanguineus* sensu lato (Acari: Ixodidae) tropical and temperate lineages: uncovering differences during *Ehrlichia canis* infection. Front Cell Infect Microbiol 2020;10:611113. https://doi.org/10.3389/fcimb.2020.611113.

25. Movilla R, Garcia C, Siebert S, et al. Countrywide serological evaluation of canine prevalence for *Anaplasma* spp., *Borrelia burgdorferi* (sensu lato), *Dirofilaria immitis* and *Ehrlichia canis* in Mexico. Parasit Vectors 2016;9(1):421. https://doi.org/10.1186/s13071-016-1686-z.

26. Taques I, Campos ANS, Kavasaki ML, et al. Geographic distribution of *Ehrlichia canis* TRP genotypes in Brazil. Vet Sci 2020;7(4). https://doi.org/10.3390/ vetsci7040165.

27. Qurollo BA, Chandrashekar R, Hegarty BC, et al. A serological survey of tick-borne pathogens in dogs in North America and the Caribbean as assessed by *Anaplasma phagocytophilum*, *A. platys*, *Ehrlichia canis*, *E. chaffeensis*, *E. ewingii*, and *Borrelia burgdorferi* species-specific peptides. Infect Ecol Epidemiol 2014;4. https://doi.org/10.3402/iee.v4.24699.

28. Jones EO, Gruntmeir JM, Hamer SA, et al. Temperate and tropical lineages of brown dog ticks in North America. Vet Parasitol Reg Stud Rep 2017;7:58–61. https://doi.org/10.1016/j.vprsr.2017.01.002.

29. Johnson EM, Ewing SA, Barker RW, et al. Experimental transmission of *Ehrlichia canis* (Rickettsiales: Ehrlichieae) by *Dermacentor variabilis* (Acari: Ixodidae). Vet Parasitol 1998;74(2–4):277–88. https://doi.org/10.1016/s0304-4017(97) 00073-3.

30. Dryden MW, Payne PA. Biology and control of ticks infesting dogs and cats in North America. *Vet Ther* Summer 2004;5(2):139–54.

31. Arroyave E, Cornwell ER, McBride JW, et al. Detection of tick-borne rickettsial pathogens in naturally infected dogs and dog-associated ticks in Medellin, Colombia. Rev Bras Parasitol Vet 2020;29(3):e005320. https://doi.org/10.1590/s1984-29612020060.

32. Ojeda-Chi MM, Rodriguez-Vivas RI, Esteve-Gasent MD, et al. *Ehrlichia canis* in dogs of Mexico: prevalence, incidence, co-infection and factors associated. Comp Immunol Microbiol Infect Dis 2019;67:101351. https://doi.org/10.1016/j.cimid.2019.101351.

33. Santamaria A, Calzada JE, Saldana A, et al. Molecular diagnosis and species identification of *Ehrlichia* and *Anaplasma* infections in dogs from Panama, Central America. Vector Borne Zoonotic Dis 2014;14(5):368–70. https://doi.org/10.1089/vbz.2013.1488.

34. Vieira RF, Biondo AW, Guimaraes AM, et al. Ehrlichiosis in Brazil. Rev Bras Parasitol Vet 2011;20(1):1–12. https://doi.org/10.1590/s1984-29612011000100002.

35. Solano-Gallego L, Trotta M, Razia L, et al. Molecular survey of *Ehrlichia canis* and *Anaplasma phagocytophilum* from blood of dogs in Italy. Ann N Y Acad Sci 2006;1078:515–8. https://doi.org/10.1196/annals.1374.101.

36. McClure JC, Crothers ML, Schaefer JJ, et al. Rapid screening and cultivation of *Ehrlichia canis* from refrigerated carrier blood. Clin Microbiol Infect : official Publ Eur Soc Clin Microbiol Infect Dis 2009;15(Suppl 2):72–3. https://doi.org/10.1111/j.1469-0691.2008.02192.x.

37. McKechnie DB, Slater KS, Childs JE, et al. Survival of *Ehrlichia chaffeensis* in refrigerated, ADSOL-treated RBCs. Transfusion 2000;40(9):1041–7. https://doi.org/10.1046/j.1537-2995.2000.40091041.x.

38. Wardrop KJ, Birkenheuer A, Blais MC, et al. Update on canine and feline blood donor screening for blood-borne pathogens. J Vet Intern Med 2016;30(1):15–35. https://doi.org/10.1111/jvim.13823.

39. Taques I, Barbosa TR, Martini AC, et al. Molecular assessment of the transplacental transmission of *Toxoplasma gondii, Neospora caninum, Brucella canis* and *Ehrlichia canis* in dogs. Comp Immunol Microbiol Infect Dis 2016;49:47–50. https://doi.org/10.1016/j.cimid.2016.09.002.

40. Lashnits E, Grant S, Thomas B, et al. Evidence for vertical transmission of *Mycoplasma haemocanis*, but not *Ehrlichia ewingii*, in a dog. J Vet Intern Med 2019;33(4):1747–52. https://doi.org/10.1111/jvim.15517.

41. Sainz A, Roura X, Miro G, et al. Guideline for veterinary practitioners on canine ehrlichiosis and anaplasmosis in Europe. Parasit Vectors 2015;8:75. https://doi.org/10.1186/s13071-015-0649-0.

42. Ueno TE, Aguiar DM, Pacheco RC, et al. *Ehrlichia canis* in dogs attended in a veterinary hospital from Botucatu, São Paulo State, Brazil. Rev Bras Parasitol Vet 2009;18(3):57–61.

43. Milanjeet HS, Singh N, Singh N, et al. Molecular prevalence and risk factors for the occurrence of canine monocytic ehrlichiosis. Vet Med 2014;59(3):129–36.

44. Piantedosi D, Neola B, D'Alessio N, et al. Seroprevalence and risk factors associated with *Ehrlichia canis, Anaplasma* spp., *Borrelia burgdorferi* sensu lato, and *D. immitis* in hunting dogs from southern Italy. Parasitol Res 2017;116(10):2651–60. https://doi.org/10.1007/s00436-017-5574-z.

45. de Castro MB, Machado RZ, de Aquino LP, et al. Experimental acute canine monocytic ehrlichiosis: clinicopathological and immunopathological findings. Vet Parasitol 2004;119(1):73–86. https://doi.org/10.1016/j.vetpar.2003.10.012.

46. Nair AD, Cheng C, Ganta CK, et al. Comparative experimental infection study in dogs with *Ehrlichia canis, E. chaffeensis, Anaplasma platys* and

A. phagocytophilum. PLoS One 2016;11(2):e0148239. https://doi.org/10.1371/journal.pone.0148239.

47. Gaunt S, Beall M, Stillman B, et al. Experimental infection and co-infection of dogs with *Anaplasma platys* and *Ehrlichia canis*: hematologic, serologic and molecular findings. Parasites & vectors 2010;3(1):33. https://doi.org/10.1186/1756-3305-3-33.

48. Gal A, Loeb E, Yisaschar-Mekuzas Y, et al. Detection of *Ehrlichia canis* by PCR in different tissues obtained during necropsy from dogs surveyed for naturally occurring canine monocytic ehrlichiosis. Vet J 2008;175(2):212–7. https://doi.org/10.1016/j.tvjl.2007.01.013.

49. Rikihisa Y. *Ehrlichia* subversion of host innate responses. Curr Opin Microbiol 2006;9(1):95–101. https://doi.org/10.1016/j.mib.2005.12.003.

50. Harrus S, Waner T, Avidar Y, et al. Serum protein alterations in canine ehrlichiosis. Vet Parasitol 1996;66(3–4):241–9. https://doi.org/10.1016/s0304-4017(96)01013-8.

51. Brandao LP, Hasegawa MY, Hagiwara MK, et al. Platelet aggregation studies in acute experimental canine ehrlichiosis. Vet Clin Pathol 2006;35(1):78–81. https://doi.org/10.1111/j.1939-165x.2006.tb00091.x.

52. Little SE. Ehrlichiosis and anaplasmosis in dogs and cats. Vet Clin North Am Small Anim Pract 2010;40(6):1121–40. https://doi.org/10.1016/j.cvsm.2010.07.004.

53. Harrus S, Waner T, Aizenberg I, et al. Amplification of ehrlichial DNA from dogs 34 months after infection with *Ehrlichia canis*. J Clin Microbiol 1998;36(1):73 6. https://doi.org/10.1128/JCM.36.1.73-76.1998.

54. Waner T, Harrus S, Bark H, et al. Characterization of the subclinical phase of canine ehrlichiosis in experimentally infected beagle dogs. Vet Parasitol 1997;69(3–4).307–17. https://doi.org/10.1016/s0304-4017(96)01130-2.

55. Liddell AM, Stockham SL, Scott MA, et al. Predominance of *Ehrlichia ewingii* in Missouri dogs. J Clin Microbiol 2003;41(10):4617–22. https://doi.org/10.1128/JCM.41.10.4617-4622.2003.

56. Qurollo BA, Buch J, Chandrashekar R, et al. Clinicopathological findings in 41 dogs (2008-2018) naturally infected with *Ehrlichia ewingii*. J Vet Intern Med Mar 2019;33(2):618–29. https://doi.org/10.1111/jvim.15354.

57. Goodman RA, Hawkins EC, Olby NJ, et al. Molecular identification of *Ehrlichia ewingii* infection in dogs: 15 cases (1997-2001). J Am Vet Med Assoc 2003;222(8):1102–7. https://doi.org/10.2460/javma.2003.222.1102.

58. Breitschwerdt EB, Hegarty BC, Hancock SI. Sequential evaluation of dogs naturally infected with *Ehrlichia canis, Ehrlichia chaffeensis, Ehrlichia equi, Ehrlichia ewingii,* or *Bartonella vinsonii.* J Clin Microbiol 1998;36(9):2645–51. https://doi.org/10.1128/JCM.36.9.2645-2651.1998.

59. Anziani OS, Ewing SA, Barker RW. Experimental transmission of a granulocytic form of the tribe Ehrlichieae by *Dermacentor variabilis* and *Amblyomma americanum* to dogs. Am J Vet Res 1990;51(6):929–31.

60. Egenvall A, Bjoersdorff A, Lilliehook I, et al. Early manifestations of granulocytic ehrlichiosis in dogs inoculated experimentally with a Swedish Ehrlichia species isolate. Vet Rec 1998;143(15):412–7. https://doi.org/10.1136/vr.143.15.412.

61. Granick JL, Armstrong PJ, Bender JB. *Anaplasma phagocytophilum* infection in dogs: 34 cases (2000-2007). J Am Vet Med Assoc 2009;234(12):1559–65. https://doi.org/10.2460/javma.234.12.1559.

62. Kohn B, Silaghi C, Galke D, et al. Infections with *Anaplasma phagocytophilum* in dogs in Germany. Res Vet Sci 2011;91(1):71–6. https://doi.org/10.1016/j.rvsc.2010.08.008.

63. Eberts MD, Diniz PPVP, Beall MJ, et al. Typical and atypical manifestations of *Anaplasma phagocytophilum* infection in dogs. J Am Anim Hosp Assoc 2011;47(6):e86–94. https://doi.org/10.5326/JAAHA-MS-5578.

64. El Hamiani Khatat S, Daminet S, Duchateau L, et al. Epidemiological and clinicopathological features of *Anaplasma phagocytophilum* infection in dogs: a systematic review. Front Vet Sci 2021;8:686644. https://doi.org/10.3389/fvets.2021.686644.

65. Chirek A, Silaghi C, Pfister K, et al. Granulocytic anaplasmosis in 63 dogs: clinical signs, laboratory results, therapy and course of disease. J Small Anim Pract 2018;59(2):112–20. https://doi.org/10.1111/jsap.12787.

66. Bouzouraa T, Rene-Martellet M, Chene J, et al. Clinical and laboratory features of canine *Anaplasma platys* infection in 32 naturally infected dogs in the Mediterranean basin. Ticks Tick Borne Dis 2016;7(6):1256–64. https://doi.org/10.1016/j.ttbdis.2016.07.004.

67. Aguirre E, Tesouro MA, Ruiz L, et al. Genetic characterization of *Anaplasma (Ehrlichia) platys* in dogs in Spain. J Vet Med B Infect Dis Vet Public Health 2006;53(4):197–200. https://doi.org/10.1111/j.1439-0450.2006.00937.x.

68. Lara B, Conan A, Thrall MA, et al. Serologic and Molecular Diagnosis of *Anaplasma platys* and *Ehrlichia canis* infection in dogs in an endemic region. Pathogens 2020;9(6). https://doi.org/10.3390/pathogens9060488.

69. Abarca K, Lopez J, Perret C, et al. *Anaplasma platys* in dogs, Chile. Emerg Infect Dis 2007;13(9):1392–5. https://doi.org/10.3201/eid1309.070021.

70. Baker DC, Simpson M, Gaunt SD, et al. Acute *Ehrlichia platys* infection in the dog. Vet Pathol 1987;24(5):449–53. https://doi.org/10.1177/030098588702400513.

71. Dawson JE, Ewing SA. Susceptibility of dogs to infection with *Ehrlichia chaffeensis,* causative agent of human ehrlichiosis. Am J Vet Res 1992;53(8):1322–7.

72. Panciera RJ, Ewing SA, Confer AW. Ocular histopathology of Ehrlichial infections in the dog. Vet Pathol 2001;38(1):43–6. https://doi.org/10.1354/vp.38-1-43.

73. Burton W, Drake C, Ogeer J, et al. Association between exposure to *Ehrlichia* spp. and risk of developing chronic kidney disease in dogs. J Am Anim Hosp Assoc 2020;56(3):159–64.

74. Eddlestone SM, Diniz PPVP, Neer TM, et al. Doxycycline clearance of experimentally induced chronic *Ehrlichia canis* infection in dogs. J Vet Intern Med 2007;21(6):1237–42. https://doi.org/10.1892/07-061.1.

75. Zhang XF, Zhang JZ, Long SW, et al. Experimental *Ehrlichia chaffeensis* infection in beagles. J Med Microbiol 2003;52(Pt 11):1021–6. https://doi.org/10.1099/jmm.0.05234-0.

76. Yu DH, Li YH, Yoon JS, et al. *Ehrlichia chaffeensis* infection in dogs in South Korea. Vector Borne Zoonotic Dis 2008;8(3):355–8. https://doi.org/10.1089/vbz.2007.0226.

77. Nair ADS, Cheng C, Jaworski DC, et al. *Ehrlichia chaffeensis* infection in the reservoir host (White-Tailed Deer) and in an incidental host (dog) is impacted by its prior growth in macrophage and tick cell environments. PLoS One 2014;9(10):e109056. https://doi.org/10.1371/journal.pone.0109056.

78. Yabsley MJ, Adams DS, O'Connor TP, et al. Experimental primary and secondary infections of domestic dogs with *Ehrlichia ewingii*. Vet Microbiol 2011;150(3–4):315–21. https://doi.org/10.1016/j.vetmic.2011.02.006.

79. Oliveira LS, Oliveira KA, Mourao LC, et al. First report of *Ehrlichia ewingii* detected by molecular investigation in dogs from Brazil. Clin Microbiol Infect 2009;15(Suppl 2):55–6. https://doi.org/10.1111/j.1469-0691.2008.02635.x.

80. Gordon WS, Brownlee A, Wilson DR, et al. Tick-borne fever (a hitherto undescribed disease of sheep). J Comp Pathol 1932;45:301–12.

81. Madigan JE, Gribble D. Equine ehrlichiosis in northern California: 49 cases (1968-1981). J Am Vet Med Assoc 1987;190(4):445–8.

82. Madewell BR, Gribble DH. Infection in two dogs with an agent resembling *Ehrlichia equi*. J Am Vet Med Assoc 1982;180(5):512–4.

83. Johansson KE, Pettersson B, Uhlen M, et al. Identification of the causative agent of granulocytic ehrlichiosis in Swedish dogs and horses by direct solid phase sequencing of PCR products from the 16S rRNA gene. Res Vet Sci 1995; 58(2):109–12.

84. Chen SM, Dumler JS, Bakken JS, et al. Identification of a granulocytotropic *Ehrlichia* species as the etiologic agent of human disease. J Clin Microbiol 1994; 32(3):589–95.

85. Bakken JS, Dumler JS, Chen SM, et al. Human granulocytic ehrlichiosis in the upper Midwest United States. A new species emerging? JAMA 1994;272(3): 212–8.

86. Greig B, Asanovich KM, Armstrong PJ, et al. Geographic, clinical, serologic, and molecular evidence of granulocytic ehrlichiosis, a likely zoonotic disease, in Minnesota and Wisconsin dogs. J Clin Microbiol 1996;34(1):44–8.

87. Centers for Disease Control and Prevention. Anaplasmosis. Centers for Disease Control and Prevention. Available at: https://www.cdc.gov/anaplasmosis/index. html. Accessed March 13, 2022.

88. Harvey JW, Simpson CF, Gaskin JM. Cyclic thrombocytopenia induced by a Rickettsia-like agent in dogs. J Infect Dis 1978;137(2):182–8. https://doi.org/ 10.1093/infdis/137.2.182.

89. Breitschwerdt EB, Hegarty BC, Qurollo BA, et al. Intravascular persistence of *Anaplasma platys, Ehrlichia chaffeensis*, and *Ehrlichia ewingii* DNA in the blood of a dog and two family members. Parasites & Vectors 2014;7(1):298. https:// doi.org/10.1186/1756-3305-7-298.

90. Maggi RG, Mascarelli PE, Havenga LN, et al. Co-infection with *Anaplasma platys, Bartonella henselae* and *Candidatus* Mycoplasma haematoparvum in a veterinarian. *Parasit Vectors* 2013;6:103. https://doi.org/10.1186/1756-3305-6-103.

91. Qurollo BA, Balakrishnan N, Cannon CZ, et al. Co-infection with *Anaplasma platys, Bartonella henselae, Bartonella koehlerae* and 'Candidatus Mycoplasma haemominutum' in a cat diagnosed with splenic plasmacytosis and multiple myeloma. J Feline Med Surg 2014;16(8):713–20. https://doi.org/10.1177/ 1098612X13519632.

92. Woldehiwet Z. The natural history of *Anaplasma phagocytophilum*. Vet Parasitol 2010;167(2–4):108–22. https://doi.org/10.1016/j.vetpar.2009.09.013.

93. Ripoche M, Bouchard C, Irace-Cima A, et al. Current and future distribution of Ixodes scapularis ticks in Quebec: field validation of a predictive model. PLoS One 2022;17(2):e0263243. https://doi.org/10.1371/journal.pone.0263243.

94. Centers for Disease Control and Prevention. Blacklegged tick (*Ixodes scapularis*) surveillance. Centers for Disease Control and Prevention. Available at: https://www.cdc.gov/ticks/surveillance/BlackleggedTick.html. Accessed March 13, 2022.

95. Eisen RJ, Eisen L, Beard CB. County-scale distribution of *Ixodes scapularis* and *Ixodes pacificus* (Acari: Ixodidae) in the Continental United States. J Med Entomol 2016;53(2):349–86. https://doi.org/10.1093/jme/tjv237.

96. Centers for Disease Control and Prevention. *Western blacklegged* tick (*Ixodes pacificus*) surveillance. Centers for Disease Control and Prevention. Available at: https://www.cdc.gov/ticks/surveillance/WesternBlackleggedTick.html. Accessed March 13, 2022.

97. Hahn MB, Disler G, Durden LA, et al. Establishing a baseline for tick surveillance in Alaska: tick collection records from 1909-2019. Ticks Tick Borne Dis 2020; 11(5):101495. https://doi.org/10.1016/j.ttbdis.2020.101495.

98. Clow KM, Leighton PA, Ogden NH, et al. Northward range expansion of *Ixodes scapularis* evident over a short timescale in Ontario, Canada. PLoS One 2017; 12(12):e0189393. https://doi.org/10.1371/journal.pone.0189393.

99. Parola P, Davoust B, Raoult D. Tick- and flea-borne rickettsial emerging zoonoses. Vet Res 2005;36(3):469–92. https://doi.org/10.1051/vetres:2005004.

100. Stuen S, Granquist EG, Silaghi C. *Anaplasma phagocytophilum*: a widespread multi-host pathogen with highly adaptive strategies. Front Cell Infect Microbiol 2013;3:31. https://doi.org/10.3389/fcimb.2013.00031.

101. Hvidsten D, Frafjord K, Gray JS, et al. The distribution limit of the common tick, *Ixodes ricinus*, and some associated pathogens in north-western Europe. Ticks Tick-borne Dis 2020;11(4):101388. https://doi.org/10.1016/j.ttbdis.2020.101388.

102. European Centre for Disease Prevention and Control and European Food Safety Authority. Tick maps. ECDC. Available at: https://ecdc.europa.eu/en/disease-vectors/surveillance-and-disease-data/tick-maps. Accessed March 13, 2022.

103. Mukhacheva TA, Shaikhova DR, Kovalev SY. Asian isolates of *Anaplasma phagocytophilum*: multilocus sequence typing. Ticks Tick Borne Dis 2019;10(4): 775–80. https://doi.org/10.1016/j.ttbdis.2019.03.011.

104. Masuzawa T, Masuda S, Fukui T, et al. PCR detection of *Anaplasma phagocytophilum* and *Borrelia burgdorferi* in *Ixodes persulcatus* ticks in Mongolia. Jpn J Infect Dis 2014;67(1):47–9. https://doi.org/10.7883/yoken.67.47.

105. Jaarsma RI, Sprong H, Takumi K, et al. *Anaplasma phagocytophilum* evolves in geographical and biotic niches of vertebrates and ticks. Parasites & Vectors 2019;12(1):328. https://doi.org/10.1186/s13071-019-3583-8.

106. Rar V, Tkachev S, Tikunova N. Genetic diversity of *Anaplasma* bacteria: twenty years later. Infect Genet Evol 2021;91:104833. https://doi.org/10.1016/j.meegid.2021.104833.

107. Keesing F, McHenry DJ, Hersh M, et al. Prevalence of human-active and variant 1 strains of the tick-borne pathogen *Anaplasma phagocytophilum* in hosts and forests of eastern North America. Am J Trop Med Hyg 2014;91(2):302–9. https://doi.org/10.4269/ajtmh.13-0525.

108. Levin ML, Nicholson WL, Massung RF, et al. Comparison of the reservoir competence of medium-sized mammals and *Peromyscus leucopus* for *Anaplasma phagocytophilum* in Connecticut. Vector Borne Zoonotic Dis Fall 2002;2(3): 125–36. https://doi.org/10.1089/15303660260613693.

109. Dugat T, Lagree AC, Maillard R, et al. Opening the black box of *Anaplasma phagocytophilum* diversity: current situation and future perspectives. Front Cell Infect Microbiol 2015;5:61. https://doi.org/10.3389/fcimb.2015.00061.

110. Nieto NC, Foley JE. Reservoir competence of the redwood chipmunk (*Tamias ochrogenys*) for *Anaplasma phagocytophilum*. Vector Borne Zoonotic Dis 2009;9(6):573–7. https://doi.org/10.1089/vbz.2008.0142.

111. Lesiczka PM, Hrazdilova K, Majerova K, et al. The role of peridomestic animals in the eco-epidemiology of *Anaplasma phagocytophilum*. Microb Ecol 2021; 82(3):602–12. https://doi.org/10.1007/s00248-021-01704-z.

112. Evason M, Stull JW, Pearl DL, et al. Prevalence of *Borrelia burgdorferi, Anaplasma* spp., *Ehrlichia* spp. and *Dirofilaria immitis* in Canadian dogs, 2008 to 2015: a repeat cross-sectional study. Parasit Vectors 2019;12(1):64. https://doi.org/10.1186/s13071-019-3299-9.

113. Little S, Braff J, Place J, et al. Canine Infect *Dirofilaria immitis, Borrelia burgdorferi, Anaplasma Ehrlichia* United States, 2013-2019. Parasit Vectors 2021;14(1): 10. https://doi.org/10.1186/s13071-020-04514-3.

114. Perez-Macchi S, Pedrozo R, Bittencourt P, et al. Prevalence, molecular characterization and risk factor analysis of *Ehrlichia canis* and *Anaplasma platys* in domestic dogs from Paraguay. Comp Immunol Microbiol Infect Dis 2019;62:31–9. https://doi.org/10.1016/j.cimid.2018.11.015.

115. Snellgrove AN, Krapiunaya I, Ford SL, et al. Vector competence of *Rhipicephalus sanguineus* sensu stricto for *Anaplasma platys*. Ticks Tick Borne Dis 2020; 11(6):101517. https://doi.org/10.1016/j.ttbdis.2020.101517.

116. Harrus S, Perlman-Avrahami A, Mumcuoglu KY, et al. Molecular detection of *Ehrlichia canis, Anaplasma bovis, Anaplasma platys, Candidatus* Midichloria mitochondrii and *Babesia canis vogeli* in ticks from Israel. Clin Microbiol Infect 2011; 17(3):459–63. https://doi.org/10.1111/j.1469-0691.2010.03316.x.

117. Javkhlan G, Enkhtaivan B, Baigal B, et al. Natural *Anaplasma phagocytophilum* infection in ticks from a forest area of Selenge province, Mongolia. West. Pac Surveill Response J 2014;5(1):21–4. https://doi.org/10.5365/WPSAR.2013.4. 3.001.

118. Papa A, Tsioka K, Kontana A, et al. Bacterial pathogens and endosymbionts in ticks. Ticks Tick Borne Dis 2017;8(1):31–5. https://doi.org/10.1016/j.ttbdis.2016. 09.011.

119. Diniz PPVP, Beall MJ, Omark K, et al. High prevalence of tick-borne pathogens in dogs from an Indian reservation in northeastern Arizona. *Vector Borne Zoonotic Dis* 2010;10(2):117–23. https://doi.org/10.1089/vbz.2008.0184.

120. Diniz PPVP, de Morais HS, Breitschwerdt EB, et al. Serum cardiac troponin I concentration in dogs with ehrlichiosis. J Vet Intern Med 2008;22(5):1136–43. https://doi.org/10.1111/j.1939-1676.2008.0145.x.

121. Ferreira RF, de Mello Figueiredo Cerqueira A, Pereira AM, et al. *Anaplasma platys* diagnosis in dogs: comparison between morphological and molecular tests. Int J Appl Res Vet Med 2007;5(3):113.

122. Pesapane R, Foley J, Thomas R, et al. Molecular detection and characterization of *Anaplasma platys* and *Ehrlichia canis* in dogs from northern Colombia. Vet Microbiol 2019;233:184–9. https://doi.org/10.1016/j.vetmic.2019.05.002.

123. Carvalho L, Armua-Fernandez MT, Sosa N, et al. *Anaplasma platys* in dogs from Uruguay. Ticks Tick Borne Dis 2017;8(2):241–5. https://doi.org/10.1016/j.ttbdis. 2016.11.005.

124. Alhassan A, Hove P, Sharma B, et al. Molecular detection and characterization of *Anaplasma platys* and *Ehrlichia canis* in dogs from the Caribbean. Ticks Tick Borne Dis 2021;12(4):101727. https://doi.org/10.1016/j.ttbdis.2021.101727.

125. Ben Said M, Belkahia H, Messadi L. *Anaplasma* spp. in North Africa: a review on molecular epidemiology, associated risk factors and genetic characteristics. Ticks Tick Borne Dis 2018;9(3):543–55. https://doi.org/10.1016/j.ttbdis.2018. 01.003.

126. Matei IA, D'Amico G, Yao PK, et al. Molecular detection of *Anaplasma platys* infection in free-roaming dogs and ticks from Kenya and Ivory Coast. *Parasit Vectors* 2016;9:157. https://doi.org/10.1186/s13071-016-1443-3.

127. Selim A, Almohammed H, Abdelhady A, et al. Molecular detection and risk factors for *Anaplasma platys* infection in dogs from Egypt. Parasit Vectors 2021; 14(1):429. https://doi.org/10.1186/s13071-021-04943-8.

128. Al–Obaidi SSA, Khalaf Al-Ani JM, Al-Shammari NB. Molecular detection of some *Anaplasma* species in blood of dogs in Baghdad Province, Iraq. Iraqi J Vet Med 2020;44(1):39–45. https://doi.org/10.30539/ijvm.v44i1.933.

129. Iatta R, Sazmand A, Nguyen VL, et al. Vector-borne pathogens in dogs of different regions of Iran and Pakistan. Parasitol Res 2021;120(12):4219–28. https://doi.org/10.1007/s00436-020-06992-x.

130. Barker EN, Langton DA, Helps CR, et al. Haemoparasites of free-roaming dogs associated with several remote Aboriginal communities in Australia. BMC Vet Res 2012;8:55. https://doi.org/10.1186/1746-6148-8-55.

131. Ybanez AP, Ybanez RH, Yokoyama N, et al. Multiple infections of *Anaplasma platys* variants in Philippine dogs. Vet World 2016;9(12):1456–60. https://doi.org/10.14202/vetworld.2016.1456-1460.

132. Sarker BR, Mitpasa T, Macotpet A, et al. First report on molecular prevalence and identification of *Anaplasma platys* in dogs in Khon Kaen, Thailand. Vet World 2021;14(10):2613–9. https://doi.org/10.14202/vetworld.2021.2613-2619.

133. Diniz PPVP, Breitschwerdt EB. *Anaplasma phagocytophilum* infection (canine granulocytotropic anaplasmosis). In: Greene CE, editor. Infectious diseases of the dog and cat. 4th edition. St. Louis (Missouri): Elsevier Saunders; 2012. p. 244–54, chap 26.

134. Scorpio DG, Dumler JS, Barat NC, et al. Comparative strain analysis of *Anaplasma phagocytophilum* infection and clinical outcomes in a canine model of granulocytic anaplasmosis. Vector Borne Zoonotic Dis 2011;11(3):223–9. https://doi.org/10.1089/vbz.2009.0262.

135. Wamsley H, Barbet A, Abbott J, et al. 2007. Experimental inoculation of dogs with a human or canine isolate of Anaplasma phagocytophilum and molecular evidence of persistent infection following doxycycline therapy. The 21st Meeting of the American Society for Rickettsiology 2007:38. Available at: http://129.130.129.21/CE/archive/2007/asr/abstracts/P_CADT_Wamsley_ExperimentalInoculation ofDogs.pdf.

136. Contreras ET, Dowers KL, Moroff S, et al. Clinical and laboratory effects of doxycycline and prednisolone in *Ixodes scapularis*-exposed dogs with chronic *Anaplasma phagocytophilum* infection. Top companion Anim Med 2018;33(4): 147–9.

137. Hovius E, de Bruin A, Schouls L, et al. A lifelong study of a pack Rhodesian ridgeback dogs reveals subclinical and clinical tick-borne *Anaplasma phagocytophilum* infections with possible reinfection or persistence. Parasit Vectors 2018;11(1):238. https://doi.org/10.1186/s13071-018-2806-8.

138. De Tommasi AS, Baneth G, Breitschwerdt EB, et al. *Anaplasma platys* in bone marrow megakaryocytes of young dogs. J Clin Microbiol 2014;52(6):2231–4. https://doi.org/10.1128/JCM.00395-14.

139. Ulutaş B, Bayramli G, Karagenç T. First case of *Anaplasma (Ehrlichia) platy*s infection in a dog in Turkey. Turkish J Vet Anim Sci 2007;31(4):279–82.

140. Sainz A, Amusategui I, Tesouro MA. *Ehrlichia platys* infection and disease in dogs in Spain. J Vet Diagn Invest 1999;11(4):382–4. https://doi.org/10.1177/104063879901100419.

141. Piratae S, Senawong P, Chalermchat P, et al. Molecular evidence of *Ehrlichia canis* and *Anaplasma platys* and the association of infections with hematological responses in naturally infected dogs in Kalasin, Thailand. Vet World 2019; 12(1):131–5. https://doi.org/10.14202/vetworld.2019.131-135.

142. Ribeiro CM, Matos AC, Azzolini T, et al. Molecular epidemiology of *Anaplasma platys, Ehrlichia canis* and *Babesia vogeli* in stray dogs in Paraná, Brazil. Pesquisa Veterinária Brasileira 2017;37:129–36.

143. Huber D, Reil I, Duvnjak S, et al. Molecular detection of *Anaplasma platys, Anaplasma phagocytophilum* and *Wolbachia* sp. but not *Ehrlichia canis* in Croatian dogs. Parasitol Res 2017;116(11):3019–26. https://doi.org/10.1007/s00436-017-5611-y.

144. Breitschwerdt EB, Abrams-Ogg AC, Lappin MR, et al. Molecular evidence supporting *Ehrlichia canis*-like infection in cats. J Vet Intern Med 2002;16(6):642–9. https://doi.org/10.1892/0891-6640(2002)016<0642:mescii>2.3.co;2.

145. Braga IA, dos Santos LG, de Souza Ramos DG, et al. Detection of *Ehrlichia canis* in domestic cats in the central-western region of Brazil. Braz J Microbiol 2014;45(2):641–5. https://doi.org/10.1590/s1517-83822014000200036.

146. Lappin MR, Breitschwerdt EB, Jensen WA, et al. Molecular and serologic evidence of *Anaplasma phagocytophilum* infection in cats in North America. J Am Vet Med Assoc 2004;225(6):893–6. https://doi.org/10.2460/javma.2004. 225.893, 879.

147. Lima M, Soares P, Ramos C, et al. Molecular detection of *Anaplasma platys* in a naturally-infected cat in Brazil. Braz J Microbiol 2010;41(2):381–5.

148. Hegarty BC, Qurollo BA, Thomas B, et al. Serological and molecular analysis of feline vector-borne anaplasmosis and ehrlichiosis using species-specific peptides and PCR. Parasit Vectors 2015;8:320. https://doi.org/10.1186/s13071-015-0929-8.

149. Braga ÍA, Taques IIGG, dos Santos Costa J, et al. *Ehrlichia canis* DNA in domestic cats parasitized by *Rhipicephalus sanguineus* sensu lato (sl) ticks in Brazil-Case report. Braz J Vet Res Anim Sci 2017;54(4):412–5.

150. Duplan F, Davies S, Filler S, et al. *Anaplasma phagocytophilum, Bartonella* spp., *Haemoplasma* species and *Hepatozoon* spp. in ticks infesting cats: a large-scale survey. Parasit Vectors 2018;11(1):201. https://doi.org/10.1186/s13071-018-2789-5.

151. Pennisi MG, Hofmann-Lehmann R, Radford AD, et al. *Anaplasma, Ehrlichia* and *Rickettsia* species infections in cats: European guidelines from the ABCD on prevention and management. J Feline Med Surg 2017;19(5):542–8. https://doi. org/10.1177/1098612X17706462.

152. Braga IA, Taques I, Grontoski EC, et al. Exposure of domestic cats to distinct *Ehrlichia canis* TRP genotypes. Vet Sci 2021;(12):8. https://doi.org/10.3390/vetsci8120310.

153. Magnarelli LA, Bushmich SL, JW IJ, et al. Seroprevalence of antibodies against *Borrelia burgdorferi* and *Anaplasma phagocytophilum* in cats. Am J Vet Res 2005;66(11):1895–9. https://doi.org/10.2460/ajvr.2005.66.1895.

154. Schafer I, Kohn B. *Anaplasma phagocytophilum* infection in cats: a literature review to raise clinical awareness. J Feline Med Surg 2020;22(5):428–41. https://dol.org/10.1177/1098612X20917600.

155. Qurollo B. Feline vector-borne diseases in North America. Vet Clin North Am Small Anim Pract 2019;49(4):687–702. https://doi.org/10.1016/j.cvsm.2019. 02.012.

156. Braga IA, dos Santos LG, Melo AL, et al. Hematological values associated to the serological and molecular diagnostic in cats suspected of *Ehrlichia canis* infection. Rev Bras Parasitol Vet 2013;22(4):470–4. https://doi.org/10.1590/S1984-29612013000400005.

157. Kidd L. Optimal vector-borne disease screening in dogs using both serology-based and polymerase chain reaction-based diagnostic panels. Vet Clin North Am Small Anim Pract 2019;49(4):703–18. https://doi.org/10.1016/j.cvsm.2019.02.011.

158. Maggi RG, Birkenheuer AJ, Hegarty BC, et al. Comparison of serological and molecular panels for diagnosis of vector-borne diseases in dogs. Parasit Vectors 2014;7:127. https://doi.org/10.1186/1756-3305-7-127.

159. Diniz PPVP. Ehrlichiosis and anaplasmosis. In: Bruyette D, editor. Clinical small animal internal medicine. Hoboken (NJ): John Wiley & Sons, Inc.; 2020. p. 903–12, chap 93.

160. Mylonakis ME, Koutinas AF, Billinis C, et al. Evaluation of cytology in the diagnosis of acute canine monocytic ehrlichiosis (*Ehrlichia canis*): a comparison between five methods. Vet Microbiol 2003;91(2–3):197–204. https://doi.org/10.1016/s0378-1135(02)00298-5.

161. Kohn B, Galke D, Beelitz P, et al. Clinical features of canine granulocytic anaplasmosis in 18 naturally infected dogs. J Vet Intern Med 2008;22(6):1289–95. https://doi.org/10.1111/j.1939-1676.2008.0180.x.

162. Rahamim M, Harrus S, Nachum-Biala Y, et al. *Ehrlichia canis* morulae in peripheral blood lymphocytes of two naturally-infected puppies in Israel. Vet Parasitol Reg Stud Rep 2021;24:100554. https://doi.org/10.1016/j.vprsr.2021.100554.

163. Iqbal Z, Chaichanasiriwithaya W, Rikihisa Y. Comparison of PCR with other tests for early diagnosis of canine ehrlichiosis. J Clin Microbiol 1994;32(7):1658–62. https://doi.org/10.1128/jcm.32.7.1658-1662.1994.

164. Qurollo BA, Stillman BA, Beall MJ, et al. Comparison of *Anaplasma* and *Ehrlichia* species–specific peptide ELISAs with whole organism–based immunofluorescent assays for serologic diagnosis of anaplasmosis and ehrlichiosis in dogs. Am J Vet Res 2021;82(1):71–80.

165. Bartsch RC, Greene RT. Post-therapy antibody titers in dogs with ehrlichiosis: follow-up study on 68 patients treated primarily with tetracycline and/or doxycycline. J Vet Intern Med 1996;10(4):271–4.

166. Neer TM, Breitschwerdt EB, Greene RT, et al. Consensus statement on ehrlichial disease of small animals from the infectious disease study group of the ACVIM. American College of Veterinary Internal Medicine. J Vet Intern Med 2002;16(3):309–15. https://doi.org/10.1892/0891-6640(2002)016<0309:csoedo>2.3.co;2.

167. Diniz PPVP, Schwartz DS, de Morais HS, et al. Surveillance for zoonotic vector-borne infections using sick dogs from southeastern Brazil. *Vector Borne Zoonotic Dis*. Winter 2007;7(4):689–97. https://doi.org/10.1089/vbz.2007.0129.

168. Mylonakis ME, Harrus S, Breitschwerdt EB. An update on the treatment of canine monocytic ehrlichiosis (*Ehrlichia canis*). Vet J 2019;246:45–53. https://doi.org/10.1016/j.tvjl.2019.01.015.

169. Stanczak J, Gabre RM, Kruminis-Lozowska W, et al. *Ixodes ricinus* as a vector of *Borrelia burgdorferi* sensu lato, *Anaplasma phagocytophilum* and Babesia microti in urban and suburban forests. Ann Agric Environ Med 2004;11(1):109–14.

170. Holman MS, Caporale DA, Goldberg J, et al. *Anaplasma phagocytophilum, Babesia microti*, and *Borrelia burgdorferi* in *Ixodes scapularis*, southern coastal Maine. Emerg Infect Dis 2004;10(4):744–6. https://doi.org/10.3201/eid1004.030566.

171. Rodriguez-Alarcon CA, Beristain-Ruiz DM, Olivares-Munoz A, et al. Demonstrating the presence of *Ehrlichia canis* DNA from different tissues of dogs with suspected subclinical ehrlichiosis. Parasit Vectors 2020;13(1):518. https://doi.org/10.1186/s13071-020-04363-0.

172. Eddlestone SM, Gaunt SD, Neer TM, et al. PCR detection of *Anaplasma platys* in blood and tissue of dogs during acute phase of experimental infection. Exp Parasitol 2007;115(2):205–10. https://doi.org/10.1016/j.exppara.2006.08.006.

173. Harrus S, Kenny M, Miara L, et al. Comparison of simultaneous splenic sample PCR with blood sample PCR for diagnosis and treatment of experimental *Ehrlichia canis* infection. Antimicrob Agents Chemother 2004;48(11):4488–90. https://doi.org/10.1128/AAC.48.11.4488-4490.2004.

174. Qurollo BA, Riggins D, Comyn A, et al. Development and validation of a sensitive and specific sodB-based quantitative PCR assay for molecular detection of *Ehrlichia* species. J Clin Microbiol 2014;52(11):4030–2. https://doi.org/10.1128/JCM.02340-14.

175. Harrus S, Waner T. Diagnosis of canine monocytotropic ehrlichiosis (*Ehrlichia canis*): an overview. Vet J 2011;187(3):292–6. https://doi.org/10.1016/j.tvjl.2010.02.001.

176. Rucksaken R, Maneeruttanarungroj C, Maswanna T, et al. Comparison of conventional polymerase chain reaction and routine blood smear for the detection of *Babesia canis, Hepatozoon canis, Ehrlichia canis*, and *Anaplasma platys* in Buriram Province, Thailand. Vet World 2019;12(5):700–5. https://doi.org/10.14202/vetworld.2019.700-705.

177. Woody BJ, Hoskins JD. Ehrlichial diseases of dogs. Vet Clin North Am Small Anim Pract 1991;21(1):75–98. https://doi.org/10.1016/s0195-5616(91)50009-7.

178. Little SE, O'Connor TP, Hempstead J, et al. *Ehrlichia ewingii* infection and exposure rates in dogs from the southcentral United States. Vet Parasitol 2010;172(3):355–60.

179. Liu J, Drexel J, Andrews B, et al. Comparative evaluation of 2 in-clinic assays for vector-borne disease testing in Dogs. Top Companion Anim Med 2018;33(4):114–8. https://doi.org/10.1053/j.tcam.2018.09.003.

180. O'Connor TP. SNAP assay technology. Top Companion Anim Med 2015;30(4):132–8. https://doi.org/10.1053/j.tcam.2015.12.002.

181. Stillman BA, Monn M, Liu J, et al. Performance of a commercially available in-clinic ELISA for detection of antibodies against *Anaplasma phagocytophilum, Anaplasma platys, Borrelia burgdorferi, Ehrlichia canis*, and *Ehrlichia ewingii* and *Dirofilaria immitis* antigen in dogs. J Am Vet Med Assoc 2014;245(1):80–6. https://doi.org/10.2460/javma.245.1.80.

182. Harrus S, Alleman AR, Bark H, et al. Comparison of three enzyme-linked immunosorbent assays with the indirect immunofluorescent antibody test for the diagnosis of canine infection with *Ehrlichia canis*. Vet Microbiol 2002;86(4):361–8. https://doi.org/10.1016/s0378-1135(02)00022-6.

183. Thomson K, Yaaran T, Belshaw A, et al. A new TaqMan method for the reliable diagnosis of *Ehrlichia* spp. in canine whole blood. Parasit Vectors 2018;11(1):350. https://doi.org/10.1186/s13071-018-2914-5.

184. Waner T, Nachum-Biala Y, Harrus S. Evaluation of a commercial in-clinic point-of-care polymerase chain reaction test for *Ehrlichia canis* DNA in artificially infected dogs. Vet J 2014;202(3):618–21. https://doi.org/10.1016/j.tvjl.2014.10.004.

185. Moroff S, Sokolchik I, Woodring T, et al. Use of an automated system for detection of canine serum antibodies against *Ehrlichia canis* glycoprotein 36. J Vet Diagn Invest 2014;26(4):558–62. https://doi.org/10.1177/1040638714534849.

186. Cárdenas AM, Doyle CK, Zhang X, et al. Enzyme-linked immunosorbent assay with conserved immunoreactive glycoproteins gp36 and gp19 has enhanced sensitivity and provides species-specific immunodiagnosis of *Ehrlichia canis* infection. Clin Vaccin Immunol 2007;14(2):123–8.

187. RE G, MJ B, AR A. Performance comparison of SNAP® 4Dx® Plus and AccuPlex® 4 for the detection of antibodies to *Borrelia burgdorferi* and *Anaplasma phagocytophilum*. Int J Appl Res Vet Med 2014;12(2).

188. Allerton F, Prior C, Bagcigil AF, et al. Overview and evaluation of existing guidelines for rational antimicrobial use in small-animal veterinary practice in Europe. Antibiotics 2021;10(4):409.

189. Weese JS, Giguere S, Guardabassi L, et al. ACVIM consensus statement on therapeutic antimicrobial use in animals and antimicrobial resistance. J Vet Intern Med 2015;29(2):487–98. https://doi.org/10.1111/jvim.12562.

190. Pedreañez A, Mosquera-Sulbaran J, Muñoz N. Increased plasma levels of nitric oxide and malondialdehyde in dogs infected by *Ehrlichia canis*: effect of doxycycline treatment. Revue Vétérinaire Clinique 2021;56(4):185–90.

191. Westfall DS, Twedt DC, Steyn PF, et al. Evaluation of esophageal transit of tablets and capsules in 30 cats. J Vet Intern Med 2001;15(5):467–70. https://doi.org/10.1892/0891-6640(2001)015<0467:eoetot>2.3.co;2.

192. German AJ, Cannon MJ, Dye C, et al. Oesophageal strictures in cats associated with doxycycline therapy. J Feline Med Surg 2005;7(1):33–41. https://doi.org/10.1016/j.jfms.2004.04.001.

193. Bissett SA, Davis J, Subler K, et al. Risk factors and outcome of bougienage for treatment of benign esophageal strictures in dogs and cats: 28 cases (1995–2004). J Am Vet Med Assoc 2009;235(7):844–50.

194. Gallo SH, McClave SA, Makk LJ, et al. Standardization of clinical criteria required for use of the 12.5 millimeter barium tablet in evaluating esophageal lumenal patency. Gastrointest Endosc 1996;44(2):181–4.

195. Papich MG, Davidson GS, Fortier LA. Doxycycline concentration over time after storage in a compounded veterinary preparation. J Am Vet Med Assoc 2013;242(12):1674–8. https://doi.org/10.2460/javma.242.12.1674.

196. Barza M, Brown RB, Shanks C, et al. Relation between lipophilicity and pharmacological behavior of minocycline, doxycycline, tetracycline, and oxytetracycline in dogs. Antimicrob Agents Chemother 1975;8(6):713–20. https://doi.org/10.1128/AAC.8.6.713.

197. Meyer FP, Specht H, Quednow B, et al. Influence of milk on the bioavailability of doxycycline: new aspects. Infection 1989;17(4):245–6. https://doi.org/10.1007/BF01639529.

198. Jenkins S, Ketzis JK, Dundas J, et al. Efficacy of minocycline in naturally occurring nonacute *Ehrlichia canis* infection in dogs. J Vet Intern Med 2018;32(1):217–21. https://doi.org/10.1111/jvim.14842.

199. Sykes JE. Ehrlichiosis. In: Sykes JE, editor. Canine and feline infectious diseases. St. Louis (Missouri): Elsevier Saunders; 2014. Chapter 28. p. 278-289.

200. Theodorou K, Mylonakis ME, Siarkou VI, et al. Efficacy of rifampicin in the treatment of experimental acute canine monocytic ehrlichiosis. J Antimicrob Chemother 2013;68(7):1619–26. https://doi.org/10.1093/jac/dkt053.

201. McClure JC, Crothers ML, Schaefer JJ, et al. Efficacy of a doxycycline treatment regimen initiated during three different phases of experimental ehrlichiosis.

Antimicrob Agents Chemother 2010;54(12):5012–20. https://doi.org/10.1128/AAC.01622-09.

202. Yancey CB, Diniz PPVP, Breitschwerdt EB, et al. Doxycycline treatment efficacy in dogs with naturally occurring *Anaplasma phagocytophilum* infection. J Small Anim Pract 2018;59(5):286–93. https://doi.org/10.1111/jsap.12799.

203. Savidge C, Ewing P, Andrews J, et al. Anaplasma phagocytophilum infection of domestic cats: 16 cases from the northeastern USA. J Feline Med Surg 2016; 18(2):85–91. https://doi.org/10.1177/1098612X15571148.

204. Schafer I, Kohn B, Muller E. Anaplasma phagocytophilum in domestic cats from Germany, Austria and Switzerland and clinical/laboratory findings in 18 PCR-positive cats (2008-2020). J Feline Med Surg 2021. https://doi.org/10.1177/1098612X211017459. 1098612X211017459.

205. Maurin M, Bakken JS, Dumler JS. Antibiotic susceptibilities of *Anaplasma (Ehrlichia) phagocytophilum* strains from various geographic areas in the United States. Antimicrob Agents Chemother 2003;47(1):413–5.

206. Sato M, Veir JK, Shropshire SB, et al. *Ehrlichia canis* in dogs experimentally infected, treated, and then immune suppressed during the acute or subclinical phases. J Vet Intern Med 2020;34(3):1214–21.

207. Shipov A, Klement E, Reuveni-Tager L, et al. Prognostic indicators for canine monocytic ehrlichiosis. Vet Parasitol 2008;153(1–2):131–8. https://doi.org/10.1016/j.vetpar.2008.01.009.

208. Silva AdCTd, Santos JRSd, Silva RMNd, et al. Prednisolone associated with doxycycline on the hematological parameters and serum proteinogram of dogs with ehrlichiosis. Ciência Rural 2021;51.

209. Leite LM, Carvalho AG, Ferreira PL, et al. Anti-inflammatory properties of doxycycline and minocycline in experimental models: an in vivo and In vitro comparative study. Inflammopharmacology 2011;19(2):99–110. https://doi.org/10.1007/s10787-011-0077-5.

210. Komnenou AA, Mylonakis ME, Kouti V, et al. Ocular manifestations of natural canine monocytic ehrlichiosis (*Ehrlichia canis*): a retrospective study of 90 cases. Vet Ophthalmol 2007;10(3):137–42. https://doi.org/10.1111/j.1463-5224.2007.00508.x.

211. Giudice E, Giannetto C, Gianesella M. Effect of desmopressin on immune-mediated haemorrhagic disorders due to canine monocytic ehrlichiosis: a preliminary study. J Vet Pharmacol Ther 2010;33(6):610–4. https://doi.org/10.1111/j.1365-2885.2010.01196.x.

212. Palacios M, Arteaga R, Calvo G. High-dose filgrastim treatment of nonregenerative pancytopenia associated with chronic canine ehrlichiosis. Top Companion Anim Med 2017;32(1):28–30. https://doi.org/10.1053/j.tcam.2017.05.005.

213. Marks SL, Kook PH, Papich MG, et al. ACVIM consensus statement: support for rational administration of gastrointestinal protectants to dogs and cats. J Vet Intern Med 2018;32(6):1823–40. https://doi.org/10.1111/jvim.15337.

214. Allen EC, Tarigo JL, LeVine DN, et al. Platelet number and function in response to a single intravenous dose of vincristine. J Vet Intern Med 2021;35(4):1754–62. https://doi.org/10.1111/jvim.16169.

215. Souza DRD, Melo ALT, Muraro LS, et al. Levamisole enhances global and differential leukocyte numbers in peripheral blood of dogs with ehrlichiosis. Turkish J Vet Anim Sci 2013;37(6):647–52.

216. Eddlestone SM, Neer TM, Gaunt SD, et al. Failure of imidocarb dipropionate to clear experimentally induced *Ehrlichia canis* infection in dogs. J Vet Intern Med 2006;20(4):840–4.

217. Dantas-Torres F. Biology and ecology of the brown dog tick, *Rhipicephalus sanguineus*. *Parasit Vectors* 2010;3:26. https://doi.org/10.1186/1756-3305-3-26.
218. Demma LJ, Eremeeva M, Nicholson WL, et al. An outbreak of Rocky Mountain Spotted Fever associated with a novel tick vector, *Rhipicephalus sanguineus*, in Arizona, 2004: preliminary report. Ann N Y Acad Sci 2006;1078:342–3. https://doi.org/10.1196/annals.1374.066.
219. Chung JK, Kim CM, Kim DM, et al. Severe fever with thrombocytopenia syndrome associated with manual de-ticking of domestic dogs. Vector Borne Zoonotic Dis 2020;20(4):285–94. https://doi.org/10.1089/vbz.2019.2463.
220. Oliveira AM, Maggi RG, Woods CW, et al. Suspected needle stick transmission of *Bartonella vinsonii* subspecies *berkhoffii* to a veterinarian. J Vet Intern Med 2010;24(5):1229–32. https://doi.org/10.1111/j.1939-1676.2010.0563.x.
221. Lin JW, Chen CM, Chang CC. Unknown fever and back pain caused by *Bartonella henselae* in a veterinarian after a needle puncture: a case report and literature review. Vector Borne Zoonotic Dis 2011;11(5):589–91. https://doi.org/10.1089/vbz.2009.0217.
222. Nichols Heitman K, Dahlgren FS, Drexler NA, et al. Increasing incidence of ehrlichiosis in the United States: a summary of national surveillance of *Ehrlichia chaffeensis* and *Ehrlichia ewingii* infections in the United States, 2008-2012. Am J Trop Med Hyg 2016;94(1):52–60. https://doi.org/10.4269/ajtmh.15-0540.
223. Dahlgren FS, Heitman KN, Drexler NA, et al. Human granulocytic anaplasmosis in the United States from 2008 to 2012: a summary of national surveillance data. Am J Trop Med Hyg 2015;93(1):66–72. https://doi.org/10.4269/ajtmh.15-0122.
224. Centers for Disease Control and Prevention. Diseases transmitted by ticks. Centers for Disease Control and Prevention. Available at: https://www.cdc.gov/ticks/diseases/index.html. Accessed March 18, 2022.
225. Blanco JR, Oteo JA. Human granulocytic ehrlichiosis in Europe. Clin Microbiol Infect 2002;8(12):763–72. https://doi.org/10.1046/j.1469-0691.2002.00557.x.
226. Tsiodras S, Spanakis N, Spanakos G, et al. Fatal human anaplasmosis associated with macrophage activation syndrome in Greece and the public health response. J Infect Public Health 2017;10(6):819–23. https://doi.org/10.1016/j.jiph.2017.01.002.
227. Dantas-Torres F. The brown dog tick, *Rhipicephalus sanguineus* (Latreille, 1806) (Acari: Ixodidae): from taxonomy to control. Vet Parasitol 2008;152(3–4):173–85. https://doi.org/10.1016/j.vetpar.2007.12.030.
228. Mathisson DC, Kross SM, Palmer MI, et al. Effect of vegetation on the abundance of tick vectors in the Northeastern United States: a review of the literature. J Med Entomol 2021;58(6):2030–7. https://doi.org/10.1093/jme/tjab098.
229. Centers for Disease Control and Prevention. Preventing ticks in the yard. Center for Disease Control and Prevention. Available at: https://www.cdc.gov/lyme/prev/in_the_yard.html. Accessed April 26, 2022.

Veterinary Chagas Disease (American Trypanosomiasis) in the United States

Sarah A. Hamer, MS, PhD, DVM[a],*, Ashley B. Saunders, DVM[b]

KEYWORDS

- *Trypanosoma cruzi* • Canine • Triatomine • Kissing bug • Cardiomyopathy

KEY POINTS

- *Trypanosoma cruzi* is transmitted by triatomine "kissing bug" insects. The parasite and vectors are endemic across the Southern United States.
- There is an increasing awareness for locally acquired human and animal Chagas disease in endemic areas, especially Texas.
- When present, clinical disease in dogs is predominately associated with cardiac rhythm disturbances, myocardial dysfunction, heart failure, and sudden death.
- Diagnosis and treatment are challenging due to a lack of awareness of disease risk, imperfect diagnostic tests, and the need for cost-effective, proven antiparasitic drug therapies with acceptable side effects.
- Increased vigilance for vectors, vector control, and habitat modifications can help reduce the risk.

INTRODUCTION

Trypanosoma cruzi is a zoonotic, protozoan parasite that causes Chagas disease in mammals. The parasite was first described by the Brazilian physician Dr Carlos Chagas in 1909 and is distributed across wide ranges in South America, Central America, Mexico, and the Southern United States. Theparasite is distributed where triatomine insect vectors, also known as "kissing bugs"occur. The burden of human Chagas disease is greatest in impoverished, rural regions of Latin America owing to vector colonization of human dwellings. Human and animal Chagas disease is increasingly diagnosed in the southern United States, owing in part to improving awareness.[1]

The authors have no conflicts to disclose.
[a] Department of Veterinary Integrative Biosciences, 4458 TAMU, College Station, TX 77843, USA; [b] Department of Small Animal Clinical Sciences, 4474 TAMU, College of Veterinary Medicine & Biomedical Sciences, College Station, TX 77843, USA
* Corresponding author.
E-mail address: shamer@cvm.tamu.edu

Vet Clin Small Anim 52 (2022) 1267–1281
https://doi.org/10.1016/j.cvsm.2022.06.008
0195-5616/22/© 2022 Elsevier Inc. All rights reserved.

TRANSMISSION AND LIFE CYCLE

Transmission of *T. cruzi* occurs by contact with the feces of infected triatomine vectors, which are obligate blood feeders. The epimastigote stage of the parasite replicates in the midgut of the insect vector. The infectious metacyclic trypomastigote stage is subsequently excreted in its feces. Fecal contamination of host mucous membranes or the bite wound during blood feeding leads to infection. Accordingly, the triatomine species that readily defecate during or shortly after feeding are likely to be more efficient vectors compared with those that have a prolonged postfeeding defecation interval.[2] The metacyclic trypomastigotes penetrate cells and transform into amastigotes. Amastigotes undergo binary fission, become trypomastigotes, and rupture host cells and enter the blood stream. Triatomines become infected by feeding on the blood of infected hosts when the trypomastigote blood stage of the parasite is circulating.

During each of their 6 life stages, triatomines blood-feed multiple times on one or more different hosts, resulting in a high level of host contact and many opportunities for parasite transmission within the life cycle of the vector. Infection of mammals can also occur vertically from infected mother to offspring. Congenital transmission is estimated to occur in approximately 5% to 10% of infected pregnant women.[3] Congenital transmission occurs in dogs[4] but its incidence is not well-documented in veterinary species. Human infection can also occur through contaminated blood products and organ transplants but the significance of these routes of transmission in veterinary medicine has not been determined. Oral transmission is likely the major route of transmission for veterinary Chagas disease. It occurs when animals ingest infected triatomines or their feces.[5] Oral *T. cruzi* transmission can also occur through consumption of infected animals through predation or scavenging.[6] In humans, the consumption of contaminated food or drink has led to devastating outbreaks of acute Chagas disease.[7] Importantly, contact with an infected dog is not recognized as a direct zoonotic risk, but rather, infected dogs can serve as sentinels for environmental (vector) exposure risk in humans.

The Vectors

Triatomines, or kissing bugs, are in the family Reduviidae, subfamily Triatominae (**Fig. 1**). In the southern United States, 11 triatomine species have been documented. The species most commonly encountered by people and dogs include *Triatoma gerstaeckeri*, *Triatoma sanguisuga*, *Triatoma rubida*, and *Triatoma protracta*.[8–10]

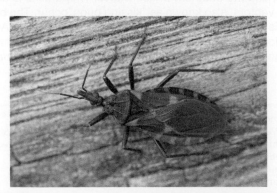

Fig. 1. *Triatoma sanguisuga* adult male from College Station, Texas. *Triatoma sanguisuga* is the most common triatomine encountered by humans across the Southeastern United States. Photo credit, Gabriel Hamer/TAMU Entomology.

Triatomines progress through 5 immature (nymph) stages before developing into the adult stage. Each stage must blood-feed from a host multiple times. Accordingly, there are dozens of interactions with host species during the life of a triatomine, each interaction potentially allowing for the insect to transmit or acquire *T. cruzi*. The Kissing Bug Community Science program at Texas A&M University, established in 2012, allows individuals to submit kissing bugs for free identification and *T. cruzi* testing. The program has received insects from the southernmost 28 states (**Fig. 2**). Approximately 75% of submitted triatomines were reportedly encountered in the outdoor environment, mostly from dog kennels, patios, and garages. Overall, 54% of adult insects were infected.[3] Dog kennels may be particularly suited to establish *T cruzi* transmission cycles.[11] High densities of dogs in confined areas are associated with heat and carbon dioxide, which attract kissing bugs.

CANINE CHAGAS DISEASE IN THE UNITED STATES–EPIDEMIOLOGY

In more than 13 years since canine Chagas disease was first reviewed in this journal by Stephen Barr,[12] several epidemiological and clinical studies of canine Chagas disease in the United States have been published, broadening our understanding of natural canine *T. cruzi* infections. The prevalence of canine Chagas disease in the United

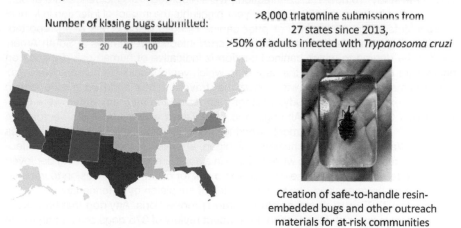

Kissing Bug Community Science Program
Texas A&M University

Engaging the community in triatomine collections while empowering participants with information to stay safe from Chagas and other vector-borne diseases

Number of kissing bugs submitted:

5   20   40   100

>8,000 triatomine submissions from 27 states since 2013, >50% of adults infected with *Trypanosoma cruzi*

Creation of safe-to-handle resin-embedded bugs and other outreach materials for at-risk communities

Project website **kissingbug.tamu.edu**: free insect identification and insect testing for *Trypanosoma cruzi* infection

Fig. 2. A Kissing Bug Community Science Program, established at Texas A&M University, encourages members of the public to submit kissing bugs they encounter to a broad research program. Veterinarians can direct clients who suspect they have encountered a kissing bug to this program, including the website: kissingbug.tamu.edu, for free insect identification and *T. cruzi* testing service. Triatomines from 28 states have been submitted to the program since its inception in 2013. Figure from Busselman et al. (2022).[53] Reproduced with permission from the Annual Review of Animal Biosciences, Volume 10 © 2022 by Annual Reviews, http://www.annualreviews.org.

States is largely unknown due to a lack of standardized surveillance. Reporting of veterinary cases of Chagas disease was mandatory only in Texas and only from 2013 to 2015. During this time, 439 cases were reported to the state health department.[13] Canine *T. cruzi* infections have been reported in at least 8 states including Texas, Louisiana, Oklahoma, Tennessee, Virginia, California, Georgia, and South Carolina.[14–21] Reported prevalence in Texas, Oklahoma, and Louisiana ranged from 3.6% to 22.1%, overall, with up to 57.6% seroprevalence in some kennel environments.[11,15,18,22–28] A study of dogs arriving to animal shelters across several ecoregions in Texas showed 18% of more than 600 dogs were seroreactive to *T. cruzi* overall, a prevalence that was statistically equivalent to that of heartworm infection in the same dogs.[25] Similarly, the seroprevalence of dogs living in impoverished Texas communities along the border with Mexico was 19.6%. Human *T. cruzi* infections were also documented in these communities.[26] In far west Texas and New Mexico, more than 45% of feral dogs were infected in one study.[4] In a survey of 540 dogs across 10 shelters in Louisiana, 6.9% of dogs were seroreactive and 15.9% were polymerase chain reaction (PCR)-positive.[23] In Oklahoma, 3.6% of more than 300 dogs sampled from the same geographic locale as an infected index case were also infected.[15]

Although prevalence studies are useful in identifying endemic areas of concern to veterinary medicine and public health, studies that measure incidence—that is, the number of new infections per year—are useful for quantifying risk. With a focus on dogs living in multidog kennel environments where triatomine vectors are endemic, Busselman and colleagues[29] monitored a cohort of 64 *T. cruzi*-infected and uninfected dogs across 10 kennels in Texas to characterize changes in infection status during a 1-year period. Among the 34 dogs testing negative for *T cruzi* based on serology and PCR at the beginning of the study, 10 new *T. cruzi* infections were recorded. This incidence rate of 30.7 new *T. cruzi* infections per 100 dogs per year highlights the impact of infection in kennel environments where triatomines or prior canine Chagas disease has been reported. Although dogs are effective sentinels for *T. cruzi* infection in humans in South America,[30,31] the degree to which canine infection is indicative of human risk depends on local vector biology, including the degree to which vectors colonize human dwellings.

As in humans, dogs infected with *T. cruzi* may travel and be diagnosed in nonendemic areas. For example, in one study, 12 dogs that resided in northern states were diagnosed with Chagas disease. All originated from Texas where triatomine vectors are common.[32] Similarly, government working dogs across several northern states including Washington, Massachusetts, Michigan, and New York had confirmed infections, likely reflecting exposure while training in a southern state before being deployed in north states.[33] Although these dogs pose no risk for onward transmission to vectors, cases can go unrecognized due to a low index of suspicion by veterinarians.

Infection with *T. cruzi* shows no strong breed predilections. Any dog that has exposure to vectors is at risk for infection. In a recent review of 375 dogs presenting to the Texas A&M Veterinary Medical Teaching Hospital during a 7-year period and tested for *T. cruzi*, 91 breeds were represented. Those with the highest prevalence of infection were nonsporting and toy breed groups.[34] The odds of infection were 13 times greater among dogs with an infected housemate or litter-mate, illustrating geographic clustering that likely reflects the presence of vectors on the property (**Box 1**).[34]

CANINE CHAGAS DISEASE—CLINICAL ASPECTS

The time course of infection and basic understanding of pathogenesis of canine Chagas disease comes in large part from the experimental infection studies of Barr and colleagues in the early 1990s.[35–37] Experimental infections of dogs have not been

---

Box 1
Risk factors for *T. cruzi* infection in dogs relate to encounters with triatomine insect vectors in the environment

- Residing in, or travel to, an area with infected insect vectors
- Lifestyles that include prolonged exposure to the outdoors, including outdoor work or housing
- Multidog kennel environments
- Having an infected littermate or dog at the same premises
- Being born to an infected mother
- Behavior of consuming insects
- Young dogs may be more likely to develop severe clinical outcomes
- Seroprevalence increases with dog age because older dogs have had a longer time for more exposures

---

repeated since then in the United States, although other natural reservoirs including racoons and opossums have been challenged with US strains of *T. cruzi*.[38] Outside the United States, dogs have been challenged with regionally important *T. cruzi* isolates.[39] Reinfections have also been investigated.[40] Chagas disease in dogs presents similarly to the disease in humans, with acute, indeterminate (ie, infected without symptoms) and chronic phases. Dogs are rarely diagnosed during the acute stage, and there are currently no guidelines for stratifying animals in their stage of infection. Given the similar disease presentation between dogs and humans, studies of clinical manifestations and disease management approaches in veterinary medicine have the potential to inform human medicine and vice versa. In infected dogs, there is a great variation in clinical outcomes. Some of this variation likely explained by the burden (load) of parasite, the distribution of the parasite within the host, the genetic strain of parasite, and host factors, including the presence of coinfections with multiple *T. cruzi* strains or other infectious agents.

Based on experimental infection models, peak parasitemia occurs approximately 17 days after infection and may be undetectable by 30 days after infection. During this time, acute disease may be characterized by generalized lymphadenopathy, lethargy, and acute myocarditis, especially in young puppies.[36] The myocarditis results from parasites rupturing from the cardiomyocytes and associated inflammation. Not all infected dogs progress to develop symptomatic chronic disease. It is estimated that approximately 20% to 30% of humans develop chronic symptomatic Chagas cardiomyopathy, and this percentage may be similar in dogs based on a few small studies.[41–43] Experimentally and naturally infected dogs with myocarditis and Chagas cardiomyopathy have documented cardiac abnormalities. Electrocardiogram (ECG) abnormalities include sinus node dysfunction, atrioventricular block and other conduction abnormalities, supraventricular and ventricular arrhythmias, decreased R-wave amplitude, and T-wave inversion[12,34,44,45] (**Fig. 3**). Ambulatory ECG recordings are more likely to detect rhythm abnormalities than short in-hospital traces.[44] Echocardiographic abnormalities in Chagas disease include right ventricular dilation with progression to include a loss of left ventricular function with decreased fractional shortening, reduced ejection fraction, reduced left ventricular free wall thickness, and increase in end-systolic volume.[12,43] Cardiac enlargement and myocardial failure lead to signs of biventricular heart failure (ascites, pleural effusion, jugular venous congestion, pulmonary edema) and in some cases, death.[12,44] The clinical findings are similar

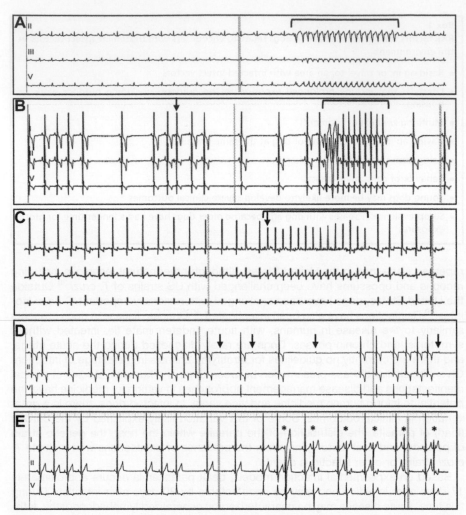

Fig. 3. Example traces taken from 24-hour ambulatory ECG (Holter, Mortara H3+ Monitor, Mortara Instrument, Inc., Milwaukee, WI) recordings of 5 dogs infected with *T. cruzi* that document the variation in abnormalities including ventricular tachycardia (*A*), supraventricular premature complexes (*arrow*) and supraventricular tachycardia (*B*, *C*), second-degree atrioventricular block characterized by nonconducted P waves (*arrows*) (*D*), and ventricular bigeminy (*asterisk*) (*E*).

to dilated cardiomyopathy seen in large breeds of dogs with idiopathic, diet-associated, and arrhythmogenic right ventricular cardiomyopathy and can also be mistaken for congenital tricuspid valve dysplasia.[44,46] Several clinical tools and approaches may be used for monitoring dogs with Chagas disease with attention to their cardiac clinical status (**Box 2**).

A recent retrospective medical records review of cardiac clinical test results among 44 dogs that tested positive for *T. cruzi* at a veterinary medical teaching hospital showed that ECG abnormalities were common, occurring in 95% of the dogs, and that ventricular arrhythmias and atrioventricular block were the most commonly identified ECG abnormalities. Thirty-three percent of dogs had more than one

---

Box 2
Clinical tools and approaches for *T. cruzi* in dogs

- ECG to monitor for arrhythmias and conduction abnormalities (in hospital recording or ambulatory 24-h Holter monitor)

- cTnI—a biomarker of cardiac injury—is used as an index of cardiac damage in dogs with Chagas disease. The utility of cTnI as a prognostic indicator is being evaluated

- Echocardiography to characterize heart size and ventricular function

- Testing for other infectious diseases

- Symptomatic management and antiparasitic treatment

---

abnormality.[44] Echocardiographic chamber enlargement was common and most often included the right ventricle and left atrium. Further, cardiac troponin I (cTnI), as an indicator of myocardial damage, was greater than or equal to twice the reference interval in more than half the dogs for which it was tested. Right ventricular enlargement was associated with a worse outcome in this population likely indicating a more advanced disease process.

The impact of Chagas disease on the US government working dogs, which perform scent detection and security functions along the borders, in airports and federal buildings and in other capacities, has been studied intensively, owing to the hardships that may be posed by morbidity or mortality in these high-value animals. Of more than 1600 government working dogs nationwide, nearly 8% were seroreactive to *T. cruzi*,[33] with a seroprevalence of up to 18.9% in dogs along the US–Mexico border.[28] Cardiac monitoring of approximately 50 dogs, approximately half *T. cruzi*-positive and half negative, showed that 70.5% of positive and 11.1% of negative dogs had one or more ECG abnormalities.[47] The most common cardiac abnormalities included supraventricular and ventricular arrhythmias and atrioventricular block. Further, positive dogs had higher serum concentrations of cTnI than negative dogs. Based on dog handler reports, only 5 of 41 (12%) noted a performance decline in their dog, 4 of those 5 dogs were seroreactive to *T. cruzi*.[47] In a case series, *T. cruzi* was the cause of death in 5 government working dogs during a 6-month period along the Texas–Mexico border. These included chronically infected dogs that were actively working at the time of their death.[48] Chagas disease presents similar hardships to military working dogs (MWDs). Deployed dogs returned to the United States due to reported clinical symptoms of cardiac issues have been subsequently diagnosed with Chagas disease.[49] MWDs at the Lackland Air Force base are screened annually and cardiovascular evaluations are performed on seroreactive dogs.[50]

BEYOND THE DOG: *TRYPANOSOMA CRUZI* INFECTIONS IN OTHER VETERINARY SPECIES

Any mammal may be susceptible to infection with *T. cruzi*, with infections noted across more than 100 wild and domestic mammal species in the Americas.[51] Although birds, reptiles, amphibians, and even invertebrate taxa may provide blood meals to triatomines and therefore be very important in maintaining vector populations, these hosts are regarded as incompetent for *T. cruzi* and do not serve as parasite reservoirs. A recent report, however, of *T. cruzi* infection in an American barn-owl (*Tyto furcata*) in Veracruz, Mexico,[52] suggests further ecological study is warranted. A recent review of the ecology of Chagas disease in the United States included a quantitative synthesis of blood feeding patterns of triatomines based on the findings of 14 studies. This synthesis of information is useful in identifying key species with which these insects interact.[53] In total, 44 different host groups were detected from analysis of blood meals from 449 insects. The most frequent hosts of the triatomines were dogs, humans, and wood rats, underscoring the importance of these hosts in the ecology of the disease, especially in areas where humans encounter triatomines.

Although diverse mammalian taxa have been reported as infected, not all play an equal role as parasite reservoirs, which can be defined as the subset of infected animals that maintain the parasite in nature and serve as a source of infection to triatomines that feed on them. A review focused on assessing T. cruzi reservoirs in the southern United States showed that raccoon (Procyon lotor), wood rat (Neotoma spp), and opossum (Didelphis virginiana) are among the most well-studied and highly infected wildlife species, with roughly one-third of individuals reported to be infected. Raccoons and striped skunk (Mephitis mephitis) were found to commonly have the parasite circulating in their blood, indicating they are likely infectious to vectors.[54] Similarly, seroprevalence studies of wildlife across the southern United States showed the highest seroprevalence is among raccoons and opossums.[55] An increasing number of exotic animals and animals in zoological collections have had T. cruzi infections identified, with a recent review reporting infections in 12 different exotic or captive species in the United States. These include including walrus, red panda, wallaby, sugar glider, among others. In many cases, clinical signs and/or histopathologic findings consistent with Chagas disease were present.[53] Additionally, T. cruzi infection has been increasingly recognized in nonhuman primates at biomedical research facilities when housed in areas endemic to triatomines, creating problems for the individual animal as well as biomedical research that requires them to be healthy.[56,57]

Although feline Chagas disease is far less studied than canine Chagas disease, cats can be infected with T. cruzi and may develop symptoms of Chagas disease. There are no standardized reports of feline Chagas disease from veterinary patients, in part because of a lack of validated serodiagnostic tests for T. cruzi antibodies in cats. However, research studies in the southern United States suggest that feline exposure may be widespread. Nearly 40% (7/24) of feral cats were infected based on PCR in western Texas and in New Mexico where infected dogs and vectors occurred.[58] In South Texas, 7.3% to 11.4% of shelter cats were seroreactive and 1.8% to 24.6% tested positive using PCR. Some infected cats had cardiac inflammation.[59] Additionally, shelter cats in Louisiana were infected with diverse T. cruzi strains.[60] Wild cats in the southern United States also are infected, including bobcats (Lynx rufus) and endangered ocelots (Leopardus pardalis), potentially raising concern for conservation of this species.[61,62]

DISCUSSION
Diagnosis

As in humans, diagnosis of Chagas disease in animals is based on the detection of the parasite or antibodies to the parasite. Direct detection of the parasite can be accomplished through visualization of the trypomastigote stage of the parasite on blood smears but this is only possible when the animal is highly parasitemic, which is most likely during acute infection. A low level or absence of circulating parasite in chronically infected animals can lead to negative results. Serologic testing is most commonly performed through the indirect fluorescent antibody test, currently available at the Texas A&M Veterinary Medical Diagnostic Laboratory. Seroreactivity often indicates active infection because infections are thought to be lifelong in the absence of antiparasitic therapy.[23] For this reason, seroreactivity is considered equivalent to active infection in epidemiologic studies. However, serologic cross-reactivity with

Leishmania is possible, and the sensitivity and specificity of this test are not firmly established. Additionally, discordance between test results occurs and has been attributed to differences between parasite strain and test antigens.[63] Molecular methods including PCR can be used to test peripheral blood or other tissues for *T. cruzi* diagnosis. For PCR testing of blood, the results are dependent on the level of circulating parasite at the time of sampling. A negative PCR result alone should not be interpreted as a lack of infection. Rapid immunochromatographic tests to detect antibodies to the parasite are widely used for dogs and wildlife in research settings[27,64] but are not currently available for veterinary diagnosis.

For postmortem diagnosis, the intracellular amastigote stage of the parasite can be seen histologically in the heart or other tissues (eg, brain, spleen, and diaphragm) of infected animals.[12,37] However, parasites are rarely seen in the hearts of chronically infected animals.[12] Histopathologic findings include mild to severe, chronic, lympho-plasmacytic to histiocytic myocarditis with variable fibrosis. Parasitic pseudocysts may be found in any of the 4 cardiac chambers.[37,65]

Prognosis

The prognosis varies highly among infected individuals. The presence of right heart enlargement and complex ventricular arrhythmias are associated with a shorter survival time.[44,66] Dogs infected at a young age seem particularly susceptible to severe disease.[46] As in humans, many infected dogs remain asymptomatic for years, whereas others will die suddenly. This may be attributed in part to living in an endemic area with increased exposure, reexposure, and parasite load. A comprehensive clinical evaluation can provide individualized patient information to identify cardiac disease associated with myocardial damage. Testing can include cTnI, 24-hour ambulatory ECG, and echocardiography.

Clinical Management

Chagas disease is particularly frustrating when it presents as sudden death or acute decompensation with heart failure in young and working dogs with little or no warning.

Asymptomatic infected dogs can be screened for cardiac disease with ECG, echocardiography, and cTnI. Management of infected dogs would ideally include addressing the clinical disease and the parasitic infection. Cardiac disease management consists of antiarrhythmics, pacemaker implantation for bradyarrhythmias, and standard heart failure therapy for myocardial failure.[67,68] Medical management of heart failure includes the use of a positive inotrope (oral pimobendan, injectable dobutamine), diuretics (furosemide, spironolactone), and centesis of the thoracic or abdominal cavity when effusions are present.

As in humans, antiparasitic therapy has been explored in dogs. Challenges include availability, side effects, and mixed outcomes. Benznidazole administered at 7 mg/kg PO q12 h can reduce inflammation and limit cardiac changes but did not result in long-term remission due to recrudescence of dormant parasites after therapy.[69] More recent study in mice suggests a modified protocol with a higher dose administered less frequently can effectively clear dormant parasites.[70] A treatment protocol combining itraconazole approximately 7.5 mg/kg PO q24h and amiodarone approximately 10 mg/kg PO q 24h administered for 12 months in seroreactive dogs was associated with improvement in clinical signs and a mean survival time of 23.19 months compared with 15.64 months in the control population.[71] Defining when treated dogs are cured is a challenge[72] because there is no single diagnostic test to declare parasitological cure in veterinary medicine. In addition, eliminating infection may not equate to improvement of clinical status. Additional study in people includes

---

Box 3
Vector control and habitat management to reduce interactions of triatomines with dogs and other veterinary species

- Turning off outdoor lights at dog kennels or in other areas where animals reside overnight may be useful because triatomines are generally nocturnal and may be attracted to lights

- Fortification of homes (sealing cracks around doors or holes in window screens) may be useful in limiting triatomine infestations

- Removal of woodpiles and animal dens and burrows from the proximity of dog kennels to reduce vector habitat

- No insecticides are labeled for triatomines in the United States but pyrethroid insecticides, specifically wettable powder or microencapsulated formulations, may be useful in areas where triatomine infestations have occurred[77]

- Host-targeted insecticides show promise against triatomines in South America,[78] and evaluations are underway to test the impact of systemic insecticides of dogs against US species of triatomines[79]

---

developing screening recommendations for individuals in endemic areas, using staging schemes to stratify patients, and optimize individual therapy, and evaluating other interventions such as vaccines and combination therapy.[41,73,74] Similar steps would certainly advance veterinary Chagas disease clinical management. Thus far, a DNA vaccine has not been effective in preventing ECG and echocardiographic abnormalities typically associated with Chagas myocarditis in dogs.[75]

SUMMARY

Veterinary Chagas disease is a concern for dogs, cats, and other mammals that can come into contact with triatomine insect vectors, which are distributed across the Southern United States. Veterinary awareness for Chagas disease should not be restricted to the south because infected pets may move to other regions with their owners. There is wide variation in clinical outcomes in infected dogs. Some remain asymptomatic, whereas others develop Chagas myocarditis, which can result in chronic disease or sudden death. Infected animals are typically managed symptomatically but promising new research suggests antiparasitic treatment options may be more readily available in the future. Vector control approaches and raising awareness among dog owners and the veterinary community for triatomines and Chagas disease is critical, especially as the vector populations are predicted to expand due to climate change.[76] Owners of infected dogs should be educated about vector control and habitat management approaches to reduce interactions of triatomines with dogs and other species (**Box 3**). Given T cruzi is a zoonotic agent, advancing our understanding of veterinary Chagas disease can provide information relevant for protecting human health and vice versa.

CLINICS CARE POINTS

- Dogs that have contact with triatomine insect vectors, which occur across the Southern United States, are at high risk for Chagas disease.

- Dogs, cats, exotic animals, and animals in zoological collections in the Southern United States are increasingly diagnosed with Chagas disease due in part to increased awareness in the veterinary community.

- Vigilance for the presence of vectors and vector control can reduce vector–host contact.

- Annual screening of dogs in high-risk settings is useful to identify dogs that need cardiac monitoring and symptomatic and/or antiparasitic treatments.

- Infected dogs may show a range of clinical manifestations ranging from no clinical signs to myocardial dysfunction resulting in sudden death or chronic heart disease.

- Challenges in preventing and controlling Chagas disease include a lack of veterinary awareness for disease risk and the need for improved diagnostics and antiparasitic treatment options.

ACKNOWLEDGMENTS

We would like to acknowledge the George A. Robinson Foundation and the Harry L. Willett Foundation for support.

REFERENCES

1. Bern C, Kjos S, Yabsley MJ, et al. *Trypanosoma cruzi* and Chagas' disease in the United States. Clin Microbiol Rev 2011;24:655–81.
2. Zeledón R, Alvarado R, Jirón LF. Observations on the feeding and defecation patterns of three triatomine species (Hemiptera: Reduviidae). Acta Trop 1977;34: 65–77.
3. Messenger LA, Bern C. Congenital Chagas disease: current diagnostics, limitations and future perspectives. Curr Opin Infect Dis 2018;31:415–21.
4. Rodriguez-Morales O, Ballinas-Verdugo MA, Alejandre-Aguilar R, et al. *Trypanosoma cruzi* connatal transmission in dogs with Chagas disease: experimental case report. Vector Borne Zoonotic Dis 2011;11:1365–70.
5. Latas PJ, Reavill D. *Trypanosoma Cruzi* Infection in sugar gliders (*Petaurus breviceps*) and hedgehogs (*Atelerix albiventris*) via ingestion. J Exot Pet Med 2019; 29:76–8.
6. Roellig DM, Ellis AE, Yabsley MJ. Oral transmission of *Trypanosoma cruzi* with opposing evidence for the theory of carnivory. J Parasitol 2009;95:360–4.
7. de Noya BA, González ON. An ecological overview on the factors that drives to *Trypanosoma cruzi* oral transmission. Acta Trop 2015;151:94–102.
8. Curtis-Robles R, Hamer SA, Lane S, et al. Bionomics and spatial distribution of triatomine vectors of *Trypanosoma cruzi* in Texas and other southern states, USA. Am J Trop Med Hyg 2018;98:113–21.
9. Reisenman CE, Savary W, Cowles J, et al. The distribution and abundance of triatomine insects, potential vectors of Chagas disease, in a metropolitan area in southern Arizona, United States. J Med Entomol 2012;49:1254–61.
10. Shender LA, Lewis MD, Rejmanek D, et al. Molecular diversity of *Trypanosoma cruzi* detected in the vector *Triatoma protracta* from California, USA. PLoS Negl Trop Dis 2016;10:e0004291.
11. Curtis-Robles R, Snowden KF, Dominguez B, et al. Epidemiology and molecular typing of *Trypanosoma cruzi* in naturally-infected hound dogs and associated triatomine vectors in Texas, USA. PLoS Negl Trop Dis 2017;11:e0005298.
12. Barr SC. Canine Chagas' disease (American trypanosomiasis) in North America. Vet Clin North Am Small Anim Pract 2009;39:1055–64.
13. Texas Department of State Health Services. Chagas Disease Data: Geographical Distribution of Chagas Disese in Texas. Available at: https://www.dshs.state.tx.us/DCU/disease/chagas/Chagas-Disease-Data.aspx. Accessed March 15, 2022.

14. Barr SC, Van Beek O, Carlisle-Nowak MS, et al. *Trypanosoma cruzi* infection in Walker hounds from Virginia. Am J Vet Res 1995;56:1037–44.
15. Bradley KK, Bergman DK, Woods JP, et al. Prevalence of American trypanosomiasis (Chagas disease) among dogs in Oklahoma. J Am Vet Med Assoc 2000;217: 1853–7.
16. Rowland ME, Maloney J, Cohen S, et al. Factors associated with Trypanosoma cruzi exposure among domestic canines in Tennessee. J Parasitol 2010;96: 547–51.
17. Snider TG, Yaeger RG, Dellucky J. Myocarditis caused by Trypanosoma cruzi in a native Louisiana dog. J Am Vet Med Assoc 1980;177:247–9.
18. Kjos SA, Snowden KF, Craig TM, et al. Distribution and characterization of canine Chagas disease in Texas. Vet Parasitol 2008;152:249–56.
19. Fox JC, Ewing SA, Buckner RG, et al. Trypanosoma cruzi infection in a dog from Oklahoma. J Am Vet Med Assoc 1986;189:1583–4.
20. Tomlinson MJ, Chapman WL Jr, Hanson WL, et al. Occurrence of antibody to Trypanosoma cruzi in dogs in the southeastern United States. Am J Vet Res 1981;42: 1444–6.
21. Navin TR, Roberto RR, Juranek DD, et al. Human and sylvatic Trypanosoma cruzi infection in California. Am J Public Health 1985;75:366–9.
22. Garcia MN, O'Day S, Fisher-Hoch S, et al. One health interactions of chagas disease vectors, canid hosts, and human residents along the texas-mexico border. PLoS Negl Trop Dis 2016;10:e0005074.
23. Elmayan A, Tu W, Duhon B, et al. High prevalence of Trypanosoma cruzi infection in shelter dogs from southern Louisiana, USA. Parasit Vectors 2019;12:322.
24. Beard CB, Pye G, Steurer FJ, et al. Chagas disease in a domestic transmission cycle, southern Texas, USA. Emerg Infect Dis 2003;9:103–5.
25. Hodo CL, Rodriguez JY, Curtis-Robles R, et al. Repeated cross-sectional study of Trypanosoma cruzi in shelter dogs in Texas, in the context of Dirofilaria immitis and tick-borne pathogen prevalence. J Vet Intern Med 2019;33:158–66.
26. Curtis-Robles R, Zecca IB, Roman-Cruz V, et al. Trypanosoma cruzi (Agent of Chagas Disease) in Sympatric Human and Dog Populations in "Colonias" of the Lower Rio Grande Valley of Texas. Am J Trop Med Hyg 2017;96:805–14.
27. Nieto PD, Boughton R, Dorn PL, et al. Comparison of two immunochromatographic assays and the indirect immunofluorescence antibody test for diagnosis of *Trypanosoma cruzi* infection in dogs in south central Louisiana. Vet Parasitol 2009;165:241–7.
28. Meyers AC, Meinders M, Hamer SA. Widespread Trypanosoma cruzi infection in government working dogs along the Texas-Mexico border: Discordant serology, parasite genotyping and associated vectors. PLoS Negl Trop Dis 2017;11: e0005819.
29. Busselman RE, Meyers AC, Zecca IB, et al. High incidence of Trypanosoma cruzi infections in dogs directly detected through longitudinal tracking at 10 multi-dog kennels, Texas, USA. PLoS Negl Trop Dis 2021;15:e0009935.
30. Gurtler RE, Cardinal MV. Reservoir host competence and the role of domestic and commensal hosts in the transmission of Trypanosoma cruzi. Acta Trop 2015;151: 32–50.
31. Travi BL. Considering dogs as complementary targets of chagas disease control. Vector Borne Zoonotic Dis 2019;19:90–4.
32. Gavic EA, Achen S, Benjamin EJ, et al. Chagas disease in 12 dogs translocated from Texas. J Vet Intern Med 2021;35:2960–1.

33. Meyers AC, Purnell JC, Ellis MM, et al. Nationwide exposure of U.S. working dogs to the Chagas disease parasite, *Trypanosoma cruzi*. Am J Trop Med Hyg 2020; 102:1078–85.

34. Meyers AC, Hamer SA, Matthews D, et al. Risk factors and select cardiac characteristics in dogs naturally infected with *Trypanosoma cruzi* presenting to a teaching hospital in Texas. J Vet Intern Med 2019;33:1695–706.

35. Barr SC, Dennis VA, Klei TR, et al. Antibody and lymphoblastogenic responses of dogs experimentally infected with *Trypanosoma cruzi* isolates from North American mammals. Vet Immunol Immunopathol 1991;29:267–83.

36. Barr SC, Gossett KA, Klei TR. Clinical, clinicopathological, and parasitological observations of Trypanosomiasis in dogs infected with North American *Trypanosoma cruzi* isolates. Am J Vet Res 1991;52:954–60.

37. Barr SC, Schmidt SP, Brown CC, et al. Pathological features of dogs inoculated with North American *Trypanosoma cruzi* isolates. Am J Vet Res 1991;52:2033–9.

38. Roellig DM, Ellis AE, Yabsley MJ. Genetically different isolates of *Trypanosoma cruzi* elicit different infection dynamics in raccoons (*Procyon lotor*) and Virginia opossums (*Didelphis virginiana*). Int J Parasitol 2009;39:1603–10.

39. Barbabosa-Pliego A, Díaz-Albiter HM, Ochoa-García L, et al. *Trypanosoma cruzi* circulating in the southern region of the State of Mexico (Zumpahuacan) are pathogenic: a dog model. Am J Trop Med Hyg 2009;81:390–5.

40. Machado EM, Fernandes AJ, Murta SM, et al. A study of experimental reinfection by *Trypanosoma cruzi* in dogs. Am J Trop Med Hyg 2001;65:958–65.

41. Bern C, Messenger LA, Whitman JD, et al. Chagas disease in the United States: a Public Health Approach. Clin Microbiol Rev 2019;33.

42. González-Vieyra SD, Ramírez-Durán N, Sandoval-Trujillo Á H, et al. *Trypanosoma cruzi* in dogs: electrocardiographic and echocardiographic evaluation, in Malinalco, State of Mexico. Res Rep Trop Med 2011;2:155–61.

43. Carvalho EB, Ramos IPR, Nascimento AFS, et al. Echocardiographic measurements in a preclinical model of chronic chagasic cardiomyopathy in dogs: validation and reproducibility. Front Cell Infect Microbiol 2019;9:332.

44. Matthews DJ, Saunders AB, Meyers AC, et al. Cardiac diagnostic test results and outcomes in 44 dogs naturally infected with *Trypanosoma cruzi*. J Vet Intern Med 2021;35:1800–9.

45. Barr SC, Holmes RA, Klei TR. Electrocardiographic and echocardiographic features of trypanosomiasis in dogs inoculated with North American *Trypanosoma cruzi* isolates. Am J Vet Res 1992;53:521–7.

46. Vitt JP, Saunders AB, O'Brien MT, et al. Diagnostic features of acute chagas myocarditis with sudden death in a family of boxer dogs. J Vet Intern Med 2016;30:1210–5.

47. Meyers AC, Ellis MM, Purnell JC, et al. Selected cardiac abnormalities in *Trypanosoma cruzi* serologically positive, discordant, and negative working dogs along the Texas-Mexico border. BMC Vet Res 2020;16:101.

48. Meyers AC, Edwards EE, Sanders JP, et al. Fatal Chagas myocarditis in government working dogs in the southern United States: Cross-reactivity and differential diagnoses in five cases across six months. Vet Parasitol Reg Stud Rep 2021;24: 100545.

49. McPhatter L, Roachell W, Mahmood F, et al. Vector surveillance to determine species composition and occurrence of *Trypanosoma cruzi* at three military installations in San Antonio, Texas. TX: US Army Medical Department Journal; 2012. p. 12–21.

50. McGraw AL, Thomas TM. Military working dogs: an overview of veterinary care of these formidable assets. Vet Clin North Am Small Anim Pract 2021;51:933–44.

51. World Health Organization. Control of chagas disease: second report of the WHO expert committee. In: World Health Organization, editor. Geneva; 2002.

52. Martínez-Hernández F, Oria-Martínez B, Rendón-Franco E, et al. *Trypanosoma cruzi*, beyond the dogma of non-infection in birds. Infect Genet Evol 2022;99: 105239.

53. Busselman RE, Hamer SA. Chagas disease ecology in the United States: recent advances in understanding *Trypanosoma cruzi* transmission among triatomines, wildlife, and domestic animals and a quantitative synthesis of vector–host interactions. Annu Rev Anim Biosciences 2022;10:325–48.

54. Hodo CL, Hamer SA. Toward an ecological framework for assessing reservoirs of vector-borne pathogens: wildlife reservoirs of *Trypanosoma cruzi* across the southern United States. ILAR J 2017;58:379–92.

55. Brown EL, Roellig DM, Gompper ME, et al. Seroprevalence of *Trypanosoma cruzi* among eleven potential reservoir species from six states across the southern United States. Vector-Borne Zoonot 2010;10:757–63.

56. Hodo CL, Wilkerson GK, Birkner EC, et al. *Trypanosoma cruzi* transmission among captive nonhuman primates, wildlife, and vectors. Ecohealth 2018;15: 426–36.

57. Dorn PL, Daigle ME, Combe CL, et al. Low prevalence of Chagas parasite infection in a nonhuman primate colony in Louisiana. J Am Assoc Lab Anim Sci 2012; 51:443–7.

58. Rodriguez F, Luna BS, Calderon O, et al. Surveillance of *Trypanosoma cruzi* infection in Triatomine vectors, feral dogs and cats, and wild animals in and around El Paso county, Texas, and New Mexico. PLoS Negl Trop Dis 2021;15:e0009147.

59. Zecca IB, Hodo CL, Slack S, et al. Prevalence of *Trypanosoma cruzi* infection and associated histologic findings in domestic cats (*Felis catus*). Vet Parasitol 2020; 278:109014.

60. Dumonteil E, Desale H, Tu W, et al. Shelter cats host infections with multiple *Trypanosoma cruzi* discrete typing units in southern Louisiana. Vet Res 2021;52:53.

61. Zecca IB, Hodo CL, Swarts HM, et al. *Trypanosoma cruzi* and Incidental *Sarcocystis* spp. in endangered ocelots (*Leopardus pardalis*) of South Texas, USA. J Wildl Dis 2021;57:667–71.

62. Curtis-Robles R, Lewis BC, Hamer SA. High *Trypanosoma cruzi* infection prevalence associated with minimal cardiac pathology among wild carnivores in central Texas. Int J Parasitol Parasites Wildl 2016;5:117–23.

63. Dumonteil E, Elmayan A, Majeau A, et al. Genetic diversity of *Trypanosoma cruzi* parasites infecting dogs in southern Louisiana sheds light on parasite transmission cycles and serological diagnostic performance. PLoS Negl Trop Dis 2020; 14:e0008932.

64. Yabsley MJ, Brown EL, Roellig DM. Evaluation of the Chagas Stat-Pak (TM) assay for detection of *Trypanosoma cruzi* antibodies in wildlife reservoirs. J Parasitol 2009;95:775–7.

65. Andrade ZA, Andrade SG, Sadigursky M, et al. The indeterminate phase of Chagas' disease: ultrastructural characterization of cardiac changes in the canine model. Am J Trop Med Hyg 1997;57:328–36.

66. Malcolm E.L., Saunders A.B., Vitt J.P., et al., Antiparasitic treatment with itraconazole and amiodarone in 2 dogs with severe, symptomatic Chagas cardiomyopathy. *J Vet Intern Med*, 36, 2022, 1100-1105.

67. Saunders AB, Gordon SG, Rector MH, et al. Bradyarrhythmias and pacemaker therapy in dogs with Chagas disease. J Vet Intern Med 2013;27:890–4.
68. Stoner CH, Saunders AB. Cardiac manifestations of *Trypanosoma cruzi* Infection in a domestic dog. CASE (Phila) 2020;4:410–4.
69. Santos FM, Mazzeti AL, Caldas S, et al. Chagas cardiomyopathy: The potential effect of benznidazole treatment on diastolic dysfunction and cardiac damage in dogs chronically infected with *Trypanosoma cruzi*. Acta Trop 2016;161:44–54.
70. Bustamante JM, Sanchez-Valdez F, Padilla AM, et al. A modified drug regimen clears active and dormant trypanosomes in mouse models of Chagas disease. Sci Transl Med 2020;12:eabb7656.
71. Madigan R, Majoy S, Ritter K, et al. Investigation of a combination of amiodarone and itraconazole for treatment of American trypanosomiasis (Chagas disease) in dogs. J Am Vet Med Assoc 2019;255:317–29.
72. Zao CL, Yang YC, Tomanek L, et al. PCR monitoring of parasitemia during drug treatment for canine Chagas disease. J Vet Diagn Invest 2019;31:742–6.
73. Forsyth CJ, Manne-Goehler J, Bern C, et al. Recommendations for screening and diagnosis of Chagas disease in the United States. J Infect Dis 2022;225:1601–10.
74. Rios LE, Vázquez-Chagoyán JC, Pacheco AO, et al. Immunity and vaccine development efforts against *Trypanosoma cruzi*. Acta Trop 2019;200:105168.
75. Arce-Fonseca M, Carbajal-Hernández AC, Lozano-Camacho M, et al. DNA vaccine treatment in dogs experimentally infected with *Trypanosoma cruzi*. J Immunol Res 2020;2020:9794575.
76. Garza M, Feria Arroyo TP, Casillas EA, et al. Projected future distributions of vectors of *Trypanosoma cruzi* in North America under climate change scenarios. PLoS Negl Trop Dis 2014;8.
77. Merchant M. Conenose or kissing bugs. insects in the city. 2022. Available at: https://citybugs.tamu.edu/factsheets/biting-stinging/others/ent-3008/. Accessed March 15, 2022.
78. Loza A, Talaga A, Herbas G, et al. Systemic insecticide treatment of the canine reservoir of *Trypanosoma cruzi* induces high levels of lethality in *Triatoma infestans*, a principal vector of Chagas disease. Parasit Vectors 2017;10:344.
79. Busselman R, Zecca I, Hamer G, Hamer S. Killer K9s: ectoparasiticide given to dogs induce high mortality in *Triatoma gerstaeckeri*, vector of *Trypanosoma cruzi*. Ontario, CA: Society of Vector Ecology; 2021.

Schistosomiasis in the United States

Audrey K. Cook, BVM&S, MRCVS, MSc Vet Ed*

KEYWORDS

- Heterobilharzia • Hypercalcemia • Enteropathy • Hepatopathy

KEY POINTS

- *Heterobilharzia americana* is a trematode parasite, endemic to the Gulf states of the United States but with an expanding intermediate host range.
- Infection in dogs occurs through exposure to skin-penetrating cercariae in fresh water.
- Infection can be subclinical or result in a chronic enteropathy and/or hepatopathy.
- Fecal PCR testing is regarded as a sensitive and specific diagnostic option.
- Treatment protocols are not well-defined but anecdotal evidence supports the use of praziquantel with fenbendazole.

INTRODUCTION

The causative agent of canine schistosomiasis in the United States is *Heterobilharzia americana* (*HA*). This trematode is part of the Schistosomatidae family and is closely related to the "blood flukes" of the genus *Schistosoma*. These parasites were first described by Theodor Bilharz in 1851 and are still a major cause of morbidity in human populations across the globe. *HA* is the only member of this group endemic to the United States and is routinely diagnosed in dogs living in the Gulf coast and southern Atlantic states.[1–5] It is sporadically identified in the central southern states, and a recent outbreak in Utah suggests that the parasite may be expanding its known range.[6–10] Small animal practitioners across the United States therefore need to be aware of this condition and have a solid understanding of the diagnosis and management of dogs with schistosomiasis.

HA has a complex life cycle, with both sexual and asexual reproduction, and vertebrate (primary) and invertebrate (intermediate) hosts (**Fig. 1**).[11] The primary host is the racoon, although infection has been reported in numerous other wildlife species including nutria, opossums, bobcats, and armadillo.[6,12,13] Eggs (**Fig. 2**) passed in the feces of infected animals are deposited or washed into streams or ponds. A single miracidium (**Fig. 3**) emerges from each egg almost immediately after contact with

Department of Small Animal Clinical Sciences, College of Veterinary Medicine and Biomedical Sciences, Texas A & M University, College Station, MS 4474, College Station, TX 77843-4474, USA
* Corresponding author.
E-mail address: akcook@cvm.tamu.edu

Vet Clin Small Anim 52 (2022) 1283–1303
https://doi.org/10.1016/j.cvsm.2022.06.009
0195-5616/22/© 2022 Elsevier Inc. All rights reserved.

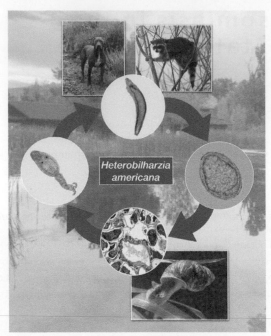

Fig. 1. The lifecycle of *HA*. Eggs are passed in the feces of the primary host (racoon). Miracidia that emerge from the eggs infect aquatic snails. Free-swimming cercariae are released after 2 cycles of asexual reproduction. Cercariae penetrate the skin of an animal as it stands in the water. Shistosomulae larvae migrate to lungs, and then mature in hepatic vessels. Adult worms then travel to the mesenteric veins to mate and eggs migrate through the walls of the intestine, completing the cycle. See text for additional information. (Image reproduced under a Creative Commons Attribution License https://creativecommons.org/licenses/by/4.0/ from Loker ES, Dolginow SZ, Pape S, et al. An outbreak of canine schistosomiasis in Utah: Acquisition of a new snail host (*Galba humilis*) by *Heterobilharzia americana*, a pathogenic parasite on the move. One Health 2021 https://doi.org/10.1016/j.onehlt.2021.100280.)

freshwater, and seeks out the intermediate host, *Galba* (or *Lymnea*) *cubensis*, a small aquatic snail. Although various species of snail may be experimentally infected with HA, *G. cubensis* was until recently the only known natural vector. However, *Galba humilis*, an amphibious snail widely distributed across North America, was implicated in the infection of 12 dogs in Utah in 2018.[10] Two cycles of asexual reproduction within the snail lead to the release of numerous cercariae (**Fig. 4**); these are free-swimming and must soon find a vertebrate host. Cercariae are able to penetrate the skin of the animal as it stands in water, after which they shed their tails and migrate through the venous system to the lungs. These larval forms are referred to as schistosomulae. Initial maturation occurs primarily within the hepatic vessels; the sexually dimorphic adult male (≈ 17 mm in length) and female (≈ 9 mm in length) worms then travel to the mesenteric veins to mate. In common with other blood schistosomes, the male holds at least one female within its gynecophoric canal. After fertilization, the female worm produces large numbers of oval eggs (approx. $70–110 \times 60–80$ μm), which are released directly into the mesenteric veins. Using proteolytic enzymes, the eggs migrate out of the vasculature and through the walls of the small and large intestines. Intact eggs are then excreted in the feces, with a prepatent period of about 10 weeks.[14]

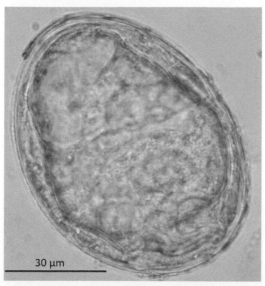

Fig. 2. Egg of *HA*. Note lack of a spine, and the miracidium within. Scale bar = 30 μm. (Image reproduced under a Creative Commons Attribution License https://creativecommons.org/licenses/by/4.0/ from Loker ES, Dolginow SZ, Pape S, et al. An outbreak of canine schistosomiasis in Utah: Acquisition of a new snail host (*Galba humilis*) by *Heterobilharzia americana*, a pathogenic parasite on the move. One Health 2021 https://doi.org/10.1016/j.onehlt.2021.100280.)

The signs reported in dogs with clinical schistosomiasis primarily reflect extensive granulomatous reactions in the gastrointestinal (GI) tract ± liver. The exuberant inflammatory reaction results in fibrosis and mineralization of affected tissues, with compromised function. Aberrant egg migration may affect other organs such as the pancreas, kidneys, spleen, and lungs, and metabolic derangements including hypercalcemia can cause significant systemic compromise. A pruritic and erythematous cutaneous reaction trigged by transdermal migration of cercariae is reported in people and is referred to colloquially as "swamp itch" or "swimmer's itch." Interestingly, cercarial dermatitis due to HA has not been reported in dogs. An acute hypersensitivity reaction attributed to the migrating schistosomulae is also described in people; this starts suddenly and is characterized by fever, myalgia, nonproductive cough, and eosinophilia.[15] This stage of infection—referred to as acute schistosomiasis or Katayama fever—resolves without treatment within 2 to 10 weeks. A similar syndrome has not been reported in canine patients.

Before 2008, establishing a diagnosis of schistosomiasis routinely depended on the identification of HA eggs using fecal saline sedimentation techniques or the visualization of eggs or adult trematodes within affected tissue(s). Antemortem diagnosis therefore required a substantial index of suspicion on the part of the practitioner, or enough compromise to the patient to merit collection of appropriate samples for histopathologic examination. The advent of a commercially available, highly sensitive, fecal polymerase chain reaction (PCR) test has simplified the diagnosis of HA, and allows practitioners to screen patients more easily for this disease.[16] It is noteworthy that the number of dogs diagnosed each year at the author's institution (Texas A&M University) increased 4-fold after the advent of the fecal PCR test.

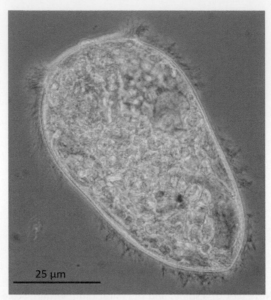

Fig. 3. Miracidium of *HA*. Scale bar = 50 μm. (Image reproduced under a Creative Commons Attribution License https://creativecommons.org/licenses/by/4.0/ from Loker ES, Dolginow SZ, Pape S, et al. An outbreak of canine schistosomiasis in Utah: Acquisition of a new snail host (*Galba humilis*) by *Heterobilharzia americana*, a pathogenic parasite on the move. One Health 2021 https://doi.org/10.1016/j.onehlt.2021.100280.)

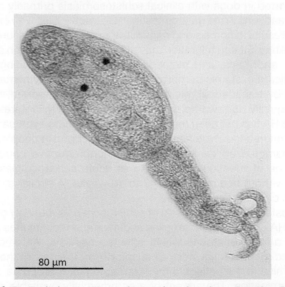

Fig. 4. Cercaria of *HA*. Scale bar = 80 μm. (Reproduced under a Creative Commons Attribution License https://creativecommons.org/licenses/by/4.0/ from Loker ES, Dolginow SZ, Pape S, et al. An outbreak of canine schistosomiasis in Utah: Acquisition of a new snail host (*Galba humilis*) by *Heterobilharzia americana*, a pathogenic parasite on the move. One Health 2021 https://doi.org/10.1016/j.onehlt.2021.100280.)

Prevalence

The prevalence of HA infection in racoons from endemic areas seems to be high, with estimates ranging from 37% to 48%.[6,17,18] Although the prevalence of infection in dogs in endemic areas has not been established, clinical disease related to schistosomiasis seems to be uncommon. A total of 39 dogs were diagnosed with HA at Texas A&M Veterinary Medical Teaching Hospital from 2010 to 2019; this represents less than 0.0005% of all canine admissions. A report describing the distribution of HA in dogs in Texas identified 238 cases diagnosed at the Texas Veterinary Medical Diagnostic Laboratory, the Veterinary Medical Teaching Hospital, and the Gastrointestinal Laboratory at Texas A&M College of Veterinary Medicine during a 22-year period.

There is mounting evidence to suggest that many infected dogs are negligibly affected, although it is unclear if these individuals have smaller parasitic burdens or are simply identified at an earlier stage of the disease. Infection seemed to be clinically silent and was diagnosed during the investigation of other issues or at necropsy for an unrelated disorder in 8/60 dogs (13.3%) in a recent retrospective study.[1] Similarly, incidental infection was reported in 7/22 dogs (31.8%) from an older case series.[2] Asymptomatic infection was identified in 2 housemates following the diagnosis of HA in a dog seen at Mississippi State University College of Veterinary Medicine in 2020. Testing of other dogs in the area identified 27 more cases, most of which were apparently well.[4]

Any dog exposed to water containing cercariae is at risk for schistosomiasis, and it is not unusual for several dogs in the same household to be simultaneously infected.[2–4,7,19] Young to middle-aged, large breed dogs do seem to be overrepresented (**Table 1**), and a recent retrospective case-controlled study found that Labrador retrievers were more likely to be diagnosed with HA (Odds ratio (OR) = 4.354; 95% CI, 1.308–12.73; P = .018) than other breeds admitted during the same time period.[28] However, this finding likely represents the influence of lifestyle and environmental rather than an innate susceptibility.

Evaluation

Infection with HA should be considered in any dog with findings suggesting a chronic enteropathy or hepatopathy. Signs commonly associated with clinical disease include lethargy, diarrhea, hematochezia, weight loss, hyporexia, and vomiting.[1,2] Polydipsia and polyuria may also be reported by the owner. Physical examination findings are generally nonspecific. Severely affected animals may be dehydrated, emaciated, or have evidence of ascites. Soft stool with frank blood may be noted on rectal examination.

Findings on the complete blood count may be within the reference ranges, although a robust eosinophil count (ie, >500/μL) may be noted. This is unexpected in clinically compromised dogs and should prompt consideration of HA. A variably regenerative anemia (hematocrit <30%) was reported in less than 20% of dogs in a recent report; this may be attributable to gastrointestinal loss or suppression of erythropoiesis secondary to chronic inflammatory disease.[1] Thrombocytopenia (<200,000/μL) was reported in greater than 50% of dogs in one case series but is usually mild and not associated with hemorrhagic tendencies.[2]

The serum biochemical profile may be similarly unremarkable or nonspecific. Changes routinely noted include hyperglobulinemia, hypoalbuminemia, and mild increases in liver enzyme activity. When present, increases in alanine aminotransferase and alkaline phosphatase are generally modest (<500 U/L), and suggestive of chronic mild hepatitis or a reactive hepatopathy.[1] Azotemia is sometimes noted in dogs with

Table 1
Summary of peer reviewed publications describing dogs with naturally occurring schistosomiasis (1980 onwards)

Author and Year	# Of Dogs	State	Method(s) of Diagnosis	Age (y)	Gender	Weight (kg)	Comments
Troy,[20] 1987	1	Texas	Biopsy	7	Male	27	Hypercalcemic
Rohrer,[5] 2000	1	Florida	Necropsy	3	Female	8	Hypercalcemic
Fradkin,[19] 2001	2	Texas	Necropsy	2.5; 3.5	Male, female	6.1; 14	Hypercalcemic; detectable PTH-rp
Flowers,[21] 2002	1	North Carolina	Biopsy	7	Male	27.7	Serum antigen capture used to monitor response to treatment
Fabrick,[2] 2010	22	Texas	Biopsy (9); necropsy (4); fecal sedimentation (9)	3.1 (median)	64% male; 36% female	24.3 (median)	Incidental finding in 7/22 Hypercalcemia in 11/22
Ruth,[22] 2010	1	Texas	Biopsy	6	Male	22.7	Associated with membranoproliferative GN; resolved with treatment
Stone,[23] 2011	1	Georgia	Biopsy	11	Male	n/r	Associated with hepatosplenic T-cell lymphoma
Kvitko-White,[24] 2011	1	Texas	Necropsy	3	Female	n/a	Histologic findings reported in Corapi et al, 2011[25]
Hanzlicek,[7] 2011	5	Kansas	Biopsy (1); necropsy (2); fecal sedimentation (2)	4	3 male 2 female	22 (median)	Severe hypercalcemia in 2 dogs
Rodriquez,[3] 2014	238	Texas	Biopsy (26); necropsy (39); fecal PCR (160); fecal sedimentation (43)	5.5 (median)	47.1% male; 52.9% female	19.6 (median)	Includes 20 dogs reported by Fabrick et al 2010[2]
Le Donne,[26] 2015	1	Louisiana	Cytology and fecal sedimentation	7	Male	n/r	HA noted on hepatic cytology

Le Roux,[27] 2015	1	Louisiana	Biopsy	n/r	n/r	n/r	Extensive gastric mineralization noted on radiographs
Rodriguez,[8] 2016	1	Indiana	Biopsy	1	Male	28.5	
Graham,[1] 2021	60	Texas	Biopsy (6); necropsy (2); Fecal PCR (49); Fecal sedimentation (3)	7.5	41.2% male; 58.3% female	23.2	Imaging findings for 55 dogs reported by Moshnikova et al 2020[28] Hypercalcemia in 4/60
Loker,[10] 2021	12	Utah	Necropsy (1); fecal PCR 10; presumptive (1)	n/r	n/r	n/r	New intermediate host identified
Cridge,[4] 2021	12	Mississippi	Fecal PCR	n/r	n/r	n/r	Asymptomatic

Abbreviations: HA, *Heterobilarzia americana*; n/r, Not reported; PTH-rp, Parathyroid hormone related peptide.

HA that are significantly hypercalcemia and likely indicates rental tubular damage related to rapid increases in ionized calcium concentrations and/or secondary renal mineralization. Serum phosphorus levels are often increased in this patient subset.

Historical reports suggest that hypercalcemia is a common finding in dogs with schistosomiasis, and an elevated serum total calcium concentration was noted in 50% of dogs in a case series published in 2010.[2,5,19,20] However, it is likely that the anecdotal association of HA with hypercalcemia influenced diagnostic decision-making, such that fecal sedimentations were traditionally more likely to be performed in dogs with gastrointestinal signs and hypercalcemia than in normocalcemic dogs with similar complaints. For many clinicians working in endemic areas, the advent of a reliable fecal PCR test has changed the diagnostic approach and resulted in the routine testing of many more dogs with appropriate clinical signs, irrespective of their calcium status. In a 2021 report of 60 dogs with HA, only 4 (6.7%) had hypercalcemia attributable to this infection, and subnormal total calcium levels were noted in 16.7% of dogs.[1]

In most cases, the hypercalcemia is a consequence of the widespread granulomatous response, in which activated macrophages secrete 1,25-dihyroxycholecalciferol (ie, calcitriol).[29] This promotes the uptake of both calcium and phosphorus by the intestinal tract and may overwhelm normal homeostatic mechanisms. However, 2 canine patients with hypercalcemia attributable to HA were found to have detectable parathyroid hormone-related peptide[19]; secretion of this fetal hormone is traditionally associated with various tumors, and it is widely regarded as a specific marker for malignancy-associated hypercalcemia.

Urine specific gravity in dogs with HA is variable and may be influenced by hydration status and calcium concentrations. Protein-losing nephropathy due to membranoproliferative glomerulonephritis was reported in one dog with HA; this resolved following treatment of schistosomiasis.[22]

Imaging

Findings on both abdominal radiography and transabdominal ultrasonography (US) may be unremarkable or essentially pathognomonic for HA. In the author's institution, findings on US have routinely prompted testing for HA in dogs being evaluated for unrelated conditions.

As a general rule, abdominal radiography provides limited diagnostic insight in dogs with HA. However, in some instances, dystrophic mineralization of various tissues may be noted. Affected sections of intestine may contain thin parallel lines of mineral opacity, which track the loops of bowel (**Fig. 5**).[24] It is important to bear in mind that this mineralization is driven by inflammation—not hypercalcemia per se—and is routinely noted in normocalcemic dogs with HA. Serosal detail may be compromised by abdominal effusion (noted in >25% of cases).[1]

Findings on US are variable but changes are noted in most infected dogs.[28] Some of the findings commonly reported are fairly nonspecific, and include effusion and changes in small intestinal wall layering (**Fig. 6**).[24,28] However, pinpoint hyperechoic foci, indicative of tissue mineralization, are often noted in small intestinal submucosal and muscularis layers of infected dogs, including those without overt clinical disease related to HA(**Figs. 7** and **8**). Mineralization may also be evident within other organs, such as the liver, mesenteric lymph nodes or pancreas, and will result in a "twinkle" artifact (**Figs. 9** and **10**). The combination of heterogenous small intestinal wall layering and pinpoint hyperechoic foci in small intestine, liver, or mesenteric nodes was found to be highly predictive of HA infection in a recent case-controlled retrospective study (OR = 36.87; positive predictive value of 94%).[27] These findings should always prompt testing for schistosomiasis.

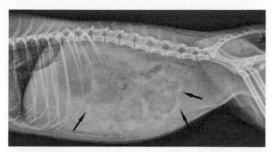

Fig. 5. Right lateral radiograph of a 3-year-old female (spayed) mixed breed dog diagnosed with *HA* on necropsy. Note the linear mineral opacities located in the wall of multiple segments of small intestine (*black arrows*). There is a loss of serosal margin detail consistent with peritoneal effusion. (Reproduced with permission from Kvitko-White HL, Sayre RS, Corapi WV, et al. Imaging diagnosis—*Heterobilharzia americana* infection in a dog. Vet Rad Ultrasound 2011;52:538-41.)

Additional Testing

Infection with HA should be confirmed definitively before treatment. Current diagnostic options include fecal saline sedimentation, fecal PCR, and histopathology of affected tissues.

Trematode eggs are first excreted in feces about 10 weeks after initial infection, and the number of HA ova is proportional to the worm burden.[30] With rare exceptions, the number of eggs present in stool is not sufficient for a diagnosis to be established by microscopic examination of a direct smear; a method relying on concentration is therefore required. The ova of HA are too dense to be supported by standard flotation solutions, and eggs must instead be concentrated by sedimentation in a saline solution.[14] This test is not technically difficult but takes considerable time. First, the feces are mixed with 1.2% saline; this slurry is then filtered through cheesecloth and allowed to settle for 30 minutes. The supernatant is subsequently discarded, and the sediment is resuspended in 1.2% saline for another 30-minute settling period. This is repeated until the supernatant is clear, at which time the sediment is examined under the microscope. Unfortunately, fecal sedimentation is not offered by large reference laboratories; some state diagnostic laboratories or facilities associated with veterinary schools may provide this test.

A miracidia hatching method has also been reported and may be used to verify findings on the sediment examination. After several saline rinses, the sediment is flooded with distilled water to trigger the hatching of viable eggs. The distinctive miracidia can then be identified microscopically.[31]

A fecal PCR test with a reported sensitivity of 1 to 2 eggs/g of feces is now commercially available (Schistosomiasis fecal PCR, Gastrointestinal Laboratory at Texas A&M University, College Station, Texas) and is routinely included by the author in the diagnostic evaluation of canine patients with chronic gastrointestinal disease or biochemical evidence of a chronic hepatopathy.[16] At least 1 gram ($\approx$1/4 tsp) of freshly collected feces is required; the submission of a pooled sample collected from 2 to 3 bowel movements is advisable because egg shedding may be intermittent. Feces may be stored for up to 1 week in the refrigerator before shipment to the laboratory on a gel ice pack. Each test run uses spiked feces (2 and 20 eggs/100 mg) as a positive control. Feces from healthy dogs and fecal DNA from dogs with roundworms, hookworms, and tapeworms are used as negative controls. During its development, the

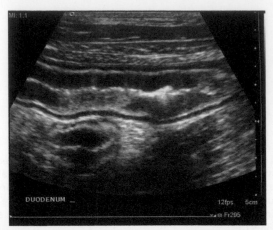

Fig. 6. Transabdominal ultrasonographic image of the duodenum of a 3-year-old male (castrated) German shorthaired pointer with vomiting and diarrhea. Note the somewhat heterogenous appearance of the mucosa. A diagnosis of HA was made using tissue samples collected endoscopically. (Image courtesy of Diagnostic Imaging Service, Veterinary Medical Teaching Hospital, Texas A&M University.)

performance of the fecal PCR was validated in-house by testing spiked fecal samples, comparisons with concurrent saline sedimentation findings, and the hatching of miracidia from positive samples. In addition, DNA sequences from positive results were compared with published sequences from HA. False-positive results are highly unlikely because the primers used in this test are not expected to cross-react with DNA from other organisms causing similar signs. Specificity with regard to other schistosome species has not been thoroughly investigated, although the fecal PCR was negative when challenged with samples from dogs infected with *Schistosoma mansoni*.[4]

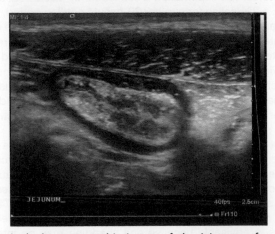

Fig. 7. Transabdominal ultrasonographic image of the jejunum of a 9-year-old female (spayed) West Highland white terrier with vomiting and diarrhea. Note the heterogenous thickening of the intestinal wall, along with pinpoint hyperechoic specks within the muscularis layer. A diagnosis of HA was made using fecal PCR. (Image courtesy of Diagnostic Imaging Service, Veterinary Medical Teaching Hospital, Texas A&M University.)

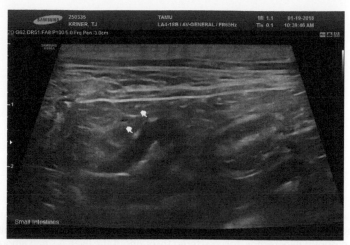

Fig. 8. Transabdominal ultrasonographic image of the small intestine of a 9-year-old male (castrated) Nova Scotia duck tolling retriever undergoing investigation for ulcerative oral lesions. Hyperechoic foci were noted in sections of the small intestine (*pointing fingers*). This dog was tested for *HA* from ultrasonographic findings and was positive on fecal PCR. Its housemate was also positive on PCR, and eggs were noted on liver biopsy. (Image courtesy of Diagnostic Imaging Service, Veterinary Medical Teaching Hospital, Texas A&M University.)

This test seems to be significantly more sensitive than fecal sedimentation. In a recent report, 12 dogs that were positive on both fecal PCR and saline sedimentation were repeatedly tested following treatment of HA.[1] Samples collected at Day 60, Day 90, and Day 120 posttreatment were all negative on sedimentation but 4/12, 5/12, and 2/12, respectively, were still positive on PCR. The diagnostic reliability of the saline sedimentation test in this study may have been impacted by using just 1 gram of feces; standard recommendations suggest the submission of 3 to 5 gram ($\approx$ 1 tsp).

Histopathology is a reliable way to confirm a diagnosis of HA, although it is prudent to screen patients for HA using the fecal PCR before considering more invasive diagnostics. The gross appearance of the liver in infected dogs is variable; it may be unremarkable or show evidence of inflammation and subsequent fibrosis. Small, white, raised granulomas may be noted on the surface of the liver lobes, along with nodular regenerative changes (**Fig. 11**). Hepatic involvement tends to be widespread, and organisms are likely to be found throughout all the lobes. The gross appearance of the gastrointestinal tract when viewed endoscopically is also variable; the mucosa may seem irregular and small erosions may be noted, particularly in the colon (**Fig. 12**). Different regions of the bowel can be less affected than others, so clinicians are encouraged to collect multiple biopsies from as many parts of the intestinal tract as possible. The author routinely collects 8 to 10 specimens from the stomach, duodenum, ileum, and colon. It is not uncommon for histiocytic and eosinophilic inflammation to be noted in every specimen, whereas eggs are only noted in 25% to 50% of the samples submitted. At laparotomy, biopsy collection should be directed to areas of the bowel with nodular plaques on the serosal surface. These represent granulomas and are expected to contain eggs.

Portions of the adult worms are occasionally identified within hepatic biopsy specimens but the eggs are routinely noted within all affected organs. These are ovoid, with a thin refractile wall, and are often found within microscopic granulomas composed of macrophages, lymphocytes, plasma cells, neutrophils, and eosinophils (**Figs. 13** and

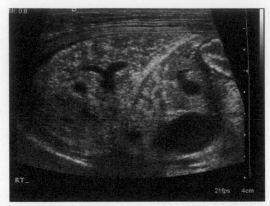

Fig. 9. Transabdominal ultrasonographic image of the liver of a 3-year-old female (spayed) mixed breed dog diagnosed with *HA* on necropsy. Note the heterogenous hepatic parenchyma and pinpoint hyperechoic foci scattered throughout the liver. A small amount of peritoneal effusion is evident between the liver and the diaphragm. (Image courtesy of Diagnostic Imaging Service, Veterinary Medical Teaching Hospital, Texas A&M University.)

14). Fibrous connective tissue often surrounds these cellular aggregates. A single miracidium is contained within each egg and may be recognized by its many thin cilia. Eggshell fragments may also be seen.

Cytology of affected organs is expected to indicate chronic inflammation, with macrophages, lymphocytes, and eosinophils. These changes are fairly nonspecific but should certainly prompt testing for HA. Evidence of schistosomiasis was identified on a hepatic aspirate in an infected dog; cytologic examination revealed eggshell fragments and the occasional ciliated miracidium, and subsequent fecal sedimentation confirmed infection with HA.[26] Failure to identify HA on an aspirate does not, however, exclude the possibility of infection.

An indirect hemagglutination test was developed several decades ago, using sheep erythrocytes sensitized to adult HA antigens.[32] Although serial dilutions less than 1:80 resulted in nonspecific agglutination in dogs with other helminth infections, titers for dogs with schistosomiasis were significantly higher than the control population by postexposure day 60. To the best of the author's knowledge, this serologic test was never made available on a commercial basis.

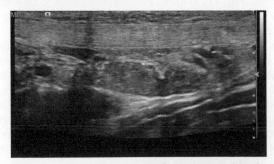

Fig. 10. Transabdominal ultrasonographic image of a mesenteric lymph node of a 4-year-old male (castrated) pit bull terrier evaluated for chronic diarrhea with intermittent hematochezia. Note the heterogenous echogenicity and pinpoint hyperechoic foci. Fecal PCR was positive for *HA*. (Image courtesy of Diagnostic Imaging Service, Veterinary Medical Teaching Hospital, Texas A&M University.)

An antigen capture enzyme-linked immunosorbent assay developed for diagnostic use in people with schistosomiasis has been used to confirm infection in a canine patient.[21] The dog had a moderate antigen concentration at the time of diagnosis; this dropped markedly following successful treatment.

Therapeutic Options

Parasitic diseases (ie, those caused by cestodes, nematodes, and trematodes) are major health concerns in both human and veterinary medicine. Early efforts to create effective anthelmintics were driven by the impact of human tropical diseases such as schistosomiasis, and the first effective agents routinely included toxic metals such as arsenic or antimony. Modern anthelmintics offer a more targeted approach; most agents have a limited spectrum of activity and cannot be used interchangeably. Mechanisms of actions often focus on disrupting neuromuscular function or altering key aspects of the parasite's metabolism. These effects may not directly or immediately kill the organism but may instead increase its susceptibility to the host's immune responses. Unlike antibiotics, which generally have easy access to their target, anthelmintic agents must penetrate the parasite's protective cuticle or gain entry via its alimentary tract. Efficacy may be compromised by the parasite's ability to pump out the drug or otherwise antagonize its action.

Human schistosomiasis has enormous socioeconomic impact in many third world countries, and efforts to control this disease rely heavily on oral praziquantel. This anthelmintic agent was introduced in the 1970s, and it remained the primary agent for the treatment and control of this condition since that time. It is estimated that tens of millions of people receive this drug every year, particularly in sub-Saharan Africa. Given at 40 to 60 mg/kg (often divided into 2–3 doses and given over the same day), praziquantel is effective against all major forms of human schistosomiasis, although it has significantly less activity against immature trematodes (schistosomula).[33,34] Its mechanism of action is incompletely understood but it is thought that praziquantel selectively targets voltage-gated calcium channels within the schistosome, resulting in the influx of calcium ions and spasmic contracture of the

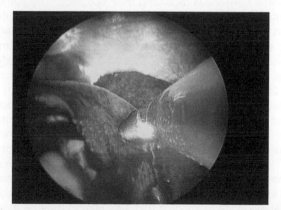

Fig. 11. Collection of a laparoscopic liver biopsy from a 9-year-old female (spayed) Labrador retriever with a persistently elevated ALT activity. Note the numerous small (1–2 mm) raised white lesions over the surface of the visible liver lobes. The distal tip of a palpation probe is visible in the ventral part of the image. A small amount of hemorrhage from a previous biopsy site is evident on the left side of the image. Histopathology revealed *HA* eggs and chronic inflammation with extensive fibrosis.

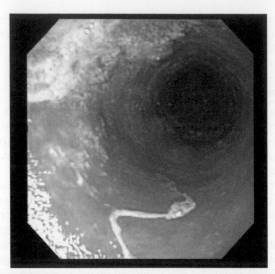

Fig. 12. Endoscopic view of the duodenum of an 8-year-old female (spayed) German shepherd dog evaluated for chronic vomiting, diarrhea, weight loss, and hyporexia. The mucosa is somewhat granular and mildly erythematous. Histopathology of multiple endoscopic biopsies revealed a severe mixed inflammatory reaction; *HA* eggs were identified in most of the specimens submitted.

musculature.[35] The worms are essentially paralyzed and slowly die. This drug also disrupts the outer covering of the schistosome, making it more vulnerable to immune attack by the host.[15]

Praziquantel is also widely used in companion animal medicine and is licensed for the management of cestodiasis (ie, tapeworm infection) in dogs (3–5 mg/kg per os, one time).[36] Based on its proven efficacy in people, it is also routinely used to treat canine schistosomiasis. Dosages used have been drawn from the human literature, although there is little consensus regarding their specifics. The author routinely prescribes 25 to 30 mg/kg PO q8 hours × 8 doses but recognizes that there is scant evidence to support this plan, and it has been suggested that fewer doses may be equally effective. Use of a human formulation (eg, Biltricide 600 mg tablet) rather than the veterinary approved product (ie, Droncit 34 mg) can simplify administration and reduce costs. In the author's hospital, the cost of the praziquantel needed for this regimen in a 20 kg patient with is more than US $600.

Side effects related to the drug itself seem to be uncommon, although vomiting has been reported and some clinicians recommend concurrent administration of an antiemetic. Praziquantel has good oral bioavailability and rapidly undergoes hepatic metabolism via oxidation to 4-hydroxy praziquantel, which is thought to be to be to be biologically active.[37] Inactive metabolites are subsequently excreted in urine. The LD50 for the oral formation is greater than 2000 mg/kg in rodent species; this has not been determined in dogs because doses greater than 200 mg/kg resulted in vomiting. There is anecdotal evidence to suggest that side effects may be more likely with the injectable formulation; pain, emesis, drowsiness, and staggering have been reported in dogs.[36]

This high dose of praziquantel is often combined with fenbendazole. Again, dosages vary but the author routinely prescribes 50 mg/kg PO q24 hours for 7 days. In a report from 1984, fenbendazole was administered at 40 mg/kg PO q24 hours for 10 days to a

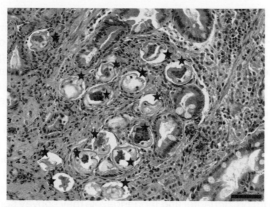

Fig. 13. Histologic section of the duodenum from the patient descried in **Fig. 12.** The specimen contains excessive numbers of inflammatory cells, consisting primary of lymphocytes, plasma cells, and eosinophils. Numerous *HA* ova (*stars*) are noted. Magnification is 200×. Scale bar = 50 μm. (Image courtesy of the Diagnostic Histology Unit, Veterinary Medical Teaching Hospital, Texas A&M University.)

beagle with a long-standing (>2 years), experimentally induced, HA infection. This dog was shown to be shedding viable eggs before treatment but no worms were found at necropsy 17 days after therapy. In contrast, more than 200 adult worms were reported in a second beagle, similarly experimentally infected, but left untreated.[38] Fenbendazole is a broad-spectrum benzimidazole anthelmintic and affects cellular function by binding to β-tubulin. In parasites, the subsequent disruption of microtubule formation impairs glucose uptake along with routine cellular division, resulting in paralysis and death. Although β-tubulin is also a key component of mammalian cells, these are

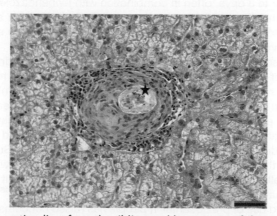

Fig. 14. Histologic section liver from the sibling and housemate of the patient described in **Fig. 8.** This dog was asymptomatic but was positive on fecal PCR. Before the treatment, a liver biopsy was collected during a cholecystectomy for an unrelated gallbladder mucocele. Multifocally and randomly within the liver are small accumulations of macrophages and eosinophils with rare multinucleated giant cells. Scattered within these areas of inflammation are 55 to 70 μm degenerate trematode eggs (*star*). Magnification is 200×. Scale bar = 50 μm. (Image courtesy of the Diagnostic Histology Unit, Veterinary Medical Teaching Hospital, Texas A&M University.)

innately resistant to fenbendazole, resulting in a greater than 300× effect within the helminth.[39] Fenbendazole is licensed for use in dogs for the management of nematode infestations, at various dosages (eg, 25 mg/kg PO q24 hours × 25 days for pregnant bitches; 50 mg/kg PO q24 hours × 7 days for lungworm; 100–200 mg/kg PO q30 days for routine parasite prophylaxis). Bioavailability is significantly enhanced by feeding. Biotransformation occurs rapidly in the liver; metabolites are subsequently conjugated and excreted via the biliary and urinary systems. Side effects are uncommon but include rare reports of idiosyncratic blood dyscrasias.[40]

There is a lack of direct evidence of a synergistic effect between praziquantel and fenbendazole, and many reports describe the use of either drug as a sole agent.[1,2,8,21,23,38] However, there is clear evidence that combinations of specific anthelmintics may be more effective than single agents for various parasitic disorders, such as giardiasis and hookworm infestation, and it is the author's opinion that combination therapy with praziquantel and fenbendazole may convey some advantages in dogs with HA.[41,42]

A recent article reported on outcomes using a lower dose of praziquantel in combination with fenbendazole (24 mg/kg PO q24 hours × 7 days) in a cohort of dogs with asymptomatic HA.[4] These dogs were given an average of 5 mg/kg (range: 3.2–6.5) of praziquantel by mouth q8 hours for 2 days. All dogs were initially positive on fecal PCR. One month after treatment, 9/12 were still positive for HA; by day 60, 4/12 were still positive. Three of these were re-treated with the same low-dose protocol and were subsequently PCR negative.

The study described above is commendable for its thorough follow-up and sincere efforts to determine treatment efficacy. Unfortunately, most single case reports and larger case series provide little information regarding this issue. Determinations of treatment outcomes are also complicated by the test(s) used, as older reports relied on the somewhat insensitive fecal sedimentation. In a recent case series, more than 65% of dogs were either PCR positive or still showing signs of infection 30 to 60 days after treatment; most of these dogs had received praziquantel at 25 mg/kg PO q8 hours for 2 to 3 days, often in combination with fenbendazole.[1] It is important to bear in mind that the initial treatment may have eradicated the adult worms but failed to kill the schistosomulae; "treatment failure" may therefore simply represent the subsequent emergence of prepatent organisms.

In people with schistosomiasis, protocols calling for the routine administration of an additional dose of praziquantel, given 2 weeks after the first, have resulted in higher cumulative cure rates.[43,44] There is an argument to adopt a similar approach in dogs with HA, and the author is aware of clinicians who routinely repeat the praziquantel/fenbendazole protocol after 3 to 4 weeks. Combining praziquantel with a drug known to eradicate the immature forms is another approach, and various options are currently under investigation for human schistosomiasis.[45] Studies in murine models support the administration of edelfosine in combination with praziquantel; this agent is an alkylphospholipid analog and kills schistosomula. It also downregulates the inflammatory response and inhibits granuloma formation.[46]

The widespread use of praziquantel in people has raised concerns about the creation of resistant strains of S. mansoni.[47–50] It seems likely that the induction of ATP-binding cassette transporters (proteins involved in the transport of toxins and xenobiotics) may play a role because changes in these proteins are commonly associated with resistance to chemotherapeutics and antibiotics. However, finding unambiguous evidence of resistance to praziquantel within Schistosoma spp is complicated because the drug is predictably less effective against the immature forms, and by the frequency of reinfection. Resistance of HA to praziquantel may explain some of the reported treatment failures in dogs, although the author is not aware of any patient with a proven persistent infection after 2 rounds of treatment with this agent.

Irrespective of the treatment protocol chosen, patients should be retested with a fecal PCR within 60 days, even if apparently normal. Housemates should also be screened for HA and treated if positive.

Clinical Outcomes

Dogs infected with HA have a wide spectrum of clinical signs and compromise; the impact on the host is likely determined by the duration of infection, the worm burden, the host's immune response to the infection, and the presence of associated conditions such as hypercalcemia. A recent case series found that almost 75% of treated dogs were alive at 180 days; this suggests an overall positive prognosis, although several animals died or were euthanized as a direct result of their infection.[1] However, because these patients were all examined at specialty hospitals, they may not provide a reliable representation of the disease.

In the author's experience, the cause of death in dogs with schistosomiasis is either kidney injury related to severe hypercalcemia; end-stage cirrhosis secondary to extensive hepatic injury; or apparent acute decompensation related to treatment of HA. The last event probably reflects an overwhelming inflammatory response related to widespread parasite death. In dogs with significant HA infection, some clinicians recommend the administration of anti-inflammatory doses of prednisone (0.3–0.5 mg/kg PO q12 hours × 3 days) when treatment is initiated. It is interesting to note that serious complications related to the treatment of human schistosomiasis seem to be exceedingly rare and were reported in less than 0.5% of greater than 25,000 people treated with praziquantel for Schistosoma japonica.[61]

Numerous Schistosoma spp have been associated with cancer in humans: Schistosoma haematobium with bladder cancer; S. japonica with colorectal cancer; and S. mansoni with lymphosarcoma.[52–54] A similar association has not been established in veterinary medicine, although a canine patient with HA and T-cell lymphoma was described in 2011.[23] Heterobilharzia ova were found embedded within sheets of neoplastic T-cell lymphocytes in both liver and mesenteric nodes; this suggested a possible causal relationship between the infection and the cancer. Lymphocytes associated with ova in the intestinal walls were also cluster of differentiation 3-positive.

SUMMARY

In endemic areas, dogs with chronic (>3 weeks) vomiting, diarrhea, and hematochezia and/or elevated alanine aminotransferase activity should be screened for HA with a fecal. To improve sensitivity, aliquots from 3 different stools should be pooled before submission. The possibility of HA infection should also be considered in dogs living elsewhere in the United States, particularly if the signs and findings listed above are accompanied by weight loss, anorexia, hyperglobulinemia, hypercalcemia, or a robust eosinophil count.

Findings on abdominal US may be unremarkable. However, the combination of heterogenous small intestinal wall layering and pinpoint hyperechoic foci in small intestine, liver, or mesenteric nodes is highly predictive with HA infection and should always prompt testing for this infection.

Treatment should include a combination of praziquantel and fenbendazole. The author recommends dosing praziquantel orally at 25 mg/kg (q8 hours for 2–3 days) in symptomatic dogs because the effect of the lower dose (5 mg/kg) has not been reported in this more vulnerable population. The response to treatment should be assessed with a follow-up PCR 1 to 2 months later. Prospective studies are needed to determine the optimal dose and duration of praziquantel because the cost of this drug can be considerable and affects owner compliance with treatment recommendations. Other canine members of the household should always be tested, because infection may be asymptomatic, at least in the initial stages.

The prognosis for clinically affected dogs is fairly positive, although sequelae such as acute kidney injury or cirrhosis may affect outcomes.

CLINICS CARE POINTS

- The discovery of a new intermediate host for HA suggests that it is likely to be diagnosed more often in areas beyond its traditional range.
- HA should be considered in any dog with chronic gastrointestinal signs or increased ALT activity.
- A recent case series suggests that hypercalcemia is an uncommon finding in dog with HA; this diagnosis should not be discounted in normocalcemic patients.
- Pinpoint hyperechoic foci the intestines, liver, or mesenteric nodes should prompt testing for HA.
- Treatment protocols vary but a combination of praziquantel and fenbendazole is widely considered to be the most appropriate approach.
- Dogs should be retested within 60 days because current treatments are less effective against the immature worms.

DISCLOSURE

The author has no disclosures related to this article.

REFERENCES

1. Graham AM, Davenport A, Moshnikova VS, et al. *Heterobilharzia americana* infection in dogs: A retrospective study of 60 cases (2010-2019). J Vet Intern Med 2021;35:1361–7.
2. Fabrick C, Bugbee A, Fosgate G. Clinical features and outcome of *Heterobilharzia americana* infection in dogs. J Vet Intern Med 2010;24:140–4.
3. Rodriguez JY, Lewis BC, Snowden KF. Distribution and characterization of *Heterobilharzia americana* in dogs in Texas. Vet Parasitol 2014;203:35–42.
4. Cridge H, Lupiano H, Nipper JD, et al. Efficacy of a low-dose praziquantel and fenbendazole protocol in the treatment of asymptomatic schistosomiasis in dogs. J Vet Intern Med 2021;35:1368–75.
5. Rohrer CR, Phillips LA, Ford SL, et al. Hypercalcemia in a dog: a challenging case. J Am Anim Hosp Assoc 2000;36:20–5.
6. McKown RD, Veatch JK, Fox LB. New locality record for *Heterobilharzia americana*. J Wildl Dis 1991;27:156–60.
7. Hanzlicek AS, Harkin KR, Dryden MW, et al. Canine schistosomiasis in Kansas: five cases (2000–2009). J Am Anim Hosp Assoc 2011;47:e95–102.
8. Rodriguez JY, Camp JW, Lenz SD, et al. Identification of *Heterobilharzia americana* infection in a dog residing in Indiana with no history of travel. J Am Vet Med Assoc 2016;248:827–30.

9. Nagamori Y, Payton ME, Looper E, et al. Retrospective survey of endoparasitism identified in feces of client-owned dogs in North America from 2007 through 2018. Vet Parasitol 2020;282:109–37.
10. Loker ES, Dolginow SZ, Pape S, et al. An outbreak of canine schistosomiasis in Utah: Acquisition of a new snail host (*Galba humilis*) by *Heterobilharzia americana*, a pathogenic parasite on the move. One Health 2021;17:100280.
11. Lee HF. Life history of *Heterobilharzia americana* Price 1929, a schistosome of the raccoon and other mammals in southeastern United States. J Parasitol 1962;48: 728–39.
12. Kaplan EH. *Heterobilharzia americana* Price, 1929, in the opossum from Louisiana. J Parasitol 1964;50:797.
13. Krotski WA, Job CK, Cogswell FB, et al. Enzootic schistosomiasis in a Louisiana armadillo. Am J Trop Med Hyg 1984;33:269–72.
14. Schistosomiasis. Available at: https://capcvet.org/guidelines/schistosomiasis/. Accessed December 31, 2021.
15. Vale N, Gouveia MJ, Rinaldi G, et al. Praziquantel for schistosomiasis: single-drug metabolism revisited, mode of action, and resistance. Antimicrob Agents Ch 2017;61:e02582.
16. Bishop MA, Suchodolski JS, Steiner JM. Development of a PCR test for the detection of *Heterobilharzia americana* DNA in dog feces. Abstract #338. J Vet Intern Med 2008;22:804–5.
17. Malek EA, Ash LR, Lee HF, et al. *Heterobilharzia* infection in the dog and other mammals in Louisiana. J Parasitol 1961;47:619–23.
18. Kelley SW. Heterobilharziasis (Trematoda: Schistosomatidae) in raccoons (*Procyon lotor*) of north-central Texas. Tex J Sci 2010;62(1):75–84.
19. Fradkin JM, Braniecki AM, Craig TM, et al. Elevated parathyroid hormone-related protein and hypercalcemia in two dogs with schistosomiasis. J Am Anim Hosp Asso 2001;37:349–55.
20. Troy GC, Forrester D, Cockburn C, et al. *Heterobilharzia americana* infection and hypercalcemia in a dog: a case report. J Am Anim Hosp Assoc 1987;23:35–40.
21. Flowers JR, Hammerberg B, Wood SL, et al. *Heterobilharzia americana* infection in a dog. J Am Vet Med Assoc 2002;220:193–6.
22. Ruth J. *Heterobilharzia americana* infection and glomerulonephritis in a dog. J Am Anim Hosp Assoc 2010;46:203–8.
23. Stone RH, Frontera-Acevedo K, Saba CF, et al. Lymphosarcoma associated with *Heterobilharzia americana* infection in a dog. J Vet Diagn Invest 2011;23: 1065–70.
24. Kvitko-White HL, Sayre RS, Corapi WV, et al. Imaging diagnosis—*Heterobilharzia americana* infection in a dog. Vet Rad Ultrasound 2011;52:538–41.
25. Corapi WV, Ajithdoss DK, Snowden KF, et al. Multi-organ involvement of Heterobilharzia americana infection in a dog presented for systemic mineralization. J Vet Diagn Invest 2011;23:826–31.
26. Le Donne V, McGovern DA, Fletcher JM, et al. Cytologic diagnosis of Heterobilharzia americana infection in a liver aspirate from a dog. Vet Pathol 2016;53: 633–6.
27. Le Roux A, Ryan K, Im Hof M, et al. What is your diagnosis? J Am Vet Med Assoc 2015;246:411–3.
28. Moshnikova VS, Gilmour LJ, Cook AK, et al. Sonographic findings of pinpoint hyperechoic foci in the small intestine, liver, and mesenteric lymph nodes are indicative of canine *Heterobilharzia americana* infection. Vet Rad Ultrasound 2019. https://doi.org/10.1111/vru.12874.

29. Sharma OP. Hypercalcemia in granulomatous disorders: a clinical review. Curr Opin Pulm Med 2000;6:442–7.
30. Malek E. Correlation analyses of cercarial exposure, worm load and egg content in stools of dogs infected with *Heterobilharzia americana.* Z Tropenmed Parasit 1969;20:333–40.
31. Goff WL, Ronald NC. Miracidia hatching technique for diagnosis of canine schistosomiasis. J Am Vet Med Assoc 1980;177:699–700.
32. Goff WL, Ronald NC. Indirect hemagglutination for the diagnosis of Heterobilharzia americana infections in dogs. Am J Vet Res 1982;43:2038–41.
33. Palha De Sousa CA, Brigham T, Chasekwa B, et al. Dosing of praziquantel by height in sub-Saharan African adults. Am J Trop Med Hyg 2014;90:634–7.
34. Pica-Mattoccia L, Cioli D. Sex- and stage-related sensitivity of *Schistosoma mansoni* to in vivo and in vitro praziquantel treatment. Int J Parasitol 2004;34:527–33.
35. Thomas CM, Timson DJ. The mechanism of action of praziquantel: six hypotheses. Curr Top Med Chem 2018;18(18):1575–84, sis: past, present and future. Chem Med Chem 2018;13:2374-1584.
36. Praziquantel VIN. Veterinary drug handbook, VIN. 2017. Available at: www.vin.com/members/cms/project/defaultadv1.aspx?pId=13468. Accessed December 31, 2021.
37. Giorgi M, Meucci V, Vaccaro E, et al. Effects of liquid and freeze-dried grapefruit juice on the pharmacokinetics of praziquantel and its metabolite 4'-hydroxy praziquantel in beagle dogs. Pharmacol Res 2003;47:87–92.
38. Ronald NC, Craig TM. Fenbendazole for the treatment of *Heterobilharzia americana* infection in dogs. J Am Vet Med Assoc 1983;182:172.
39. Ritter JM, Flower R, Henderson G, et al. Anthelmintic drugs. In: Rang and dale pharmacology. 9th edition. Elsevier; 2020. p. 710–5.
40. Gary AT, Kerl ME, Wiedmeyer CE, et al. Bone marrow hypoplasia associated with fenbendazole administration in a dog. J Am Anim Hosp Assoc 2004;40:224–9.
41. Olson ME, Heine J. Synergistic effect of febantel and pyrantel embonate in elimination of Giardia in a gerbil model. Parasitol Res 2009;105:135–40.
42. Hess LB, Millward LM, Rudinsky A, et al. Combination anthelmintic treatment for persistent *Ancylostoma caninum* ova shedding in greyhounds. J Am Anim Hosp Assoc 2019;55:160–6.
43. N'Goran EK, Gnaka HN, Tanner M, et al. Efficacy and side-effects of two praziquantel treatments against *Schistosoma haematobium* infection, among schoolchildren from Côte d'Ivoire. Ann Trop Med Parasitol 2003;97:37–51.
44. King CH, Olbrych SK, Soon M, et al. Utility of repeated praziquantel dosing in the treatment of schistosomiasis in high-risk communities in Africa: a systematic review. Plos Negl Trop Dis 2011;5(9):e1321.
45. Gouveia MJ, Brindley PJ, Gärtner F, et al. Drug repurposing for schistosomiasis: combinations of drugs or biomolecules. Pharmaceuticals 2018;11:15.
46. Yepes E, Varela -MRE, López-Abán J, et al. Inhibition of granulomatous inflammation and prophylactic treatment of schistosomiasis with a combination of edelfosine and praziquantel. Plos Negl Trop Dis 2015;9(7):e0003893.
47. Wang W, Wang L, Liang YS. Susceptibility or resistance of praziquantel in human schistosomiasis: a review. Parasitol Res 2012;111:1871–7.
48. Doenhoff MJ, Cioli D, Utzinger J. Praziquantel: mechanisms of action, resistance and new derivatives for schistosomiasis. Curr Opin Infect Dis 2008;21:659–67.
49. Sanchez MC, Cupit PM, Bu L, et al. Transcriptomic analysis of reduced sensitivity to praziquantel in *Schistosoma mansoni.* Mol Biochem Parasit 2019;228:6–15.

50. Mäder P, Rennar GA, Ventura AMP, et al. Chemotherapy for fighting schistosomiasis: past, present and future. ChemMedChem 2018;13:2374–89.
51. Chen MG, Fu S, Hua XJ, et al. A retrospective survey on side effects of praziquantel among 25,693 cases of schistosomiasis japonica. SE Asian J Trop Med 1983;14:495–500.
52. Botelho MC, Machado JC, Correia da Costa JM. *Schistosoma haematobium* and bladder cancer: what lies beneath? Virulence 2010;1:84–7.
53. Hamid HK. Schistosoma japonicum–associated colorectal cancer: a review. Am J Trop Med Hyg 2019;100:501.
54. Zanelli M, Zizzo M, Mengoli MC, et al. Diffuse large B cell lymphoma and schistosomiasis: a rare simultaneous occurrence. Ann Hematol 2019;98:1511–2.

Emerging Spotted Fever Rickettsioses in the United States

Linda Kidd, DVM, PhD*

KEYWORDS

- *Rickettsia* • Canine • Feline • Vasculitis • Thrombocytopenia

KEY POINTS

- Rocky Mountain spotted fever (RMSF), caused by *Rickettsia rickettsii*, causes acute, potentially fatal, febrile disease in dogs, similar to the disease it causes in people.
- Both PCR and serology may be negative at the time of presentation when dogs are ill.
- Empiric treatment of suspected cases with doxycycline before confirming the diagnosis is important.
- The role of other spotted fever group rickettsia as disease-causing agents in dogs, cats, and people in the United States is being elucidated.
- Preventing parasitism of dogs and cats by fleas and ticks is important for human and animal health.

Abbreviations	
RMSF	Rocky Mountain Spotted Fever
PCR	Polymerase Chain Reaction
SFG	Spotted Fever Group
TG	Typhus Group
CDC	Center for Disease Control and Prevention
aPTT	activated Partial Thromboplastin Time
PT	Prothrombin Time
DIC	Disseminated Intravascular Coagulation

Western University of Health Sciences, College of Veterinary Medicine, 309 East Second Street, Pomona, CA 91766, USA
* Corresponding author
E-mail address: lkidd@westernu.edu

Vet Clin Small Anim 52 (2022) 1305–1317
https://doi.org/10.1016/j.cvsm.2022.07.003
0195-5616/22/© 2022 Elsevier Inc. All rights reserved.

INTRODUCTION

Rickettsia species are obligately intracellular alpha-proteobacteria belonging to the genus *Rickettsia,* family *Rickettsiaceae,* and order *Rickettsiales*. There are currently 29 named species of *Rickettsia,* with many more proposed species based primarily on genotypic characterization (http://www.bacterio.net/)[1]. *Rickettsia* spp. have historically been divided into the spotted fever group (SFG) the typhus group (TG), and an ancestral group. The division between the spotted fever and typhus groups is based on clinically relevant genotypic and phenotypic characterIstIcs. These include, but are not limited to, differences in disease manifestations, the host's serologic response to the organisms, and the types of vectors that transmit them.

Most of the SFG *Rickettsia* are tick-transmitted, while members of the TG are flea or louse transmitted. *Rickettsia felis* and *Rickettsia akari* have been considered, and are still referred to by some, as members of the SFG. However, they share genotypic and clinically relevant features with both the SFG and TG *Rickettsia*. For example, *R. felis* and *R. akari* are flea and mite transmitted, respectively, and the diseases they cause in people are distinct from other spotted fever rickettsioses. In 2008 it was proposed that be placed in a separate "transitional" group based on phylogenomic analysis.[2] A recent analysis of genomic evolution of arthropod-associated *Rickettsia* suggests that these organisms may belong to a phylogenetically distinct spotted fever group.[3]

Historically, SFG *Rickettsia* have been considered pathogenic or nonpathogenic. The most well-described pathogenic SFG *Rickettsia* that infects people and dogs in the Americas is *R. rickettsii*, the cause of Rocky Mountain spotted fever (RMSF). In Europe, Africa, Asia, and the Middle East, *Rickettsia conorii* is responsible for causing similarly severe spotted fever rickettsioses, Mediterranean spotted fever. Mediterranean Spotted Fever has also been described in dogs.[4,5] Infections with several other species of SFG *Rickettsia* have been described in people with spotted-fever-like illnesses in recent years.[1,6–14] Thus, the spotted fever rickettsioses are considered important emerging infectious diseases in the United States and globally.[1,15] Some of these novel rickettsioses are caused by newly discovered species while others have been associated with species previously thought to be nonpathogenic endosymbionts of ticks. Disease caused by "classic" SFG *Rickettsia* like *R. rickettsii* is also considered "emerging" due to increasing prevalence in expanding geographic locales.[13,14,16]

CANINE ROCKY MOUNTAIN SPOTTED FEVER
Epidemiology

Illness caused by *R. rickettsii* is very well characterized in dogs and is quite similar to Rocky Mountain spotted fever (RMSF) in people. *Rickettsia rickettsii* is transmitted by several hard (Ixodid) ticks including *Dermacentor variabilis* (American dog tick), *Dermacentor andersoni* (Rocky Mountain wood tick), *Amblyomma americanum* (lone star tick), *Amblyomma cajennense* (Cayenne tick), and *Rhipicephalus sanguineus* (brown dog tick). Historically, the geographic distribution of RMSF in the United States has primarily followed that of its primary tick vectors in the region, *D. variabilis* and *D. andersoni*. According to the Center for Disease Control and Prevention (CDC), Arkansas, Missouri, North Carolina, Tennessee, and Virginia account for most cases (cdc.gov and **Fig. 1**).Most cases of canine and human RMSF are reported from spring to late summer, months of peak *Dermacentor* tick activity. Dogs living outdoors, particularly those with access to shrubs and high grass, are at increased risk.

Increasing travel and the effects of climate change on tick populations and habitats are changing the geographic distribution of RMSF and other emerging infectious

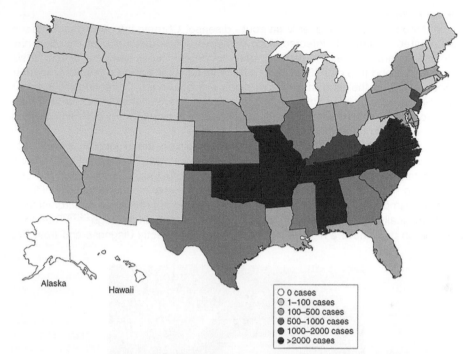

Fig. 1. Geographic distribution of the incidence of spotted fever group rickettsioses in people in the United States, 2010 to 2019. (Used with permission from Ch 46. Spotted Fever Rickettsioses, Flea-borne rickettsioses and Typhus. Kidd L., Breitschwerdt EB. Greene's Infectious Diseases of the Dog and Cat 5th Edition. Ed. JE Sykes Elsevier 2022.)

diseases. For example, in the early 2000s, a fatal outbreak of RMSF in people occurred in a nonendemic area of Arizona.[16] The outbreak was caused by *Rh. sanguineus*. Retrospectively, it was shown that infection existed in the dog population before the fatal outbreak in people.[17] The seasonal incidence of cases in this region is longer than in other regions of the United States.(cdc.gov/rmsf/stats) This is thought to be due to differences in the activity of *Rh. sanguineus* compared with *Dermacentor* ticks.

Rhipicephalus sanguineus is also the primary vector of *R. rickettsii* in Mexico. In South America, *Amblyomma* species are the main vectors. *Amblyomma* ticks are also potential vectors in the United States.[18,19] Veterinarians should consider the possibility of transmission by novel vectors if dogs present with clinical signs of RMSF in nonendemic areas or at an unusual time of year.

Pathophysiology
Rickettsia rickettsii infects endothelial cells. The resulting vasculitis contributes to the development of disordered primary hemostasis, tissue edema, hypovolemia, and microthrombosis. Thrombocytopenia is common and occurs due to vasculitis and possibly immune-mediated platelet destruction.[20] Increased vascular permeability and associated edema and hypovolemia result from the disruption of adherens junctions, endothelial cell death, and expression of inflammatory cytokines. Organisms also induce changes in platelet adherence to endothelium, increased tissue factor expression, increased plasminogen activator inhibitor and cause the release of von-Willebrand factor, all of which likely contribute to microthrombosis.[21,22]

Clinical findings

Rocky Mountain spotted fever is an acute disease. Chronic infection has not been documented in naturally infected dogs. However, recrudescence of infection has been documented in experimentally infected dogs.[23] Low numbers of *Rickettsia* circulate in blood free or in detached endothelial cells for a short period of time after infection. This is the time that clinical signs are observed. Coinfection with other vector-borne agents is common and should be considered if the clinical presentation is atypical, there is an incomplete response to doxycycline therapy or if clinical signs have been present chronically.

Because *R. rickettsii* infects endothelial cells, vasculitis is the major clinical sign associated with infection. Due to variation in the extent and severity of vascular injury among dogs, a range of signs can occur, and disease manifestations are initially mild and nonspecific. The nonspecific nature of the clinical signs makes diagnosis difficult. This is very important because a delay in diagnosis and appropriate antimicrobial therapy dramatically increases morbidity and mortality in people and in dogs.[24,25] Therefore, the clinician must have a high index of suspicion to correctly diagnose and treat this

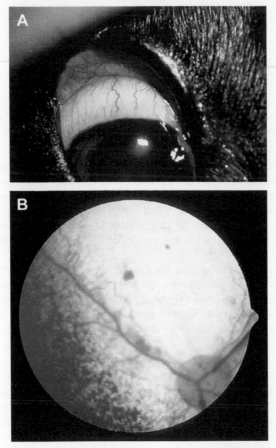

Fig. 2. Ocular complications in dogs with RMSF. *(A)*, Conjunctival hyperemia and scleral injection. *(B)*, Retinal hemorrhages. (Used with permission from Ch 46. Spotted Fever Rickettsioses, Flea-borne rickettsioses and Typhus. Kidd L., Breitschwerdt EB. Greene's Infectious Diseases of the Dog and Cat 5th Edition. Ed. JE Sykes Elsevier 2022.)

disease. This can be difficult because there is often no known history of a tick bite.[24] Lethargy and anorexia are common and may be the only clinical signs. Vomiting and diarrhea occur frequently, which is case context that unfortunately can lead clinicians down a diagnostic path that does not include testing for vector-borne disease. Melena may also occur. Central nervous system abnormalities including vestibular disease and seizures may be observed. Dramatic and rapid weight loss has been described.

Fever and ocular abnormalities are common physical examination findings. Ocular signs may include mucopurulent discharge, scleral and conjunctival injection and hemorrhage, conjunctivitis, uveitis, retinal hemorrhage, and retinitis (**Fig. 2**). Lymphadenomegaly, splenomegaly, nasal discharge, epistaxis, tachypnea, dyspnea, petechiae, ecchymosis, peripheral edema, hyperemia, and necrosis may occur. Cutaneous lesions are not always present in dogs or people. Orchitis and scrotal edema, hyperemia, and epididymal pain are common in intact male dogs. Generalized myalgia and arthralgia can be observed. Central nervous system abnormalities can be focal or generalized and include paraparesis, tetraparesis, ataxia, hyperesthesia, central or peripheral vestibular signs, stupor, seizures, and/or coma. Arrhythmias may be noted. Microvascular hemorrhage, thrombosis, hypotension, oliguric renal failure, cardiovascular collapse, and brain death can occur in severe cases. Thoracic radiographs may show an unstructured interstitial pattern.[26]

Laboratory testing
Importantly, treatment must be instituted before definitive diagnostic tests confirm infection. Because direct inoculation into blood or aerosolization can cause infection, all specimens should be handled with care and marked clearly as biohazards. Avoid needle sticks, contact with cuts in the skin, and aerosolization of rickettsemic blood.

Complete blood counts commonly show thrombocytopenia but it does not occur in all dogs with RMSF. Leukopenia or leukocytosis may be observed. Neutrophils may have toxic change. Nonregenerative anemia may be present. Serum biochemical abnormalities may include hypoalbuminemia, elevated alkaline phosphatase, hyponatremia, and mild hyperbilirubinemia. Prolonged aPTT, PT, and elevated fibrinogen and fibrin degradation products may occur. DIC is uncommon. Urinalysis results are variable and may include proteinuria, hematuria, bilirubinuria, and pyuria. Granular casts can be observed. Cerebral spinal fluid analysis may reveal a mixed cellular, neutrophilic, or lymphocytic pleocytosis. Arthrocentesis may reveal neutrophilic polyarthritis.

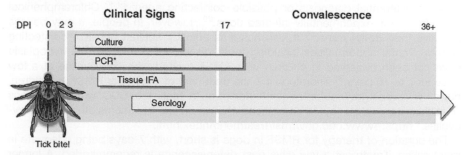

Fig. 3. Timing in relation to day postinfection (DPI) that clinical signs and diagnostic tests for *Rickettsia rickettsii* may be positive in an infected dog. *Further studies are needed to determine exactly how DNA can be detected in peripheral blood after infection. (Used with permission from Ch 46. Spotted Fever Rickettsioses, Flea-borne rickettsioses and Typhus. Kidd L., Breitschwerdt EB. Greene's Infectious Diseases of the Dog and Cat 5th Edition. Ed. JE Sykes Elsevier 2022.)

Cytologic examination of enlarged lymph nodes is consistent with reactive lymphoid hyperplasia.

Active infection with an SFG *Rickettsia* is confirmed in a patient with compatible acute clinical signs and demonstration of the organism using PCR or immunohistochemistry, or documentation of seroconversion. Importantly, serology and PCR can be negative at the time of testing because clinical signs can occur before seroconversion, and organisms circulate transiently in blood in low number (**Fig. 3**).[27] Infection also cannot be definitively diagnosed by documenting a single positive titer because of cross-reactivity with nonpathogenic SFG *Rickettsia* and the potential for long-lived antibody levels after infection. Therefore, documenting a four-fold change in titer is necessary to confirm acute infection with SFG *Rickettsia* using serology. That said, a single high titer in the context of acute and compatible clinical signs and appropriate response to therapy is suggestive of infection.[24] It is important to note that most antibody-based diagnostic tests do not differentiate among species of SFG *Rickettsia*. Some PCR tests can differentiate among species infecting *Rickettsia* while others only amplify conserved rickettsial DNA targets. Veterinarians should check with their laboratory regarding the sensitivity and specificity of a given PCR, keeping in mind that in vitro (absolute) sensitivity is higher than in vivo sensitivity due to the low circulating copy number of *Rickettsia* in blood (see **Fig. 3**). Importantly, a negative PCR test and negative serologic test do not rule out infection or the need for immediate antimicrobial treatment.

Treatment

Appropriate antibiotic therapy must be immediately instituted based on clinical suspicion before diagnostic tests confirm infection. Inappropriate or delayed antibiotic therapy may increase morbidity and mortality.[24] A recent analysis of the human literature showed mortality increased from 4% for patients receiving doxycycline within the first 5 days of illness to 35% when treatment was delayed beyond day five.[28] Treating with an antibiotic that is not effective also allows rapid progression. Some antibiotics such as trimethoprim sulfa may worsen disease in people. Doxycycline (5 mg/kg PO BID) is the treatment of choice. It is highly effective at eliminating *R. rickettsii* in dogs. Furthermore, doxycycline provides effective empiric therapy for *A. phagocytophilum*, *Ehrlichia spp*, and *Borrelia burgdorferi,* agents that are differential diagnoses or may coinfect patients with RMSF. Enrofloxacin has been shown to be effective against *R. rickettsii* in experimentally infected dogs, but it is not effective against *Ehrlichia canis*, a differential diagnosis or possible coinfecting agent.[29,30] Chloramphenicol was effective in experimentally infected dogs.[29] However, in people, it may be less effective than doxycycline.[25] It also has less efficacy against possible coinfecting agents. Dental abnormalities including tooth discoloration and enamel hypoplasia have not been observed in children with RMSF treated with doxycycline at a low dose for 7 to 10 days.[31] Therefore, it is the treatment of choice for RMSF in children. https://www.cdc.gov/rmsf/treatment/index.html In fact, the CDC warns clinicians "Healthcare providers should be cautions when exploring treatments other than doxycycline." https://www.cdc.gov/rmsf/treatment/index.html.

The duration of therapy for RMSF in dogs is short, with 7 days being adequate in most cases. Treatment a few days past defervescence is recommended. A longer course of (doxycycline) therapy is recommended for patients coinfected with an *E spp.* or *B. burgdorferi*. Owners should be warned of the potential, yet possibly low, risk of dental abnormalities if doxycycline is used short term to treat RMSF in puppies.

Many patients require hospitalization. Intravenous antibiotic therapy may be necessary for debilitated patients. Aggressive supportive care for complications such as thrombosis, central nervous system deficits, and gastrointestinal signs may be necessary. Due to the loss in vascular integrity, fluids should be administered with caution and colloids may be warranted in some cases.

The use of corticosteroids in dogs with RMSF is controversial. Anti-inflammatory and immunosuppressive doses did not affect the overall outcome of experimentally infected dogs, but rickettsemia was longer in dogs concurrently treated with doxycycline and immunosuppressive doses of corticosteroids.[32] Of note, the duration of rickettsemia, which was documented using a culture technique, was not determined beyond 10 days postinfection in that study. Anti-inflammatory doses of corticosteroids have been used in dogs with severe CNS manifestations and may be necessary topically or systemically for the treatment of ocular abnormalities.

Response to appropriate antibiotic therapy is very rapid (24–48 hours). Coinfection with *B. burgdorferi*, *Ehrlichia spp*, *Babesia spp*, and *Bartonella spp* or other agents should be considered in dogs with severe or prolonged clinical signs and dogs that fail to respond to doxycycline. Residual central nervous system and other deficits may occur in severely affected patients. A convalescent serum sample should be drawn 2 to 3 weeks after the initial serologic sample in PCR-negative patients to confirm infection.

Prognosis

The prognosis is good to excellent if the disease is diagnosed and treated with appropriate antibiotics and supportive care early in the course of illness.

Public health implications

Human spotted fever rickettsioses are reportable diseases in the United States. The same is true for dogs in some counties. Dogs are sentinels for spotted fever rickettsloses In people. It Is Important for veterinarians to communicate with owners and physicians that infection in a dog may precede tick-transmitted infection to owners or neighbors. It is well established that people living near dogs and with dogs in endemic areas are at increased risk for acquiring RMSF. This results from human exposure to the same environments whereby the dogs acquire ticks, and through interactions with tick-infested dogs. Instruct clients to remove ticks properly and avoid crushing to prevent exposure to infected hemolymph. See http://www.cdc.gov/ticks/removing_a_tick.html for CDC guidelines on appropriate tick removal. Educating owners regarding the importance of tick control and prevention for people, pets, and the environment is critical. In cases whereby *Rh. sanguineus* is the vector, environmental control is particularly important given its proclivity to live within housing structures.

EMERGING SPOTTED FEVER GROUP RICKETTSIOSES IN THE UNITED STATES

The classic geographic distribution of RMSF has been changing, and novel vectors may be contributing to this phenomenon. As mentioned above, RMSF is now present in the Southwest due to *Rh. sanguineus*, a novel vector for *R. rickettsii* in the United States. *Rh. sanguineus* is the primary vector of *R. rickettsii* in Mexico, and an ongoing outbreak in people in Mexicali Mexico, which borders southern California was associated with this tick species, and again, dogs.[33,34] Interestingly, no *R. rickettsii* DNA was amplified from *Rh. sanguineus* ticks collected from dogs at an animal shelter in Imperial county California, just North of the Mexico/California border.[35] In contrast, SFG *Rickettsia*, including *R. rickettsii*, *Rickettsia massiliae*, and *Rickettsia parkeri*, were amplified from *Rh. sanguineus* ticks parasitizing dogs participating in a Mexican government sterilization program near the same region.[36] In addition, a recent serosurvey showed that 12.2% of 752 dogs residing in Imperial county California were seroreactive to SFG *Rickettsia*.[33] Dogs close to the border and taken across the border were significantly more likely to be seroreactive. Genetic differences among lineages of *Rh. sanguineus* and environmental factors may contribute to differences in the prevalence of SFG *Rickettsia* infecting ticks in different, but relatively close, geographic locales.[37]

In South America, *Amblyomma* species are the main vector for *R. rickettsii*. In 2011, *A. americanum* was implicated in the transmission of *R. rickettsii* to a person in North Carolina, and recently this tick was shown to be a competent vector.[18,19] As mentioned above, veterinarians should consider the possibility of transmission by novel vectors if dogs present with clinical signs of RMSF in nonendemic areas or at an unusual time of year.

Spotted fever group (SFG) *Rickettsia* other than *R. rickettsii* have also been implicated as spotted-fever like illness causing agents in people in the United States. Clinical signs of infection with other SFG *Rickettsia* can differ from RMSF. *Rickettsia parkeri* is an SFG *Rickettsia* that is most commonly found in the United States in *Amblyomma maculatum* (Gulf Coast tick). Infection has been increasingly recognized in people in the United States. Because diagnosis is often based on serologic testing, which is not species specific, it is thought that some cases reported to the CDC in previous years as being RMSF were actually infections with this agent.[13] In contrast to RMSF, infection in people is usually associated with the formation of an eschar, a localized inflammatory and necrotic skin lesion with a black crust that forms at the site of the tick bite. The formation of eschars has been associated with other SFG *Rickettsia* infections, and their formation is inversely associated with disease severity.[38] Generally speaking, *R. parkeri* is thought to cause a milder illness than *R. rickettsii* in people. *Rickettsia parkeri* was also recently amplified from ill people after hiking in southern Arizona.[39] The suspected vector was *Amblyomma triste*, a Neotropical species recently recognized in the United States. *Rickettsia parkeri* was amplified using PCR from 13% of 93 dogs residing in shelters in Southern Louisiana.[40] The dogs did not have clinical signs of illness, whether hematologic or other abnormalities were present was not investigated. DNA from *R. parkeri* has also been recently amplified from *Rh. sanguineus* parasitizing dogs at the United States Mexico border.[36]

R. massiliae, another *SFG Rickettsia* has been implicated as a disease-causing agent in people in the United States and elsewhere. Recently, infection with *R. massiliae* was suspected in ill, seropositive dogs infested with *R. massiliae* infected *Rh. sanguineus* ticks in Los Angeles county California.[11] This species of SFG *Rickettsia* has also been amplified from *Rh. sanguineus* ticks in Arizona, the US–Mexico Border, and the Eastern United States.[36,41,42]

Rickettsia amblyommatis (formerly *Can.* Rickettsia amblyommii), and *R. montanensis*, (Formerly *Rickettsia montana*) are thought to be nonpathogenic endosymbionts of ticks. Exposure is common in dogs in areas endemic to *R. rickettsii*, which can complicate serodiagnosis of RMSF due to crossreactivity.[43] Recent evidence suggests that these organisms may be capable of causing illness in some people.[44,45] Experimental infection of beagles with *R. montana* (*R. montanensis*) did not result in seroconversion or illness.[46] DNA from *R. amblyommii* and *R. montanensis* was recently amplified from the blood of 2 naturally infected dogs who did not seem clinically ill.[47] Taken together, these data suggest that if these organisms can cause disease in dogs it is uncommon.

Pacific Coast Fever is another spotted fever rickettsioses of increasing importance in the Western United States' people.[38] It is caused by *Rickettsia* strain 364D (proposed name *R. philipii*), and transmitted by *Dermacentor occidentalis*, the Pacific

Coast Tick. The disease is less severe than RMSF and, like other milder spotted fever rickettsioses, is often associated with an eschar at the region of the tick bite. Whether this organism infects or causes illness in dogs is not known.

Recently, infection with a novel SFG *Rickettsia* closely related to *R. massiliae* and *R. heilongjiangensis* was documented in three dogs in the United States with clinical signs and laboratory abnormalities associated with RMSF.[48] In addition, several SFG *Rickettsia* were identified in large study of *Dermacentor* ticks parasitizing dogs and cats in the United States.[49] *Rickettsia* species were identified in 12.5% of ticks and included *R. montanensis*, *R. bellii*, *R. rhipicephali*, *R. peacocki*, *R. amblyommatis*, *R. cooleyi*, and unclassified *Rickettsia* species. Whether these agents might cause disease in individual patients continues to be elucidated.

SPOTTED FEVER RICKETTSIOSES IN CATS

Although antibodies to *R. rickettsii* are detected in cats in endemic areas, active infection and associated clinical signs have not been documented. Antibodies to several other SFG *Rickettsia* have been detected in cats, and recently, DNA from some SFG *Rickettsia* species most closely resembling *R. massiliae* Bar29 and *R. conorii* has been amplified from naturally infected cats.[50] DNA from "*Candidatus* Rickettsia senegalensis" was also recently amplified from the blood of 2 cats in Riverside county CA.[51] The ability of SFG *Rickettsia* to cause disease in cats is not known.

RICKETTSIA AKARI AND *RICKETTSIA FELIS* INFECTIONS IN DOGS AND CATS

Although there is an ongoing debate over whether *R. akari* and *R. felis* belong in the same phylogenetic group as other SFG rickettsia, the disease they cause in people is similar to other spotted fever rickettsioses.[2,3] *Rickettsia akari* is transmitted by mites primarily in urban areas. Exposure to *R. akari* has been documented in dogs from New York City.[52] In addition, *R. akari* DNA was amplified from the peripheral blood of an 8-month old dog from Mexico with clinical and laboratory abnormalities similar to RMSF that were rapidly doxycycline responsive.[53] The organism was also amplified from 2 *Rh. sanguineus* ticks parasitizing the dog, prompting the authors to suggest that a vector other than mites may be possible.

Rickettsia felis is primarily transmitted by *Ctenocephalides felis* in the continental United States. The disease is endemic in Southern and Central Texas and California. In people, it causes disease similar to that caused by a typhus group *Rickettsia*, *R. typhi*. However, despite its vector, as mentioned above, it is more closely genetically related to SFG *Rickettsia* so it is included in this article. Opossums are an important reservoir as they live in close proximity to humans and cats and harbor high loads of cat fleas. Indoor/outdoor cats may be infested with cat fleas which then infect the cat's human companions.[54] Although experimental and natural exposure and infection have been documented in cats and dogs, the role of it as a disease-causing agent in companion animals is not well defined.[51,55,56] However, it is clear that flea control and reducing exposure to opossums is absolutely essential to reduce the zoonotic risk of illness in people.

SUMMARY

Rocky Mountain spotted fever causes an acute febrile illness in dogs and people. Both PCR and serology may be negative at the time of presentation. Doxycycline therapy must be initiated based on clinical suspicion to prevent death and morbidity. Response to therapy is very rapid. Dogs are sentinels for disease in people. The geographic distribution of RMSF is expanding. The role of other SFG *Rickettsia* as disease-causing agents in cats and dogs continues to be elucidated. Flea and tick control is important from a One Health perspective to protect dogs, cats, and their human companions.

CLINICS CARE POINTS

- Rocky Mountain spotted fever, caused by *R. rickettsii* causes a febrile, acute illness in dogs.
- Dogs are sentinels for infection in their human companions; therefore, notify clients to contact a physician immediately if they feel ill when RMSF is suspected in a canine patient.
- Both PCR and serologic testing may be negative when dogs are clinically ill.
- Doxycycline must be started immediately based on clinical suspicion.
- Combining PCR with serologic testing, repeat testing using PCR, and testing convalescent serum for seroconversion may be necessary to confirm the diagnosis.
- The prognosis is excellent if appropriate antimicrobial therapy is begun in a timely fashion.
- Infection from exposure to novel vectors or with novel agents should be considered if cases present in unusual geographic locales or times of year.

DISCLOSURE

Paid speaker and consultant for Zoetis and IDEXX laboratories. Currently employed at Zoetis.

REFERENCES

1. Fang R, Blanton LS, Walker DH. Rickettsiae as Emerging Infectious Agents. Clin Lab Med 2017;37:383–400.
2. Gillespie JJ, Williams K, Shukla M, et al. Rickettsia phylogenomics: unwinding the intricacies of obligate intracellular life. PLoS One 2008;3:e2018.
3. El Karkouri K, Ghigo E, Raoult D, et al. Genomic evolution and adaptation of arthropod-associated Rickettsia. Sci Rep 2022;12:3807.
4. Solano-Gallego L, Kidd L, Trotta M, et al. Febrile illness associated with Rickettsia conorii infection in dogs from Sicily. Emerg Infect Dis 2006;12:1985–8.
5. Solano-Gallego L, Capri A, Pennisi MG, et al. Acute febrile illness is associated with Rickettsia spp infection in dogs. Parasit Vectors 2015;8:216.
6. Shapiro MR, Fritz CL, Tait K, et al. Rickettsia 364D: a newly recognized cause of eschar-associated illness in California. Clin Infect Dis 2010;50:541–8.
7. Parola P, Paddock CD, Raoult D. Tick-borne rickettsioses around the world: emerging diseases challenging old concepts. Clin Microbiol Rev 2005;18: 719–56.
8. Cragun WC, Bartlett BL, Ellis MW, et al. The expanding spectrum of eschar-associated rickettsioses in the United States. Arch Dermatol 2010;146:641–8.
9. Raoult D, Parola P. Rocky Mountain spotted fever in the USA: a benign disease or a common diagnostic error? Lancet Infect Dis 2008;8:587–9.
10. Padgett KA, Bonilla D, Eremeeva ME, et al. The Eco-epidemiology of Pacific Coast Tick Fever in California. Plos Negl Trop Dis 2016;10:e0005020.
11. Beeler E, Abramowicz KF, Zambrano ML, et al. A focus of dogs and Rickettsia massiliae-infected Rhipicephalus sanguineus in California. Am J Trop Med Hyg 2011;84:244–9.

12. Johnston SH, Glaser CA, Padgett K, et al. Rickettsia spp. 364D causing a cluster of eschar-associated illness, California. Pediatr Infect Dis J 2013;32:1036–9.

13. Parola P, Labruna MB, Raoult D. Tick-borne rickettsioses in America: unanswered questions and emerging diseases. Curr Infect Dis Rep 2009;11:40–50.

14. Parola P, Paddock CD, Socolovschi C, et al. Update on tick-borne rickettsioses around the world: a geographic approach. Clin Microbiol Rev 2013;26:657–702.

15. Drexler NA, Dahlgren FS, Heitman KN, et al. National Surveillance of Spotted Fever Group Rickettsioses in the United States, 2008-2012. Am J Trop Med Hyg 2016;94:26–34.

16. Demma LJ, Traeger MS, Nicholson WL, et al. Rocky Mountain spotted fever from an unexpected tick vector in Arizona. N Engl J Med 2005;353:587–94.

17. Nicholson WL, Gordon R, Demma LJ. Spotted fever group rickettsial infection in dogs from eastern Arizona: how long has it been there? Ann N Y Acad Sci 2006; 1078:519–22.

18. Breitschwerdt EB, Hegarty BC, Maggi RG, et al. Rickettsia rickettsii Transmission by a Lone Star Tick, North Carolina. Emerg Infect Dis 2011;17:873–5.

19. Levin ML, Zemtsova GE, Killmaster LF, et al. Vector competence of Amblyomma americanum (Acari: Ixodidae) for Rickettsia rickettsii. Ticks Tick Borne Dis 2017; 8:615–22.

20. Grindem CB, Breitschwerdt EB, Perkins PC, et al. Platelet-associated immunoglobulin (antiplatelet antibody) in canine Rocky Mountain spotted fever and ehrlichiosis. J Am Anim Hosp Assoc 1999;35:56–61.

21. Sahni SK, Rydkina E. Host-cell interactions with pathogenic Rickettsia species. Future Microbiol 2009;4:323–39.

22. Mansueto P, Vitale G, Cascio A, et al. New insight into immunity and immunopathology of Rickettsial diseases. Clin Dev Immunol 2012;2012:967852.

23. Levin ML, Killmaster LF, Zemtsova GE, et al. Clinical presentation, convalescence, and relapse of rocky mountain spotted fever in dogs experimentally infected via tick bite. PLoS One 2014;9:e115105.

24. Gasser AM, Birkenheuer AJ, Breitschwerdt EB. Canine Rocky Mountain Spotted fever: a retrospective study of 30 cases. J Am Anim Hosp Assoc 2001;37:41–8.

25. Biggs HM, Behravesh CB, Bradley KK, et al. Diagnosis and Management of Tickborne Rickettsial Diseases: Rocky Mountain Spotted Fever and Other Spotted Fever Group Rickettsioses, Ehrlichioses, and Anaplasmosis - United States. MMWR Recomm Rep 2016;65:1–44.

26. Drost WT, Berry CR, Breitschwerdt EB, et al. Thoracic radiographic findings in dogs infected with Rickettsia rickettsii. Vet Radiol Ultrasound 1997;38:260–6.

27. Kidd L, Maggi R, Diniz PP, et al. Evaluation of conventional and real-time PCR assays for detection and differentiation of Spotted Fever Group Rickettsia in dog blood. Vet Microbiol 2008;129:294–303.

28. Jay R, Armstrong PA. Clinical characteristics of Rocky Mountain spotted fever in the United States: A literature review. J Vector Borne Dis 2020;57:114–20.

29. Breitschwerdt EB, Davidson MG, Aucoin DP, et al. Efficacy of chloramphenicol, enrofloxacin, and tetracycline for treatment of experimental Rocky Mountain spotted fever in dogs. Antimicrob Agents Chemother 1991;35:2375–81.

30. Neer TM, Eddlestone SM, Gaunt SD, et al. Efficacy of enrofloxacin for the treatment of experimentally induced Ehrlichia canis infection. J Vet Intern Med 1999;13:501–4.

31. Todd SR, Dahlgren FS, Traeger MS, et al. No visible dental staining in children treated with doxycycline for suspected Rocky Mountain Spotted Fever. J Pediatr 2015;166:1246–51.

32. Breitschwerdt EB, Davidson MG, Hegarty BC, et al. Prednisolone at anti-inflammatory or immunosuppressive dosages in conjunction with doxycycline does not potentiate the severity of Rickettsia rickettsii infection in dogs. Antimicrob Agents Chemother 1997;41:141–7.

33. Estrada I, Balagot C, Fierro M, et al. Spotted fever group rickettsiae canine serosurveillance near the US-Mexico border in California. Zoonoses Public Health 2020;67:148–55.

34. Alvarez-Hernandez G, Roldan JFG, Milan NSH, et al. Rocky Mountain spotted fever in Mexico: past, present, and future. Lancet Infect Dis 2017;17:e189–96.

35. Fritz CL, Kriner P, Garcia D, et al. Tick infestation and spotted-fever group Rickettsia in shelter dogs, California, 2009. Zoonoses Public Health 2012;59:4–7.

36. Pieracci EG, De La Rosa JDP, Rubio DL, et al. Seroprevalence of spotted fever group rickettsiae in canines along the United States-Mexico border. Zoonoses Public Health 2019;66:918–26.

37. Rene-Martellet M, Minard G, Massot R, et al. Bacterial microbiota associated with Rhipicephalus sanguineus (s.l.) ticks from France, Senegal and Arizona. Parasit Vectors 2017;10:416.

38. Drexler N, Nichols Heitman K, Cherry C. Description of Eschar-Associated Rickettsial Diseases Using Passive Surveillance Data - United States, 2010-2016. MMWR Morb Mortal Wkly Rep 2020;68:1179–82.

39. Herrick KL, Pena SA, Yaglom HD, et al. Rickettsia parkeri Rickettsiosis, Arizona, USA. Emerg Infect Dis 2016;22:780–5.

40. Grasperge BJ, Wolfson W, Macaluso KR. Rickettsia parkeri infection in domestic dogs, Southern Louisiana, USA, 2011. Emerg Infect Dis 2012;18:995–7.

41. Fornadel CM, Smith JD, Zawada SE, et al. Detection of Rickettsia massiliae in Rhipicephalus sanguineus from the eastern United States. Vector Borne Zoonotic Dis 2013;13:67–9.

42. Eremeeva ME, Bosserman EA, Demma LJ, et al. Isolation and identification of Rickettsia massiliae from Rhipicephalus sanguineus ticks collected in Arizona. Appl Environ Microbiol 2006;72:5569–77.

43. Hoskins JD, Breitschwerdt EB, Gaunt SD, et al. Antibodies to Ehrlichia canis, Ehrlichia platys, and spotted fever group rickettsiae in Louisiana dogs. J Vet Intern Med 1988;2:55–9.

44. Billeter SA, Blanton HL, Little SE, et al. Detection of Rickettsia amblyommii in association with a tick bite rash. Vector Borne Zoonotic Dis 2007;7:607–10.

45. Delisle J, Mendell NL, Stull-Lane A, et al. Human Infections by Multiple Spotted Fever Group Rickettsiae in Tennessee. Am J Trop Med Hyg 2016;94:1212–7.

46. Breitschwerdt EB, Walker DH, Levy MG, et al. Clinical, hematologic, and humoral immune response in female dogs inoculated with Rickettsia rickettsii and Rickettsia montana. Am J Vet Res 1988;49:70–6.

47. Barrett A, Little SE, Shaw E. Rickettsia amblyommii" and R. montanensis infection in dogs following natural exposure to ticks. Vector Borne Zoonotic Dis 2014;14:20–5.

48. Wilson JM, Breitschwerdt EB, Juhasz NB, et al. Novel Rickettsia Species Infecting Dogs, United States. Emerg Infect Dis 2020;26:3011–5.

49. Duncan KT, Grant A, Johnson B, et al. Identification of Rickettsia spp. and Babesia conradae in Dermacentor spp. Collected from Dogs and Cats Across the United States. Vector Borne Zoonotic Dis 2021;21:911–20.

50. Segura F, Pons I, Miret J, et al. The role of cats in the eco-epidemiology of spotted fever group diseases. Parasit Vectors 2014;7:353.
51. Mullins KE, Maina AN, Krueger L, et al. Rickettsial Infections among Cats and Cat Fleas in Riverside County, California. Am J Trop Med Hyg 2018;99:291–6.
52. Comer JA, Vargas MC, Poshni I, et al. Serologic evidence of Rickettsia akari infection among dogs in a metropolitan city. J Am Vet Med Assoc 2001;218: 1780–2.
53. Zavala-Castro JE, Zavala-Velazquez JE, del Rosario Garcia M, et al. A dog naturally infected with Rickettsia akari in Yucatan, Mexico. Vector Borne Zoonotic Dis 2009;9:345–7.
54. Anstead GM. History, Rats, Fleas, and Opossums. II. The Decline and Resurgence of Flea-Borne Typhus in the United States, 1945-2019. Trop Med Infect Dis 2020;6.
55. Hoque MM, Barua S, Kelly PJ, et al. Identification of Rickettsia felis DNA in the blood of domestic cats and dogs in the USA. Parasit Vectors 2020;13:581.
56. Nelson K, Maina AN, Brisco A, et al. A 2015 outbreak of flea-borne rickettsiosis in San Gabriel Valley, Los Angeles County, California. Plos Negl Trop Dis 2018;12: e0006385.

Hemotropic Mycoplasma

Séverine Tasker, BSc (Hons), BVSc (Hons), DSAM, PhD, FHEA, FRCVS

KEYWORDS

- Hemoplasma • Hemoparasite • Infectious anemia • Vector-borne disease
- Zoonosis

KEY POINTS

- Hemoplasma infections are erythrocytic infections found in both cats and dogs but are more common, and more often associated with disease, in cats.
- *Mycoplasma haemofelis* is the most pathogenic species in cats, causing hemolytic anemia and fever in immunocompetent hosts, whereas *Mycoplasma haemocanis* usually only results in hemolytic anemia in dogs that are splenectomized or immunocompromised.
- Diagnosis is by polymerase chain reaction on blood samples because cytology is unreliable.
- Prompt treatment of clinical disease with supportive care and at least 2 weeks of doxycycline is usually successful.
- Transmission pathways have not been confirmed, but indirect, via vectors, and direct via bites/fights/predation are likely.

INTRODUCTION

The hemotropic mycoplasmas (hemoplasmas) are small (0.3–1.0 μm) wall-less gram-negative bacteria that infect erythrocytes; most species live on the erythrocyte surface (**Fig. 1**), but a porcine hemoplasma species has been shown to reside intracellularly within erythrocytes. Hemoplasmas infect a wide range of hosts worldwide including cats, dogs, rodents, pigs, cattle, sheep, horses, bats, beetles, and people. Infection can result in a hemolytic anemia of variable severity, depending on the host and the infecting hemoplasma species. Individual hemoplasma species can also comprise several genotypes,[1] so it is possible that different genotypes of a species influence pathogenicity.

HEMOPLASMA CLASSIFICATION

The hemoplasmas were initially classified as rickettsial organisms within the Haemobartonella and Eperythrozoon genera, but sequence analysis of the 16S rRNA gene of hemoplasmas resulted in their reclassification within the genus *Mycoplasma*.[2–4]

Bristol Veterinary School, University of Bristol, Langford, Bristol BS40 5DU, United Kingdom & Linnaeus Veterinary Limited, Shirley, B90 4BN, United Kingdom
E-mail address: s.tasker@bristol.ac.uk

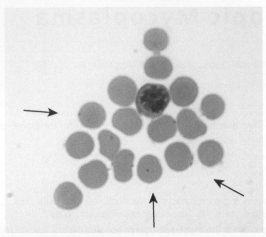

Fig. 1. Romanowsky-stained blood smear from an 8-year-old male neutered domestic short-hair cat showing epierythrocytic bacteria typical of *Mycoplasma haemofelis* (*arrows*), reproduced with permission.[159]

Although hemoplasmas share similarities with the mycoplasmas, such as small size, fastidious in vitro growth requirements, and absence of a cell wall, they also differ in their target cell (erythrocyte rather than mucosal cells). It has been proposed that hemoplasmas warrant being in a separate genus to that of the *Mycoplasma* species within the family Mycoplasmatale.[5]

HEMOPLASMA SPECIES INFECTING CATS AND DOGS

Several different species of hemoplasma exist, which vary in pathogenicity (**Table 1**). Three major species infect cats:

- *Mycoplasma haemofelis*
- '*Candidatus* Mycoplasma haemominutum'
- '*Candidatus* Mycoplasma turicensis'

Two major species infect dogs:

- *Mycoplasma haemocanis*
- '*Candidatus* Mycoplasma haematoparvum'

Occasionally '*Ca* M turicensis',[6,7] '*Ca*. M. haemominutum',[6,8–10] and a species similar to the latter,[11] have been detected in dogs, as has the ovine *Mycoplasma ovis*,[12] the bovine '*Candidatus* Mycoplasma haemobos',[13–15] and the porcine *Mycoplasma suis*.[16] A '*Ca*. M. haematoparvum'-like organism has also been reported in a small number of cats.[17,18] Of these species *M. haemofelis* and *M. haemocanis* are the most pathogenic and important species in cats and dogs, respectively.

PREVALENCE OF HEMOPLASMAS IN CATS AND DOGS

Hemoplasma prevalence figures vary greatly in different studies; this may be due to differences in geography/climate (which may influence possible vector distribution), whether the cats and dogs sampled are healthy and/or anemic, sample types (eg, blood or tissue samples) and detection methods used (eg, cytology, polymerase chain reaction [PCR], and whether PCR assays detect/distinguish all hemoplasma species

Table 1
Hemoplasma species infecting cats and dogs, their prevalences determined by polymerase chain reaction (PCR) in global studies, and an outline of their pathogenicity

Hemoplasma Species Name	Host Species	Reported PCR Prevalence Range (Median)	Outline of Pathogenicity
Mycoplasma haemofelis	Cat	0.0%–28.6% (4.8%)	Acute infection can result in hemolytic anemia and fever in immunocompetent cats
'Candidatus Mycoplasma haemominutum'[a]	Cat	0.0%–66.7% (14.6%)	Acute infection induces a decrease in erythrocyte values, but hemolytic anemia does not usually result unless cat has comorbidities or is immunocompromised, eg, retrovirus infection, neoplasia
'Candidatus Mycoplasma turicensis'[a]	Cat	0.0%–10.0% (1.4%)	
Mycoplasma haemocanis	Dog	0.0%–52.4% (7.6%)	Infection can result in hemolytic anemia in splenectomized dogs
'Candidatus Mycoplasma haematoparvum'[a]	Dog	0.0%–33.3% (2.0%)	Hemolytic anemia does not usually result unless dog has concurrent disease or is immunocompromised, eg, chemotherapy

[a] Some species have the status Candidatus, which is the name used for newly described species for which genetic sequence data are available but which cannot be phenotypically characterized to the level required by the International Code of Nomenclature of Bacteria due to the inability to grow them in vitro.[160] The species M. haemofelis and M. haemocanis do not have the Candidatus status, even though they have not yet been grown in vitro, because they represent the previously existing Haemobartonella felis and Haemobartonella canis species, respectively. Bacterial nomenclature forbids the "demotion" of any bacterial species, including during renaming.

in that host animal). **Table 1** shows the major published prevalence ranges for each hemoplasma species based on the use of PCR as diagnosis:

- In cats, 'Ca. M. haemominutum' is the most common species, followed by M. haemofelis and then 'Ca M turicensis'
- In dogs, M. haemocanis is usually the more common species, then 'Ca. M. haematoparvum'
- Dual, and triple in cats, hemoplasma species infections can occur. 'Ca. M. turicensis'-infected cats are often dual infected with another hemoplasma species, especially 'Ca. M. haemominutum'

WHAT RISK FACTORS EXIST FOR HEMOPLASMA INFECTION?
Feline Hemoplasmas

In cats, many studies have found that male, older, nonpedigrees with outdoor access are more likely to be infected with feline hemoplasmas (especially 'Ca. M. haemominutum').[1,17,19–32] Some studies have also shown significant associations for all or some hemoplasma species and retrovirus infection,[17,18,20,22,23,28,29,33–35] especially feline immunodeficiency virus [FIV],[21,27,36–42] whereas others have not.[31,43,44] An association between anemia/reduced erythrocyte values and hemoplasma infection (especially *M. haemofelis*) is sometimes seen in studies[24–26,32,33,38,40,42,45–47] but is often not present,[18–21,28,31,37,38,48–52] probably due to the existence of chronic subclinical infections. In one US study, '*Ca*. M. haemominutum'-infected cats were less likely to be anemic than non-'*Ca*. M. haemominutum'-infected cats.[17] Only a few studies have looked at the presence of vectors as risk factors for feline hemoplasma infection, and in these, no association has been found with either fleas[18,53] or ticks.[18]

Canine Hemoplasmas

In one large study, in dogs, kenneled, young crossbreeds and those with mange were more likely to be hemoplasma infected,[54] whereas other studies have found no association with age[21,55–62] or found that dogs older than one[63,64] or two[7] years were more likely to be infected. An association between being male and hemoplasma status has only been reported in a few canine studies,[7,56,65] whereas most do not find an association with gender,[11,15,21,41,54–62,66–68] in contrast to feline hemoplasmas. An association with anemia is not commonly found,[21,54–59,69,70] with pathogenicity largely confined to case reports of symptomatic dogs.

Hemoplasma infection is said to be common in fighting dogs,[70–72] which suggests that horizontal transmission may be possible between dogs. Potential vectors are also implicated as risk factors for canine hemoplasma infections. In some studies, associations exist between canine hemoplasma infections and both other vector-borne infections,[21,67] particularly *Babesia* spp (notably *Babesia vulpis* and *Babesia gibsoni*),[70,72–74] and the presence of ticks[15,65,67] or ectoparasites in general.[11,68] Other studies have failed to show any association with ticks,[56,57,63] so results are variable. Living in a rural[7,63] or free-roaming[13,41,67] setting may also be a risk factor for canine hemoplasma infection.

PATHOGENESIS OF HEMOPLASMA INFECTION
Mycoplasma haemofelis

This is the most pathogenic of the feline hemoplasma species, with acute infection causing severe hemolytic anemia (primarily extravascular, but occasionally intravascular is reported[75]) in immunocompetent cats with no other comorbidities. Osmotic fragility[75,76] and reduced erythrocyte lifespan[77] occur. Younger cats are likely to develop severe clinical disease.[78] A regenerative response with reticulocytosis occurs following anemia.[29] Acute *M. haemofelis* infection can also be associated with the development of erythrocyte-bound antibodies, demonstrable by the presence of persistent autoagglutination or a positive Coombs' tests,[76,80,81] although the role of these antibodies in the development of anemia is not known[81] and cats with erythrocyte-bound antibodies respond to antibiotic and supportive treatment alone, without the need for specific glucocorticoid treatment. Experimental infections have shown that *M. haemofelis* blood organism numbers can markedly fluctuate over the course of a day or two in the first few weeks of infection, possibly due to antigenic variation and evasion of host immunity,[82] important to consider when interpreting PCR results. In addition, chronic *M. haemofelis* infection is usually subclinical with no anemia.[31]

'*Ca*. M. haemominutum'

This species is less pathogenic, rarely causing clinical anemia, but infection is associated with a small fall in erythrocyte numbers.[81] Cats with comorbidities (eg, lymphoma, immunosuppression or feline leukemia virus [FeLV] infection)[83,84] are more likely to develop anemia following '*Ca*. M. haemominutum' infection; however, splenectomized cats do not seem to be at an increased risk of developing disease.[85]

Nevertheless, there are reports of primary 'Ca. M. haemominutum' anemia in cats without comorbidities.[86]

'Ca M. turicensis'

Our understanding of the pathogenesis of 'Ca. M. turicensis' is more limited. Experimental infection can result in anemia[75] or a small decrease in erythrocyte numbers,[81] but generally clinical anemia is not common. Comorbidities are both thought to be involved in the pathogenesis of 'Ca. M. turicensis' disease,[32,75] as for 'Ca. M. haemominutum'.

M. haemocanis and 'Ca. M. Haematoparvum'

Less data are available on the pathogenesis of canine hemoplasma species, and anemia is not commonly associated with infection.[87] Infection with M. haemocanis and 'Ca. M. haematoparvum' usually only results in hemolytic anemia in splenectomized or immunocompromised dogs.[88–96]

Subclinical Carrier Status of Hemoplasmas

Long-term subclinical carrier status can occur in both cats and dogs with hemoplasma infections.[30,55,97] Subclinical infections are particularly common with 'Ca. M. haemominutum' infection, although clearance of infection can occur with and without antibiotic treatment.[31] Some M. haemofelis- and 'Ca. M. turicensis'-infected cats spontaneously clear infection a few months following acute infection. The host immune response, as well as infecting species, is likely to be play a role in the outcome of hemoplasma infection. Reactivation of infection can result in clinical disease, but this seems to be rare.[78,98–100]

Immunity to Hemoplasmas

The existence of dual and triple hemoplasma infections in hosts suggests that cross protection across the hemoplasma species does not occur. Indeed, a study has shown that not only were 'Ca. M. turicensis'-recovered cats not protected against M. haemofelis challenge, they became PCR-positive for M. haemofelis significantly earlier than the naive cats, suggesting possible antibody-dependent enhancement.[101] Furthermore, passive immunization via transfusion of a small volume of pooled plasma from M. haemofelis-recovered cats failed to provide protection from infection with M. haemofelis and may have exacerbated clinical disease.[102] M. haemofelis- and 'Ca. M. turicensis'-recovered cats are protected against rechallenge with the same species,[103,104] suggesting immunity due to previous infection; this may suggest that if animals do clear infection after acute hemoplasmosis, they may be immune to reinfection with the same species but still susceptible to infection by other hemoplasma species infections, possibly with more severe disease.

HOW ARE HEMOPLASMA SPECIES TRANSMITTED?
Multiple Modes of Transmission

The natural route of transmission of feline and canine hemoplasma species in the field has not yet been determined, and it may be that different routes predominate for different host and hemoplasma species. Indeed, recent pioneering work on the transmission of 'Ca. M. haemominutum' in domestic and wild felids[1] suggests that multiple transmission pathways exist concurrently. These pathways include indirect spread (ie, vector-borne) and direct spread (via predation, of larger cats over smaller cats, or fighting), and it will be interesting for future work to evaluate other hemoplasmas using a similar approach.

Indirect Vector-Borne Transmission

Evidence for the presence of canine and feline hemoplasmas, usually via PCR studies amplifying hemoplasma DNA, has been found in fleas, ticks, and mosquitoes[53,79,105–113], although the numbers of samples testing positive vary widely. However, this does not confirm that these vectors mediate transmission, because the presence of hemoplasmas could simply reflect the vectors' hematophagous activity on infected hosts.

Fleas

Although *Ctenocephalides felis* has been implicated in hemoplasma transmission in cats, evidence for this is very limited. Only very transient *M. haemofelis* (and not '*Ca.* M. haemominutum') infection has been reported in a small study of cats experimentally infected via the hematophagous activity of fleas, and clinical and hematologic signs of *M. haemofelis* infection were not induced in the recipient cat.[114] Another study did not detect any evidence of transmission of either *M. haemofelis* or '*Ca.* M. haemominutum' to cats by the ingestion of hemoplasma-infected fleas.[115] In addition, there was no evidence of hemoplasma transmission when fleas were introduced into groups of cats housed together.[116]

Ticks

Published studies do support ticks being a vector for canine hemoplasma transmission. Experimental transmission of *M. haemocanis* by the brown dog tick, *Rhipicephalus sanguineus,* has been reported, although this study was performed before the development of sensitive and specific molecular diagnostic methods to confirm transmission.[106] The clustered geographic distribution of infection in some studies supports the role of an arthropod vector in feline hemoplasma transmission,[17] and hemoplasma prevalences in dogs can vary according to the presence of *R. sanguineus*.[54,55,61,65] Associations also exist between canine hemoplasma infections and other vector-borne infections, particularly *Babesia vulpis* and *Babesia gibsoni*, and ticks and other ectoparasites, also supporting vector transmission.

Direct Spread via Fighting

Fights and biting are likely to transmit hemoplasmas. Studies have found that subcutaneous inoculation of '*Ca.* M. turicensis'-containing blood resulted in infection transmission, whereas '*Ca.* M. turicensis'-containing saliva did not. A high prevalence of hemoplasma infection has also been reported in fighting dogs.[70,71] Thus hemoplasma transmission by social contact (saliva via mutual grooming, and so on) is less likely than transmission by aggressive interactions (blood transmission during a cat bite incident).[117]

Vertical Transmission

Vertical transmission of hemoplasmas in dogs and cats has not been definitively proven using molecular methods but has been strongly suggested for *M haemocanis*.[118]

Blood Transfusion

Fresh blood transfusions can transmit hemoplasmas[119] so blood donors should be screened for all hemoplasma species infection.[120–122]

CLINICAL SIGNS AND PHYSICAL EXAMINATION

When anemia results from hemoplasma infection, common clinical signs reported include lethargy, pallor, weakness, inappetence, dehydration, weight loss, and intermittent fever. Splenomegaly may also be evident on physical examination, although dogs with clinical hemoplasmosis usually have a history of splenectomy (a predisposing factor in the development of clinical disease). Severe anemia may result in tachycardia, tachypnea, and weak or bounding femoral pulses with hemic cardiac murmurs. Icterus is uncommon despite the severe nature of the hemolytic anemia involved.

DIFFERENTIAL DIAGNOSIS

Hemoplasmosis should be considered as a differential diagnosis in cats or dogs presenting with regenerative anemia, especially with fever. Other diagnoses to consider are primary (nonassociative) immune-mediated hemolytic anemia,[93,94] secondary (associative) immune-mediated hemolytic anemia (eg, to drugs, neoplasia, other infectious diseases including feline infectious peritonitis), babesiosis, cytauxzoonosis (cats), retroviral infection (cats), Heinz body-associated hemolysis (cats), hypophosphatemia, and inherited red blood cell disorders (eg, pyruvate kinase deficiency, and red cell fragility disorders).

DIAGNOSIS
Hematology

Hematology typically reveals a macrocytic hypochromic regenerative anemia, although sometimes the reticulocytosis is minimal.[123] Nucleated erythrocytes may also feature on hematology. Other features of hematology tend to remain within the reference range. Manual reticulocyte counts should be interpreted with care because hemoplasma-infected erythrocytes can appear like reticulocytes in blood smears stained with new methylene blue. As mentioned earlier, cases with erythrocyte-bound antibodies can give positive Coombs' test results or show persistent autoagglutination.

Blood Smear Cytology

Cytologic examination of blood smears may show hemoplasmas on the surface of erythrocytes, but cytology, although quick and possible in-house, is unreliable especially for those without experience of reading blood smears. Specificity is an issue because it is difficult to differentiate hemoplasma organisms from stain precipitate (careful staining with filtered Romanowsky-type stain solutions [eg, Wright-Giemsa or Diff-Quik] is essential), Howell-Jolly bodies, and basophilic stippling. Specificity is good at 84% to 98% when smears are examined by specialist clinical pathologists.[26,30,45,124] Cytology is very insensitive (0%–37.5%),[26,30,45,124,125] and only when huge numbers of organisms are present in the blood (likely only early in acute infections) can they be visualized on blood smears; indeed 'Ca. M. turicensis' has never been seen on blood smears due to the low numbers of organisms present in the blood during infection.[31,126] Blood smear examination cannot differentiate between hemoplasma species.[127] It is advisable to submit blood smears to an external laboratory with expertise in their interpretation to maximise specificity, despite the delay in reporting results that this may bring. As M. haemocanis organisms tend to form chains (Fig. 2), they can be more readily recognized on cytology because chain formation allows differentiation from stain precipitate and erythrocyte morphologic changes.

Serum Biochemistry

Biochemistry may reveal hyperbilirubinemia, due to hemolysis, although this is not usually severe. Hypoxic damage to the liver may result in increased activities of alanine

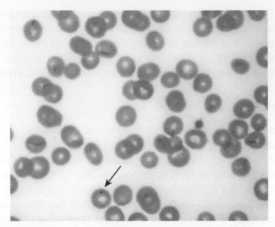

Fig. 2. Romanowsky-stained blood smear showing chains of epierythrocytic bacteria typical of *M. haemocanis*. A Howell-Jolly body is also present (*arrow*), reproduced with permission.[159]

aminotransferase and aspartate transaminase. Hyperproteinemia, due to a polyclonal gammopathy, sometimes occurs.[7,101]

Retrovirus Testing

Tests for FeLV and FIV infection may be positive, especially in cats showing more severe clinical signs than expected.

Urinalysis

Urinalysis is usually unremarkable. Bilirubinuria may be present where hyperbilirubinemia is present.

Culture

Despite numerous attempts by researchers, it has not been possible to culture veterinary hemoplasmas in vitro,[128,129] thus culture (and antimicrobial sensitivity) testing cannot be used diagnostically.

Polymerase Chain Reaction

PCR assays, performed on DNA extracted from ethylenediaminetetraacetic acid blood samples, are the most reliable diagnostic test for hemoplasma infection due to their sensitivity and specificity. Blood samples should ideally be taken before any antibiotic treatment is started because organisms can decrease rapidly if antibiotic treatment is successful.[130]

Many PCR assays exist, both conventional and real-time quantitative PCR (qPCR), which are generally based on detection of segments of the 16S rRNA gene; increasingly, hemoplasma PCR assays are duplexed with a host housekeeping gene PCR[56,131] as an internal control, so that false-negative results due to the failure of DNA extraction, presence of PCR inhibitors, or setup errors are recognized. Others amplify host housekeeping genes in a separate PCR (ie, not duplexed),[7] which is less optimal. Well-designed PCR assays, run in high-quality laboratories, can detect low numbers of organisms in the blood, allowing for detection of subclinical carrier cats and dogs. Samples need to be sent to an external laboratory for analysis, which typically takes a few days. The detection of subclinical carrier status by PCR means that a positive PCR result does not equate with hemoplasmosis being the cause of disease in the animal being tested. Thus, positive PCR results must be interpreted in conjunction with the clinical signs shown by the animal being tested (anemia, pyrexia), clinicopathological results, any concurrent disease or immunosuppression, and the pathogenicity of the hemoplasma species detected by PCR. Last, large numbers of hemoplasmas (reported by qPCR) may be more consistent with clinical hemoplasmosis, but the marked fluctuations in organism numbers in acute *M. haemofelis* infection makes qPCR interpretation more difficult. However, the detection of low numbers of organisms in an animal with appropriate clinical signs, in the absence of another cause of the anemia, could well be reflective of clinical hemoplasmosis, warranting treatment.

Isothermal Assay

A new point-of-care machine, using isothermal nonquantitative amplification of DNA to diagnose *M. haemofelis* infection has been evaluated in a small study.[132] However, in-house extraction of DNA from blood is needed, and the extraction kit used affects the sensitivity of the assay, possibly limiting the usefulness of this assay.

Serology

Although serologic assays to detect antibodies against hemoplasmas were more sensitive than PCR in detecting exposure to 'Ca. M. turicensis' in one study,[133] and have been used in research,[133,134] none are commercially available.

TREATMENT
Overview

Prompt antibiotic treatment (**Table 2**) is indicated for cats and dogs with clinical signs and clinicopathological abnormalities consistent with clinical hemoplasmosis. However, although clinical improvement in the anemia is seen, clearance of infection is rare. Most studies evaluating antibiotics have centered on *M. haemofelis* infection, and information is then extrapolated to guide treatment for other hemoplasma species. However, the response of different hemoplasma species, and indeed probably different strains/genotypes of the same species, to antibiotics varies, so clinicians should always be aware that a change in treatment may be required if a clinical response is not seen within a few days.

Tetracyclines

Tetracyclines, particularly doxycycline,[92,135] are indicated as first-line antibiotic treatment of clinical hemoplasmosis. Because of the possibility of esophagitis in cats, administration of the hyclate preparation of doxycycline should always be followed by food or water. Doxycycline is typically given for 2 weeks, with clinical improvement within 3 days. In simple cases that show a rapid response, the 2-week course of doxycycline is usually adequate with no further monitoring required. However, if the hemoplasmosis is a reactivated infection, or comorbidities are present and/or clinical signs do not improve within 3 days, ideally blood organism numbers should be monitored by qPCR to determine if they are decreasing with doxycycline. The results of qPCR, alongside repeat hematology, can guide whether a longer doxycycline course (up to 4 weeks) is required if only a partial response has occurred, or whether a second-line antibiotic is needed if little response is seen. In one study, 'Ca. M. haemominutum' infection was not as effectively treated by doxycycline as *M. haemofelis*,[85] highlighting the varying response of different hemoplasma species to the same antibiotic.

Table 2
Suggested drug dosages for antibiotic treatment of acute clinical hemoplasmosis in cats and dogs

Antibiotic Class & Name	Dosage (mg/kg)[a]	Route & Frequency[b]	Comments
Tetracycline: doxycycline	5 10	PO q 12 h PO q 24 h	Commonly used first-line antibiotic for acute hemoplasmosis. Can be associated with gastrointestinal side effects when dosed q 24 h. Can be associated with esophagitis if incompletely swallowed so always follow with food or water
Fluoroquinolone: marbofloxacin	2–5.5	PO q 24 h	Reserve fluoroquinolones as second-line antibiotics. Reported use in combination (sequentially) with doxycycline to clear *M haemofelis*[140]
Fluoroquinolone: pradofloxacin	3–5	PO q 24 h	Reserve fluoroquinolones as second-line antibiotics. May be more efficacious at clearing *M haemofelis* than doxycycline[139]
Fluoroquinolone: enrofloxacin	5	PO q 24 h	Reserve fluoroquinolones as second-line antibiotics. Enrofloxacin is not a preferred fluoroquinolone in cats as it has potential for irreversible retinal toxicity as idiosyncratic reaction

Abbreviations: PO, by mouth; q, every.
[a] Licensed dosages (eg, for marbofloxacin) and drug availability vary by formulation and country.
[b] Two-week courses are usually adequate for treatment of uncomplicated hemoplasmosis: courses can be extended if only a partial clinical response occurs.

Fluoroquinolones

Fluoroquinolones, notably marbofloxacin and pradofloxacin,[135–139] are also effective but are reserved as second-line treatments. Again, these are given typically for 2 weeks with improvement occurring within a few days. Pradofloxacin may be more efficacious at clearing *M. haemofelis* infection than doxycycline.[139] Although marbofloxacin treatment is known to result in a marked and sustained decrease in blood *M haemofelis* organisms in cats and clinical response,[138] it only caused a temporary decrease of '*Ca.* M. haemominutum' organisms[137] and PCR positive results for '*Ca.* M. haemominutum' have remained following either enrofloxacin or doxycycline treatment,[18] thus highlighting the varying response of different hemoplasma species.

Treatment of Hemoplasmosis in the Absence of a Published Evidence Base

Little evidence exists on the response of *M. haemocanis*, '*Ca.* M. haematoparvum' and '*Ca.* M. turicensis' to antibiotics, but one report described a successful response of '*Ca.* M. turicensis' to doxycycline,[31] and doxycycline is generally used as a first-line treatment of all infections. Some cases seem to be refractory to tetracyclines, and in 1 *M. haemocanis* case report,[91] oxytetracycline, and subsequent enrofloxacin, did not markedly reduce organism numbers, although clinical signs did improve. It is important to focus on the clinical response to treatment but to be prepared to try an alternative antibiotic if the clinical response is inadequate, preferably alongside qPCR results if finances allow, to document hemoplasma organism numbers to further help assess response to treatment.

Low numbers of hemoplasma organisms are often detectable by qPCR following antibiotic treatment, even if a good clinical response is seen. Some have suggested using longer courses of antibiotics (eg, 6 weeks) to try and clear infection and obtain a negative qPCR result, although antibiotic stewardship should always be considered to limit inappropriate antibiotic use. Recently a protocol to clear chronic *M. haemofelis* infection in cats has been described,[140] comprising a 4-week course of doxycycline (5 mg/kg by mouth every 12 hours) and then, if still qPCR positive (repeated testing on multiple occasions), a 2-week course of marbofloxacin (2 mg/kg by mouth every 24 hours). Treatment breaks of up to 4 weeks between the courses of antibiotics did not influence the outcome. This protocol is an option for cases in which reactivation of infection or particularly severe disease (eg, with comorbidities) has occurred.

Supportive Treatment

As well as antibiotics, supportive therapy is important for the successful management of acute hemoplasmosis in cats and dogs. Intravenous fluid therapy to correct dehydration and blood products (packed red blood cells if available, or whole blood) for severe anemia may be required if tachycardia, weakness, and/or tachypnea are present.

Glucocorticoids

Glucocorticoids are not usually required for hemoplasmosis treatment, even if erythrocyte-bound antibodies are documented. Efficacious antibiotic treatment is adequate in these cases[81] and immunosuppressive glucocorticoids have actually been used experimentally to enhance bacteremia and to try and induce reactivation of subclinical hemoplasma infection.[78,135,139–141] Glucocorticoids would only be indicated in cases in which the response to antibiotics was not appropriate and primary immune-mediated hemolytic anemia was a likely diagnosis.

PROGNOSIS

The prognosis for acute hemoplasmosis is generally good if effective antibiotic and supportive treatment is started promptly, with clinical improvement occurring within 3 days of starting treatment. Many animals remain subclinical hemoplasma carriers following recovery, and reactivation of disease is possible months or years later.

PREVENTION

The lack of definitive knowledge on how hemoplasmas are transmitted in the field makes it difficult to make firm recommendations to prevent infection, but risk factors for hemoplasma infection should be avoided if possible. Prevention of fighting, control measures for flea and tick infestations, and screening of blood donors by PCR should be helpful.

PUBLIC HEALTH ASPECTS

Molecular techniques have confirmed infections in humans with hemoplasma species already reported in animal hosts such as cats,[142] dogs,[143,144] pigs,[145–147] and sheep,[144,148] suggesting that zoonotic transmission is possible. Most reports have suggested that hemoplasma-associated clinical signs are more likely in immunocompromised humans, and clinically ill people have often had coinfections with *Bartonella henselae*.[142,143,148] Further investigation is warranted into the effects of *B. henselae* coinfection on transmission and disease.[149]

More recently, human infections with a novel hemoplasma species have been described[144,150–153]; this species was named '*Candidatus* Mycoplasma haemohominis,' and has since been found in bats[153–158] with zoonotic transmission by direct contact with bats believed to have occurred. '*Flying fox hemoytic fever*' is the name recently given to the '*Ca* M haemohominis'-associated syndrome in humans, characterized by febrile splenomegaly, weight loss, life-threatening autoimmune hemolytic anemia, and hemophagocytosis in New Caledonia.[153] These patients usually had a history of contact with bats (via hunting/food preparation primarily), and '*Ca*. M. haemohominis' was found in a significant number of bats tested. Interestingly, these patients were not immunocompromised before succumbing to '*Ca*. M. haemohominis' disease and usually recovered if treated promptly with a 3-week course of doxycycline.

Until further information is available on zoonotic potential and transmission, veterinarians should handle blood and tissues from animals suspected to be hemoplasma infected with caution.

SUMMARY

Hemotropic mycoplasmas (hemoplasmas) exist worldwide and are wall-less bacteria. The main pathogenic species in dogs and cats are *M. haemocanis* and *M. haemofelis*, respectively. The species infect erythrocytes and induce hemolytic anemia and fever. Their natural mode of transmission has not been confirmed, but likely includes vertical, fighting/biting, and vector-borne transmission. Reliable diagnosis is by PCR on blood samples because cytology is insensitive. Prompt treatment of clinical disease with supportive care and at least 2 weeks of doxycycline is usually successful. Subclinical carrier status is common, but reactivation of clinical disease is rare. Zoonotic infection is possible, most likely via direct contact with bats.

CLINICS CARE POINTS

- Consider hemoplasmosis in cats and splenectomized or immunocompromised dogs presenting with a regenerative anemia and fever
- In-house blood smear examination (cytology) for diagnosis is generally unreliable unless interpreted by someone with experience in cytology
- PCR is the diagnostic method of choice, performed on EDTA blood samples collected before antibiotic treatment is started
- A 2-week course of doxycycline is usually successful for treatment, with supportive care (including a blood transfusion) if needed; an improvement is usually seen within 3 days. If the response is inadequate to doxycycline, pradofloxacin or marbofloxacin treatment can be used as a second-line treatment
- Glucocorticoid treatment is not usually required
- Despite a clinical response to treatment, clearance of infection may not result from treatment; subclinical-infected animals remain at risk of reactivation of infection, but this seems to be rare

DISCLOSURE

S. Tasker has received financial support for infectious disease research from BSAVA PetSavers, Journal of Comparative Pathology Educational Trust, Langford Trust, Langford Vets Clinical Research Fund, Morris Animal Foundation, NERC/BBSRC/

MRC, Petplan Charitable Trust, South-West Biosciences DTP, The Wellcome Trust, and Zoetis Animal Health and has received speaker honoraria or consultancy fees in the past from Elanco (Bayer) and veterinary associations such as BSAVA, WSAVA, and ISFM. S. Tasker is also a member of the Companion Animal Vector-Borne World Forum, supported by Elanco, and the European Advisory Board for Cat Diseases, a scientifically independent committee whose activities have been supported by Boehringer Ingelheim, the founding sponsor, and by Virbac and Idexx.

REFERENCES

1. Kellner A, Carver S, Scorza V, et al. Transmission pathways and spillover of an erythrocytic bacterial pathogen from domestic cats to wild felids. Ecol Evol 2018;8(19):9779–92.

2. Messick JB, Walker PG, Raphael W, et al. 'Candidatus Mycoplasma haemodidelphidis' sp. nov., 'Candidatus Mycoplasma haemolamae' sp. nov and Mycoplasma haemocanis comb. nov., haemotrophic parasites from a naturally infected opossum (Didelphis virginiana), alpaca (Lama pacos) and dog (Canis familiaris): phylogenetic and secondary structural relatedness of their 16S rRNA genes to other mycoplasmas. Int J Syst Evol Microbiol 2002;52:693–8.

3. Neimark H, Johansson KE, Rikihisa Y, et al. Proposal to transfer some members of the genera Haemobartonella and Eperythrozoon to the genus Mycoplasma with descriptions of 'Candidatus Mycoplasma haemofelis', 'Candidatus Mycoplasma haemomuris', 'Candidatus Mycoplasma haemosuis' and 'Candidatus Mycoplasma wenyonii. Int J Syst Evol Microbiol 2001;51(Pt 3):891–9.

4. Neimark H, Johansson KE, Rikihisa Y, et al. Revision of haemotrophic Mycoplasma species names. Int J Syst Evol Microbiol 2002;52:683.

5. Hicks CA, Barker EN, Brady C, et al. Non-ribosomal phylogenetic exploration of Mollicute species: new insights into haemoplasma taxonomy. Infect Genet Evol 2014;23:99–105.

6. Biondo AW, Dos Santos AP, Guimaraes AM, et al. A review of the occurrence of hemoplasmas (hemotrophic mycoplasmas) in Brazil. Rev Bras Parasitol Vet 2009;18(3):1–7.

7. Soto F, Walker R, Sepulveda M, et al. Occurrence of canine hemotropic mycoplasmas in domestic dogs from urban and rural areas of the Valdivia Province, southern Chile. Comp Immunol Microbiol Infect Dis 2017;50:70–7.

8.. Zhuang QJ, Zhang HJ, Lin RQ, et al. The occurrence of the feline "Candidatus Mycoplasma haemominutum" in dog in China confirmed by sequence-based analysis of ribosomal DNA. Trop Anim Health Prod 2009;41(4):689–92.

9.. Obara H, Fujihara M, Watanabe Y, et al. A feline hemoplasma, 'Candidatus Mycoplasma haemominutum', detected in dog in Japan. J Vet Med Sci 2011;73(6):841–3.

10. Liu M, Ruttayaporn N, Saechan V, et al. Molecular survey of canine vector-borne diseases in stray dogs in Thailand. Parasitol Int 2016;65(4):357–61.

11. Valle SD, Messick JB, dos Santos AP, et al. Identification, occurrence and clinical findings of canine hemoplasmas in southern Brazil. Comp Immunol Microb 2014;37(4):259–65.

12.. Varanat M, Maggi RG, Linder KE, et al. Molecular prevalence of Bartonella, Babesia, and hemotropic Mycoplasma sp. in dogs with splenic disease. J Vet Intern Med 2011;25(6):1284–91.

13. Barker EN, Langton DA, Helps CR, et al. Haemoparasites of free-roaming dogs associated with several remote Aboriginal communities in Australia. BMC Vet Res 2012;8(1):55.

14. Hii SF, Kopp SR, Thompson MF, et al. Canine vector-borne disease pathogens in dogs from south-east Queensland and north-east Northern Territory. Aust Vet J 2012;90(4):130–5.

15. Happi AN, Toepp AJ, Ugwu CA, et al. Detection and identification of blood-borne infections in dogs in Nigeria using light microscopy and the polymerase chain reaction. Vet Parasitol Reg Stud Rep 2018;11:55–60.

16.. Mascarelli PE, Tartara GP, Pereyra NB, et al. Detection of *Mycoplasma haemocanis*, *Mycoplasma haematoparvum*, *Mycoplasma suis* and other vector-borne pathogens in dogs from Cordoba and Santa Fe, Argentina. Parasit Vectors 2016;9(1):642.

17. Sykes JE, Drazenovich NL, Ball LM, et al. Use of conventional and real-time polymerase chain reaction to determine the epidemiology of hemoplasma infections in anemic and nonanemic cats. J Vet Intern Med 2007;21(4):685–93.

18. Martinez-Diaz VL, Silvestre-Ferreira AC, Vilhena H, et al. Prevalence and co-infection of haemotropic mycoplasmas in Portuguese cats by real-time polymerase chain reaction. J Feline Med Surg 2013;15(10):879–85.

19. Aquino LC, Hicks CA, Scalon MC, et al. Prevalence and phylogenetic analysis of haemoplasmas from cats infected with multiple species. J Microbiol Methods 2014;107:189–96.

20. Bauer N, Balzer HJ, Thure S, et al. Prevalence of feline haemotropic mycoplasmas in convenience samples of cats in Germany. J Feline Med Surg 2008;10(3):252–8.

21. Roura X, Peters IR, Altet L, et al. Prevalence of hemotropic mycoplasmas in healthy and unhealthy cats and dogs in Spain. J Vet Diagn Invest 2010;22(2):270–4.

22. Luria BJ, Levy JK, Lappin MR, et al. Prevalence of infectious diseases in feral cats in Northern Florida. J Feline Med Surg 2004;6(5):287–96.

23. Stojanovic V, Foley P. Infectious disease prevalence in a feral cat population on Prince Edward Island, Canada. Can Vet J 2011;52(9):979–82.

24. Tasker S, Braddock JA, Baral R, et al. Diagnosis of feline haemoplasma infection in Australian cats using a real-time PCR assay. J Feline Med Surg 2004;6:345–54.

25. Lobetti R, Lappin MR. Prevalence of Toxoplasma gondii, Bartonella species and haemoplasma infection in cats in South Africa. J Feline Med Surg 2012;14(12):857–62.

26. Ghazisaeedi F, Atyabi N, Zahrai Salehi T, et al. A molecular study of hemotropic mycoplasmas (hemoplasmas) in cats in Iran. Vet Clin Pathol 2014;43(3):381–6.

27. Tanahara M, Miyamoto S, Nishio T, et al. An epidemiological survey of feline hemoplasma infection in Japan. J Vet Med Sci 2010;72(12):1575–81.

28. Georges K, Ezeokoli C, Auguste T, et al. A comparison of real-time PCR and reverse line blot hybridization in detecting feline haemoplasmas of domestic cats and an analysis of risk factors associated with haemoplasma infections. BMC Vet Res 2012;8:103.

29. Sykes JE, Terry JC, Lindsay LL, et al. Prevalences of various hemoplasma species among cats in the United States with possible hemoplasmosis. J Am Vet Med Assoc 2008;232(3):372–9.

30. Tasker S, Binns SH, Day MJ, et al. Use of a PCR assay to assess prevalence and risk factors for *Mycoplasma haemofelis* and '*Candidatus* Mycoplasma haemominutum' in cats in the United Kingdom. Vet Rec 2003;152:193–8.

31. Willi B, Boretti FS, Baumgartner C, et al. Prevalence, risk factor analysis, and follow-up of infections caused by three feline hemoplasma species in cats in Switzerland. J Clin Microbiol 2006;44(3):961–9.

32. Willi B, Tasker S, Boretti FS, et al. Phylogenetic Analysis of '*Candidatus* Mycoplasma turicensis' Isolates from Pet Cats in the United Kingdom, Australia and South Africa, with Analysis of Risk Factors for Infection. J Clin Microbiol 2006;44:4430–5.

33. Diaz-Reganon D, Villaescusa A, Ayllon T, et al. Epidemiological study of hemotropic mycoplasmas (hemoplasmas) in cats from central Spain. Parasit Vectors 2018;11(1):140.

34. Attipa C, Papasouliotis K, Solano-Gallego L, et al. Prevalence study and risk factor analysis of selected bacterial, protozoal and viral, including vector-borne, pathogens in cats from Cyprus. Parasite Vector 2017;10(1):130.

35.. Wang X, Cui Y, Zhang Y, et al. Molecular characterization of hemotropic mycoplasmas (*Mycoplasma ovis* and '*Candidatus* Mycoplasma haemovis') in sheep and goats in China. BMC Vet Res 2017;13(1):142.

36. Sabat G, Rose P, Hickey WJ, et al. Selective and sensitive method for PCR amplification of *Escherichia coli* 16S rRNA genes in soil. Appl Environ Microbiol 2000;66(2):844–9.

37. Macieira DB, de Menezes RD, Damico CB, et al. Prevalence and risk factors for hemoplasmas in domestic cats naturally infected with feline immunodeficiency virus and/or feline leukemia virus in Rio de Janeiro - Brazil. J Feline Med Surg 2008;10:120 9.

38. Gentilini F, Novacco M, Turba ME, et al. Use of combined conventional and real-time PCR to determine the epidemiology of feline haemoplasma infections in northern Italy. J Feline Med Surg 2009;11(4):277–85.

39. Walker Vergara R, Morera Galleguillos F, Gomez Jaramillo M, et al. Prevalence, risk factor analysis, and hematological findings of hemoplasma infection in domestic cats from Valdivia, Southern Chile. Comp Immunol Microbiol Infect Dis 2016;46:20–6.

40. Sarvani E, Tasker S, Kovac evic Filipovic M, et al. Prevalence and risk factor analysis for feline haemoplasmas in cats from Northern Serbia, with molecular subtyping of feline immunodeficiency virus. JFMS Open Rep 2018;4(1). 2055116918770037.

41. Ravagnan S, Carli E, Piseddu E, et al. Prevalence and molecular characterization of canine and feline hemotropic mycoplasmas (hemoplasmas) in northern Italy. Parasite Vector 2017;10:132.

42. Persichetti MF, Pennisi MG, Vullo A, et al. Clinical evaluation of outdoor cats exposed to ectoparasites and associated risk for vector-borne infections in southern Italy. Parasite Vector 2018;11(1):136.

43. Marcondes M, Hirata KY, Vides JP, et al. Infection by Mycoplasma spp., feline immunodeficiency virus and feline leukemia virus in cats from an area endemic for visceral leishmaniasis. Parasit Vectors 2018;11(1):131.

44. Imre M, Vaduva C, Darabus G, et al. Molecular detection of hemotropic mycoplasmas (hemoplasmas) in domestic cats (Felis catus) in Romania. BMC Vet Res 2020;16(1):399.

45. Jensen WA, Lappin MR, Kamkar S, et al. Use of a polymerase chain reaction assay to detect and differentiate two strains of *Haemobartonella felis* infection in naturally infected cats. Am J Vet Res 2001;62:604–8.

46. Lobetti RG, Tasker S. Diagnosis of feline haemoplasma infection using a real-time PCR. J South Afr Vet Assoc 2004;75(2):94–9.

47. Nibblett BM, Waldner C, Taylor SM, et al. Hemotropic mycoplasma prevalence in shelter and client-owned cats in Saskatchewan and a comparison of polymerase chain reaction (PCR) - Results from two independent laboratories. Can J Vet Res 2010;74(2):91–6.

48. Juvet F, Lappin MR, Brennan S, et al. Prevalence of selected infectious agents in cats in Ireland. J Feline Med Surg 2010;12(6):476–82.

49. Ural K, Kurtdede A, Ulutas B. Prevalence of haemoplasma infection in pet cats from 4 different provinces in Turkey. Rev Med Vet-toulouse 2009;160(5):226–30.

50. Makino H, de Paula DAJ, Sousa VRF, et al. Natural hemoplasma infection of cats in Cuiaba, Mato Grosso, Brazil. Semin-Cienc Agrar 2018;39(2):875–80.

51. Munhoz AD, Simoes I, Calazans APF, et al. Hemotropic mycoplasmas in naturally infected cats in Northeastern Brazil. Rev Bras Parasitol Vet 2018;27(4): 446–54.

52. Berzina I, Capligina V, Namina A, et al. Haemotropic Mycoplasma species in pet cats in Latvia: a study, phylogenetic analysis and clinical case report. J Feline Med Surg Open Rep 2021;7(2). 20551169211028088.

53. Assarasakorn S, Veir JK, Hawley JR, et al. Prevalence of *Bartonella* species, hemoplasmas, and *Rickettsia felis* DNA in blood and fleas of cats in Bangkok, Thailand. Res Vet Sci 2012;93:1213–6.

54. Novacco M, Meli ML, Gentilini F, et al. Prevalence and geographical distribution of canine hemotropic mycoplasma infections in Mediterranean countries and analysis of risk factors for infection. Vet Microbiol 2010;142:276–84.

55. Wengi N, Willi B, Boretti FS, et al. Real-time PCR-based prevalence study, infection follow-up and molecular characterization of canine hemotropic mycoplasmas. Vet Microbiol 2008;126(1–3):132–41.

56. Barker EN, Tasker S, Day MJ, et al. Development and use of real-time PCR to detect and quantify *Mycoplasma haemocanis* and "*Candidatus* Mycoplasma haematoparvum" in dogs. Vet Microbiol 2010;140(1–2):167–70.

57. Tennant KV, Barker EN, Polizopoulou Z, et al. Real-time quantitative polymerase chain reaction detection of haemoplasmas in healthy and unhealthy dogs from Central Macedonia, Greece. J Small Anim Pract 2011;52(12):645–9.

58. Aquino LC, Kamani J, Haruna AM, et al. Analysis of risk factors and prevalence of haemoplasma infection in dogs. Vet Parasitol 2016;221:111–7.

59. Hasiri MA, Sharifiyazdi H, Moradi T. Molecular detection and differentiation of canine hemoplasma infections using RFLP-PCR in dogs in southern Iran. Vet Arhiv 2016;86(4):529–40.

60. Aktas M, Ozubek S. Molecular survey of haemoplasmas in shelter dogs and associations with Rhipicephalus sanguineus sensu lato. Med Vet Entomol 2017; 31(4):457–61.

61. Abd Rani PA, Irwin PJ, Coleman GT, et al. A survey of canine tick-borne diseases in India. Parasit Vectors 2011;4:141.

62. Inpankaew T, Hii SF, Chimnoi W, et al. Canine vector-borne pathogens in semi-domesticated dogs residing in northern Cambodia. Parasit Vectors 2016; 9(1):253.

63. Vieira RF, Vidotto O, Vieira TS, et al. Molecular Investigation of Hemotropic Mycoplasmas in Human Beings, Dogs and Horses in a Rural Settlement in Southern Brazil. Rev Inst Med Trop Sao Paulo 2015;57(4):353–7.

64. Hamel D, Shukullari E, Rapti D, et al. Parasites and vector-borne pathogens in client-owned dogs in Albania. Blood pathogens and seroprevalences of parasitic and other infectious agents. Parasitol Res 2016;115(2):489–99.

65.. Barbosa MV, Paulino PG, Camilo TA, et al. Spatial distribution and molecular epidemiology of hemotropic *Mycoplasma* spp. and *Mycoplasma haemocanis* infection in dogs from Rio de Janeiro, Brazil. Infect Genet Evol 2021;87. 104660.

66.. Hosseini SR, Sekhavatmandi A, Khamesipour F. PCR based analysis of Haemobartonellosis (*Candidatus* Mycoplasma haematoparvum and *Mycoplasma haemocanis*) and its prevalence in dogs in Isfahan, Iran. Biosci Biotechno Res 2017;10(2):187–91.

67. Aktas M, Ozubek S. A molecular survey of hemoplasmas in domestic dogs from Turkey. Vet Microbiol 2018;221:94–7.

68.. Torkan S, Aldavood SJ, Sekhavatmandi A, et al. Detection of haemotropic *Mycoplasma* (*Haemobartonella*) using multiplex PCR and its relationship with epidemiological factors in dogs. Comp Clin Pathol 2014;23(3):669–72.

69.. Kaewmongkol G, Lukkana N, Yangtara S, et al. Association of *Ehrlichia canis*, Hemotropic *Mycoplasma* spp. and *Anaplasma platys* and severe anemia in dogs in Thailand. Vet Microbiol 2017;201:195–200.

70. Cannon SH, Levy JK, Kirk SK, et al. Infectious diseases in dogs rescued during dogfighting investigations. Vet J 2016;211:64–9.

71. Sasaki M, Ohta K, Matsuu A, et al. A molecular survey of *Mycoplasma haemocanis* in dogs and foxes in Aomori Prefecture, Japan. J Protozoology Res 2008; 18(2):57–60.

72. Levy JK, Lappin MR, Glaser AL, et al. Prevalence of infectious diseases in cats and dogs rescued following Hurricane Katrina. J Am Vet Med Assoc 2011; 238(3):311–7.

73. Bouzouraa T, Cadore JL, Chene J, et al. Implication, clinical and biological impact of vector-borne haemopathogens in anaemic dogs in France: a prospective study. J Small Anim Pract 2017;58(9):510–8.

74.. Barash NR, Thomas B, Birkenheuer AJ, et al. Prevalence of *Babesia* spp. and clinical characteristics of *Babesia vulpes* infections in North American dogs. J Vet Intern Med 2019;33(5):2075–81.

75. Willi B, Boretti FS, Cattori V, et al. Identification, molecular characterisation and experimental transmission of a new hemoplasma isolate from a cat with hemolytic anaemia in Switzerland. J Clin Microbiol 2005;43(6):2581–5.

76. Maede Y, Hata R. Studies on feline haemobartonellosis. II. The mechanism of anemia produced by infection with *Haemobartonella felis*. Jap J Vet Sci 1975; 37(1):49–54.

77. Maede Y. Studies on feline haemobartonellosis. IV. Lifespan of erythrocytes of cats infected with *Haemobartonella felis*. Jap J Vet Sci 1975;37(5):269–72.

78. Harvey JW, Gaskin JM. Feline haemobartonellosis: attempts to induce relapses of clinical disease in chronically infected cats. J Am Anim Hosp Assoc 1978;14: 453–6.

79. Shaw SE, Kenny MJ, Tasker S, et al. Pathogen carriage by the cat flea *Ctenocephalides felis* (Bouché) in the United Kingdom. Vet Microbiol 2004;102(3–4): 183–8.

80. Zulty JC, Kociba GJ. Cold agglutinins in cats with haemobartonellosis. J Am Vet Med Assoc 1990;196(6):907–10.

81. Tasker S, Peters IR, Papasouliotis K, et al. Description of outcomes of experimental infection with feline haemoplasmas: copy numbers, haematology, Coombs' testing and blood glucose concentrations. Vet Microbiol 2009; 139(3–4):323–32.

82. Barker EN, Darby AC, Helps CR, et al. Molecular characterization of the uncultivatable hemotropic bacterium *Mycoplasma haemofelis*. Vet Res 2011;42(1):83.

83. De Lorimier LP, Messick JB. Anemia Associated With '*Candidatus* Mycoplasma haemominutum' in a Feline Leukemia Virus-Negative Cat With Lymphoma. J Am Anim Hosp Assoc 2004;40(5):423–7.

84. George JW, Rideout BA, Griffey SM, et al. Effect of preexisting FeLV infection or FeLV and feline immunodeficiency virus coinfection on pathogenicity of the small variant of *Haemobartonella felis* in cats. Am J Vet Res 2002;63(8):1172–8.

85. Sykes JE, Henn JB, Kasten RW, et al. *Bartonella henselae* infection in splenectomized domestic cats previously infected with hemotropic Mycoplasma species. Vet Immunol Immunopathol 2007;116(1–2):104–8.

86.. Reynolds CA, Lappin MR. '*Candidatus* Mycoplasma haemominutum' infections in 21 client-owned cats. J Am Anim Hosp Assoc 2007;43(5):249–57.

87. Warman SM, Helps CR, Barker EN, et al. Haemoplasma infection is not a common cause of canine immune-mediated haemolytic anaemia in the UK. J Small Anim Pract 2010;51(10):534–9.

88. Lester SJ, Hume JB, Phipps B. *Haemobartonella canis* infection following splenectomy and transfusion. Can Vet J 1995;36(7):444–5.

89. Sykes JE, Bailiff NL, Ball LM, et al. Identification of a novel hemotropic mycoplasma in a splenectomized dog with hemic neoplasia. J Am Vet Med Assoc 2004;224(12):1946–51.

90. Kemming G, Messick JB, Mueller W, et al. Can we continue research in splenectomized dogs? *Mycoplasma haemocanis*: old problem–new insight. Eur Surg Res 2004;36(4):198–205.

91. Hulme-Moir KL, Barker EN, Stonelake A, et al. Use of real-time quantitative polymerase chain reaction to monitor antibiotic therapy in a dog with naturally acquired *Mycoplasma haemocanis* infection. J Vet Diagn Invest 2010;22(4):582–7.

92. Pitorri F, Dell'Orco M, Carmichael N, et al. Use of real-time quantitative PCR to document successful treatment of *Mycoplasma haemocanis* infection with doxycycline in a dog. Vet Clin Pathol 2012;41(4):493–6.

93. Bellamy JE, MacWilliams PS, Searcy GP. Cold-agglutinin hemolytic anaemia and *Haemobartonella canis* infection in a dog. J Am Vet Med Assoc 1978; 173(4):397–401.

94. Bundza A, Lumsden JH, McSherry BJ, et al. Haemobartonellosis in a dog in association with Coombs' positive anaemia. Can Vet J 1976;17(10):267–70.

95. Pryor WH Jr, Bradbury RP. *Haemobartonella canis* infection in research dogs. Lab Anim Sci 1975;25(5):566–9.

96. Sykes JE, Ball LM, Bailiff NL, et al. '*Candidatus* Mycoplasma haematoparvum' sp.nov., a Novel Small Haemotropic Mycoplasma from a Dog. Int J Syst Evol Microbiol 2004;55(1):27–30.

97. Novacco M, Boretti FS, Wolf-Jackel GA, et al. Chronic "*Candidatus* Mycoplasma turicensis" infection. Vet Res 2011;42(1):59.

98. Harvey JW, Gaskin JM. Experimental feline haemobartonellosis. J Am Anim Hosp Assoc 1977;13:28–38.

99. Foley JE, Harrus S, Poland A, et al. Molecular, clinical, and pathologic comparison of two distinct strains of *Haemobartonella felis* in domestic cats. Am J Vet Res 1998;59(12):1581–8.
100. Weingart C, Tasker S, Kohn B. Infection with haemoplasma species in 22 cats with anaemia. J Feline Med Surg 2016;18(2):129–36.
101.. Baumann J, Novacco M, Willi B, et al. Lack of cross-protection against *Mycoplasma haemofelis* infection and signs of enhancement in "*Candidatus* Mycoplasma turicensis"-recovered cats. Vet Res 2015;46:104.
102.. Sugiarto S, Spiri AM, Riond B, et al. Passive immunization does not provide protection against experimental infection with *Mycoplasma haemofelis*. Vet Res 2016;47(1):79.
103.. Novacco M, Boretti FS, Franchini M, et al. Protection from reinfection in "*Candidatus* Mycoplasma turicensis"-infected cats and characterization of the immune response. Vet Res 2012;43(1):82.
104. Hicks CA, Willi B, Riond B, et al. Protective immunity against infection with *Mycoplasma haemofelis*. Clin Vaccin Immunol 2014;22(1):108–18.
105.. Lappin MR, Griffin B, Brunt J, et al. Prevalence of *Bartonella* species, haemoplasma species, *Ehrlichia* species, *Anaplasma phagocytophilum*, and *Neorickettsia risticii* DNA in the blood of cats and their fleas in the United States. J Feline Med Surg 2006;8(2):85–90.
106. Seneviratna P, Weerasinghe N, Ariyadasa S. Transmission of *Haemobartonella canis* by the dog tick, *Rhipicephalus sanguineus*. Res Vet Sci 1973;14(1):112–4.
107. Taroura S, Shimada Y, Sakata Y, et al. Detection of DNA of '*Candidatus* Mycoplasma haemominutum' and *Spiroplasma* sp. in unfed ticks collected from vegetation in Japan. J Vet Med Sci 2005;67(12):1277–9.
108. Willi B, Boretti FS, Meli ML, et al. Real-time PCR investigation of potential vectors, reservoirs and shedding patterns of feline hemotropic mycoplasmas. Appl Environ Microbiol 2007;73(12):3798–802.
109.. Barrs VR, Beatty JA, Wilson BJ, et al. Prevalence of *Bartonella* species, *Rickettsia felis*, haemoplasmas and the *Ehrlichia* group in the blood of cats and fleas in eastern Australia. Aust Vet J 2010;88(5):160–5.
110.. Reagan KL, Clarke LL, Hawley JR, et al. Assessment of the ability of Aedes species mosquitoes to transmit feline *Mycoplasma haemofelis* and '*Candidatus* Mycoplasma haemominutum'. J Feline Med Surg 2017;19(8):798–802.
111.. Duplan F, Davies S, Filler S, et al. *Anaplasma phagocytophilum*, *Bartonella* spp., haemoplasma species and *Hepatozoon* spp. in ticks infesting cats: a large-scale survey. Parasit Vectors 2018;11(1):201.
112. Abdullah S, Helps C, Tasker S, et al. Pathogens in fleas collected from cats and dogs: distribution and prevalence in the UK. Parasit Vectors 2019;12(1):71.
113. Hamel D, Silaghi C, Zapadynska S, et al. Vector-borne pathogens in ticks and EDTA-blood samples collected from client-owned dogs, Kiev, Ukraine. Ticks Tick Borne Dis 2013;4(1–2):152–5.
114. Woods JE, Brewer MM, Hawley JR, et al. Evaluation of experimental transmission of '*Candidatus* Mycoplasma haemominutum' and *Mycoplasma haemofelis* by *Ctenocephalides felis* to cats. Am J Vet Res 2005;66(6):1008–12.
115. Woods JE, Wisnewski N, Lappin MR. Attempted transmission of *Candidatus* Mycoplasma haemominutum and *Mycoplasma haemofelis* by feeding cats infected *Ctenocephalides felis*. Am J Vet Res 2006;67(3):494–7.
116. Lappin M.R., Feline haemoplasmas are not transmitted by Ctenocephalides felis, Paper presented at: 9th Symposium of the CVBD World Forum 24th March 2014; Lisbon, Portugal.

117. Museux K, Boretti FS, Willi B, et al. *In vivo* transmission studies of *'Candidatus* Mycoplasma turicensis'* in the domestic cat. Vet Res 2009;40(5):45.
118. Lashnits E, Grant S, Thomas B, et al. Evidence for vertical transmission of *Mycoplasma haemocanis*, but not *Ehrlichia ewingii*, in a dog. J Vet Intern Med 2019;33(4):1747–52.
119. Gary AT, Richmond HL, Tasker S, et al. Survival of *Mycoplasma haemofelis* and *'Candidatus* Mycoplasma haemominutum' in blood of cats used for transfusions. J Feline Med Surg 2006;8(5):321–6.
120. Tasker S. Haemotropic mycoplasmas: what's the real significance in cats? J Feline Med Surg 2010;12(5):369–81.
121. Nury C, Blais MC, Arsenault J. Risk of transmittable blood-borne pathogens in blood units from blood donor dogs in Canada. J Vet Intern Med 2021;35(3):1316–24.
122. Mesa-Sanchez I, Ferreira RRF, Cardoso I, et al. Transfusion transmissible pathogens are prevalent in healthy cats eligible to become blood donors. J Small Anim Pract 2021;62(2):107–13.
123. Kewish KE, Appleyard GD, Myers SL, et al. *Mycoplasma haemofelis* and *Mycoplasma haemominutum* detection by polymerase chain reaction in cats from Saskatchewan and Alberta. Can Vet J 2004;45(9):749–52.
124. Westfall DS, Jensen WA, Reagan WJ, et al. Inoculation of two genotypes of *Haemobartonella felis* (California and Ohio variants) to induce infection in cats and the response to treatment with azithromycin. Am J Vet Res 2001;62(5):687–91.
125. Firmino FP, Aquino LC, Marçola TG, et al. Frequency and hematological alterations of different hemoplasma infections with retrovirusis co-infections in domestic cats from Brazil. Pesq Vet Bras 2016;36(8):731–6.
126. Willi B, Museux K, Novacco M, et al. First morphological characterization of 'Candidatus Mycoplasma turicensis' using electron microscopy. Vet Microbiol 2011;149(3–4):367–73.
127. Tasker S, Helps CR, Belford CJ, et al. 16S rDNA comparison demonstrates near identity between a United Kingdom *Haemobartonella felis* strain and the American California strain. Vet Microbiol 2001;81:73–8.
128.. Baumann J, Novacco M, Riond B, et al. Establishment and characterization of a low-dose *Mycoplasma haemofelis* infection model. Vet Microbiol 2013;167(3–4):410–6.
129.. Schreiner SA, Hoelzle K, Hofmann-Lehmann R, et al. Nanotransformation of the haemotrophic *Mycoplasma suis* during in vitro cultivation attempts using modified cell free *Mycoplasma* media. Vet Microbiol 2012;160(1–2):227–32.
130. Tasker S, Helps CR, Day MJ, et al. Use of Real-Time PCR to detect and quantify *Mycoplasma haemofelis* and *'Candidatus* Mycoplasma haemominutum' DNA. J Clin Microbiol 2003;41:439–41.
131. Peters IR, Helps CR, Willi B, et al. The prevalence of three species of feline haemoplasmas in samples submitted to a diagnostics service as determined by three novel real-time duplex PCR assays. Vet Microbiol 2008;126(1–3):142–50.
132. Hawley J, Yaaran T, Maurice S, et al. Amplification of *Mycoplasma haemofelis* DNA by a PCR for point-of-care use. J Vet Diagn Invest 2018;30(1):140–3.
133. Novacco M, Wolf-Jackel G, Riond B, et al. Humoral immune response to a recombinant hemoplasma antigen in experimental 'Candidatus Mycoplasma turicensis' infection. Vet Microbiol 2012;157(3–4):464–70.
134. Barker EN, Helps CR, Heesom KJ, et al. Detection of humoral response using a recombinant heat shock protein 70, DnaK, of *Mycoplasma haemofelis* in

experimentally and naturally hemoplasma-infected cats. Clin Vaccin Immunol 2010;17(12):1926–32.

135. Dowers KL, Olver C, Radecki SV, et al. Use of enrofloxacin for treatment of large-form *Haemobartonella felis* in experimentally infected cats. J Am Vet Med Assoc 2002;221(2):250–3.

136. Ishak AM, Dowers KL, Cavanaugh MT, et al. Marbofloxacin for the treatment of experimentally induced *Mycoplasma haemofelis* infection in cats. J Vet Intern Med 2008;22(2):288–92.

137. Tasker S, Caney SMA, Day MJ, et al. Effect of chronic FIV infection, and efficacy of marbofloxacin treatment, on 'Candidatus Mycoplasma haemominutum' infection. Microbes Infect 2006;8(3):653–61.

138. Tasker S, Caney SMA, Day MJ, et al. Effect of chronic FIV infection, and efficacy of marbofloxacin treatment, on *Mycoplasma haemofelis* infection. Vet Microbiol 2006;117:169–79.

139. Dowers KL, Tasker S, Radecki SV, et al. Use of pradofloxacin to treat experimentally induced *Mycoplasma hemofelis* infection in cats. Am J Vet Res 2009;70(1): 105–11.

140. Novacco M, Sugiarto S, Willi B, et al. Consecutive antibiotic treatment with doxy-cycline and marbofloxacin clears bacteremia in *Mycoplasma haemofelis*-infected cats. Vet Microbiol 2018;217:112–20.

141. Yuan C, Yang Z, Zhu J, et al. Effect of an immunosuppressor (dexamethasone) on eperythrozoon infection. Vet Res Commun 2007;31(6):661–4.

142. Santos AP, Santos RP, Biondo AW, et al. Hemoplasma infection in HIV-positive patient, Brazil. Emerg Infect Dis 2008;14(12):1922–4.

143.. Maggi RG, Mascarelli PE, Havenga LN, et al. Co-infection with *Anaplasma platys*, *Bartonella henselae* and *Candidatus* Mycoplasma haematoparvum in a veterinarian. Parasit Vectors 2013;6:103.

144.. Maggi RG, Compton SM, Trull CL, et al. Infection with Hemotropic *Mycoplasma* Species in Patients with or without Extensive Arthropod or Animal Contact. J Clin Microbiol 2013;51(10):3237–41.

145.. Congli Y, Zhibiao Y, Ningyu Z, et al. The 1.8kb DNA fragment formerly confirmed as *Mycoplasma suis (M. suis)* specific was originated from the porcine genome. Vet Microbiol 2009;138(1–2):197–8 [author reply: 199].

146. Yuan C, Liang A, Yu F, et al. *Eperythrozoon* infection identified in an unknown aetiology anaemic patient. Ann Microbiol 2007;57(3):467–9.

147. Yuan CL, Liang AB, Yao CB, et al. Prevalence of *Mycoplasma suis* (*Eperythrozoon suis*) infection in swine and swine-farm workers in Shanghai, China. Am J Vet Res 2009;70(7):890–4.

148. Sykes JE, Lindsay LL, Maggi RG, et al. Human co-infection with *Bartonella henselae* and two hemotropic mycoplasma variants resembling *Mycoplasma ovis*. J Clin Microbiol 2010;48(10):3782–5.

149. Manvell C, Ferris K, Maggi R, et al. Prevalence of Vector-Borne Pathogens in Reproductive and Non-Reproductive Tissue Samples from Free-Roaming Domestic Cats in the South Atlantic USA. Pathogens 2021;10(9).

150. Steer JA, Tasker S, Barker EN, et al. A novel hemotropic Mycoplasma (hemoplasma) in a patient with hemolytic anemia and pyrexia. Clin Infect Dis 2011; 53(11):e147–51.

151. Hattori N, Kuroda M, Katano H, et al. 'Candidatus Mycoplasma haemohominis' in Humans, Japan. Emerg Infect Dis 2020;26(1):11–9.

152. Alcorn K, Gerrard J, Cochrane T, et al. First report of *Candidatus* Mycoplasma haemohominis infection in Australia causing persistent fever in an animal carer. Clin Infect Dis 2020. https://doi.org/10.1093/cid/ciaa089.
153.. Descloux E, Mediannikov O, Gourinat AC, et al. Flying Fox Hemolytic Fever, Description of a New Zoonosis Caused by *Candidatus* Mycoplasma haemohominis. Clin Infect Dis 2021;73(7):e1445–53.
154. Hornok S, Szoke K, Meli ML, et al. Molecular detection of vector-borne bacteria in bat ticks (Acari: Ixodidae, Argasidae) from eight countries of the Old and New Worlds. Parasit Vectors 2019;12(1):50.
155.. Mascarelli PE, Keel MK, Yabsley M, et al. Hemotropic mycoplasmas in little brown bats (*Myotis lucifugus*). Parasite Vector 2014;7:117.
156. Millan J, Cevidanes A, Sacristan I, et al. Detection and Characterization of Hemotropic Mycoplasmas in Bats in Chile. J Wildl Dis 2019;55(4):977–81.
157.. Millan J, Lopez-Roig M, Delicado V, et al. Widespread infection with hemotropic mycoplasmas in bats in Spain, including a hemoplasma closely related to "*Candidatus* Mycoplasma hemohominis". Comp Immunol Microb 2015; 39:9–12.
158. Volokhov DV, Becker DJ, Bergner LM, et al. Novel hemotropic mycoplasmas are widespread and genetically diverse in vampire bats. Epidemiol Infect 2017; 145(15):3154–67.
159. Barker EN, Tasker S. Hemotropic Mycoplasma Infections. In: Sykes JE, ed. Greene's Infectious Diseases of the Dog and Cat, Expert Consult. 5th Edition. In print.
160. Murray RG, Stackebrandt E. Taxonomic note: implementation of the provisional status *Candidatus* for incompletely described procaryotes. Int J Syst Bacteriol 1995;45(1):186–7.

Hepatozoonosis of Dogs and Cats

Gad Baneth, DVM, PhD[a],*, Kelly Allen, MS, PhD[b]

KEYWORDS

- *Hepatozoon canis* • *Hepatozoon americanum* • *Hepatozoon felis*
- *Hepatozoon silvestris* • American canine hepatozoonosis

KEY POINTS

- *Hepatozoon* species are not transmitted by the saliva of their arthropod vectors. Dogs are infected when licking or grooming and ingesting ticks containing mature parasite oocysts.
- *Hepatozoon* spp affect a variety of specific target organs in their hosts and elicit subclinical to severe life-threatening infections with considerable diversity between the infecting species.
- According to PCR surveys, *H canis* is probably the most prevalent vector-borne parasite of dogs in Africa, Eurasia, and Latin America.
- *Hepatozoon americanum* causes severe myositis, and treatment of infected dogs must be continued for a long term to arrest the development of tissue parasite forms, which are not eliminated by antiprotozoal drugs.
- Three species of *Hepatozoon* infect domestic cats and although infection is often subclinical, it may be associated with severe clinical disease.

INTRODUCTION

Canine and feline hepatozoonosis is caused by protozoon parasites from the genus *Hepatozoon*. There are more than 340 species in this genus, and so far 2 have been found to infect dogs, *Hepatozoon canis* and *Hepatozoon americanum,* and 3 infect domestic cats, *Hepatozoon felis, Hepatozoon silvestris,* and *Hepatozoon canis.*[1,2] The life cycle of *Hepatozoon* spp involves transmission by hematophageous arthropod vectors, ixodid ticks in the case of the *Hepatozoon* spp that infect dogs. The arthropod vector harbors the oocyst stage of the parasite and is consumed by the vertebrate host when transmission occurs.[1] Different *Hepatozoon* spp affect a variety of target

[a] The Koret School of Veterinary Medicine, The Hebrew University of Jerusalem, PO Box 12, Rehovot 7610001, Israel; [b] Department of Veterinary Pathobiology, Oklahoma State University's College of Veterinary Medicine, 250 McElroy Hall, Stillwater, OK 74078, USA
* Corresponding author.
E-mail address: gad.baneth@mail.huji.ac.il

Vet Clin Small Anim 52 (2022) 1341–1358
https://doi.org/10.1016/j.cvsm.2022.06.011
vetsmall.theclinics.com

organs in carnivores and elicit subclinical to severe life-threatening infections with considerable diversity between the infecting species (**Table 1**).[3]

Hepatozoon canis

Etiology and epidemiology

Hepatozoon canis was described initially in India in 1905[4] and is probably the most prevalent vector-borne parasite of dogs in Africa, Eurasia, and Latin America, with epidemiologic surveys showing 59% prevalence by polymerase chain reaction (PCR) in dogs from 6 countries in Africa, 54% in Turkey, 53% in Brazil, 48% in Cuba, 47% in Iran and Pakistan, 30% in India, and 20% in Portugal.[5–11]

Hepatozoon canis forms a clade of closely related genetic variants that infect domestic dogs and wild carnivores including red foxes (*Vulpes vulpes*), gray wolves (*Canis lupus*), golden jackals (*Canis aureus*), black-backed jackals (*Canis mesomelas*), African wild dogs, and coyotes (*Canis latrans*) with high infection rates in some areas.[12–17] *Hepatozoon canis* has also been reported in some noncanine carnivores including domestic cats, tigers (*Panthera tigris*), raccoons (*Procyon lotor*), beech martens (*Martes fiona*) and opossums (*Didelphis albiventris*) in Brazil.[18–22]

Hepatozoon canis has also been reported to infect domestic dogs in North America, mostly in areas where *Hepatozoon americanum* is prevalent, and in some cases as coinfection with *H. americanum*.[23] Furthermore, an *Ixodes scapularis* tick with *H. canis* DNA has been reported in eastern Canada suggesting that the parasite may also be circulating in Canada.[24]

Pathogenesis

H canis is transmitted by the brown dog tick *Rhipicepahlus sanguineus* sensu lato and also by *Rhipicephalus turanicus* and by *Amblyomma ovale* in Brazil.[25–27] Transstadial transmission from the larva to the nymph stage, and also from the nymph to the adult stage, has been demonstrated in *R. sanguineus;* however, no transovarial transmission from the tick to its eggs has been reported. *H. canis* is also transmitted transplacentally during gestation from dams to their pups.[28] After tick ingestion, *H. canis* sporozoites cross the dog's gut and are carried by blood or lymph to the spleen, bone marrow, lymph nodes, and other organs such as the lungs, kidney and liver, where they form meronts (**Fig. 1**).[25] Merozoites that develop in meronts release and invade neutrophils and monocytes to transform into gamonts, which circulate in the blood within their host cells and can then be ingested by feeding ticks (**Fig. 2**). The life cycle of *H. canis,* including both tick and dog parts of the cycle, is completed within 81 days.[25] Adult-stage *R. sanguineus* ticks were infective to dogs by ingestion 53 days after the ticks fed as nymphs on a naturally infected dog in an experimental study. Meronts were first detected in the experimentally infected dog's bone marrow 13 days postinoculation, and gamonts were evident in the blood in 28 days, thereby completing the parasite's life cycle.[25]

Most dogs infected with *H. canis* have a subclinical infection; however, a variety of clinical abnormalities, which range in severity from a mild anemia to a debilitating and life-threatening illness, are possible.[29] The severity of the disease has been correlated with the degree of *H. canis* parasitemia and number of circulating gamonts.[29,30] Most infected dogs have a low parasitemia, with less than 5% of circulating leukocytes infected with gamonts. Dogs with a high level of parasitemia (>800 gamonts/μL) in some cases approaching 100% of infected circulating segmented leukocytes have very high tissue parasite loads and may develop hepatitis, glomerulonephritis, or pneumonitis associated with *H. canis* meronts, in addition to severe anemia, fever, and cachexia.[29]

Table 1
Characteristics of the *Hepatozoon* species that infect domestic dogs and cats

Species	Domestic Animal Host	Vector	Geographic Distribution	Main Target Organs and Systems
Hepatozoon canis	Dog (also infects cats)	*Rhipicephalus sanguineus* s.l.; *Rhipicephalus turanicus*; *Amblyomma ovale*	Africa, Eurasia, Latin America, Southeastern United States	Lymph node, spleen, bone marrow, liver, kidney, lungs
Hepatozoon americanum	Dog	*Amblyomma maculatum*	Southeastern United States spreading north and west	Skeletal and cardiac muscle, extraocular muscles
Hepatozoon felis	Cat	Unknown	Africa, Southern and central Europe, Asia, Brazil, United States	Skeletal and cardiac muscles
Hepatozoon silvestris	Cat	Unknown	Southern and central Europe	Cardiac muscles

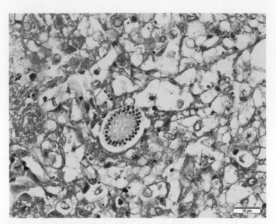

Fig. 1. A wheel-spoke-shaped *Hepatozoon canis* meront in the lung of a dog (hematoxylin-eosin stain). (Image courtesy of Dr. Shelly Hahn.)

Other infections and immune-suppressive conditions increase the susceptibility to new *H. canis* infection or permit existing dormant infections to reactivate. Coinfections with pathogens such as *Ehrlichia canis, Anaplasma* spp, *Babesia* spp, *Toxoplasma gondii, Leishmania infantum,* canine parvovirus, and canine distemper have been reported in dogs with *H. canis* infection.[1] *Ehrlichia canis, Anaplasma platys,* and *Babesia vogeli* are transmitted by the same tick vector as *H. canis, R. sanguineus* s.l., and therefore it is common to find concurrent infections with these canine pathogens.

Clinical signs
No sex or breed predilection has been confirmed as predisposing for infection with *H. canis,* and dogs of all age groups, from pups younger than 3 months to old dogs, are susceptible to disease. Dogs with *H. canis* infection are more likely to be from a rural area when compared with an urban setting, possibly due to a higher tick exposure rate.

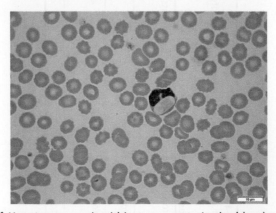

Fig. 2. Gamont of *Hepatozoon canis* within a monocyte in the blood of a dog. Note the thick capsule visible around the parasite and the compression of the host cell lobulated nucleus (May-Grunwald Giemsa stain).

Dogs infected with *H. canis* may not have any apparent clinical signs or present with mild disease with pale mucous membranes and lethargy; however, dogs with high parasitemia frequently exhibit fever, extreme lethargy, lymphadenomegaly, spleno-megaly, and severe weight loss.[1]

Laboratory findings
Anemia, usually normocytic normochromic, is the most common hematologic abnor-mality found in *H. canis* infection.[29,31,32] The leukocyte count is frequently within the reference ranges when the parasitemia level is low, and is frequently elevated with a high parasitemia. Extreme leukocytosis reaches even up to 150,000 white blood cells/μL in some dogs with high gamont loads.[29,32–34] Mild to moderate thrombocyto-penia is found in about a third of the dogs infected with *H. canis*.[35] Serum chemistry abnormalities include elevated total proteins with polyclonal hyperglobulinemia, hypo-albuminemia, and increased activities of alkaline phosphatase (ALP) and creatine ki-nase (CK).[1]

Diagnosis
Hepatozoon canis gamonts are ellipsoid corpuscles enveloped in thick membranes that measure approximately 11 × 4 μm and can be readily detected in the cytoplasm of neutrophils and monocytes by light microscopy of Giemsa- or Diff-Quik-stained blood smears (see **Fig. 2**). The gamonts often compress the lobulated nuclei of their host cells toward the cell membrane.[25] Examination of buffy coat smears is more sen-sitive than routine blood smear evaluation; however, PCR of blood is by far more sen-sitive. Population studies comparing detection of *H. canis* by blood smear microscopy versus PCR have shown that PCR is up to 22 times more sensitive.[36]

The meront stage of *H. canis* can be detected in cytologic preparations from lymph nodes, the spleen, and bone marrow. Meronts are round to oval, approximately 30 μm in diameter, and contain merozoites in different stages of development (see **Fig. 1**). Histopathology of affected tissues shows typical "wheel-spoke" meronts in which developing merozoites are aligned in a circle around a central opaque core.[25]

Serologic testing using enzyme-linked immunosorbent assay and IFA has been used mostly for epidemiologic studies because anti-*H. canis* antibodies indicate expo-sure and not necessarily persistent infection.[1]

Treatment
Antiprotozoal treatment of *H. canis* results in clinical improvement with gradual decrease of parasitemia but often not in complete elimination of parasites as indicated by the persistence of a positive blood PCR.[37,38] Imidocarb dipropionate, currently considered the drug of choice for *H. canis* infection, is injected intramuscularly or sub-cutaneously at 5 to 6 mg/kg, every 14 days, until gamonts are no longer detected in blood smears. The elimination of gamonts in heavy infections may require treatment for 8 weeks or longer. Doxycycline at 10 mg/kg/d orally for 21 days is often used in combination with imidocarb dipropionate to treat rickettsial vector-borne coinfections such as ehrlichiosis and anaplasmosis.[1] Oral treatment with the anticoccidial toltra-zuril at 10 mg/kg/d for 5 days followed by 5 mg/kg/d for an additional 10 days, com-bined with trimethoprim-sulfonamide at 15 mg/kg orally every 12 hours for 30 days was described to be successful in a case report involving a single dog.[39]

Prevention
Prevention of *H. canis* infection consists of tick control using topical and environmen-tally active commercial ectoparasiticides. Dogs should be prevented from ingesting ticks while grooming or scavenging. *Hepatozoon* canis has not been reported to be

transmitted by blood transfusion from donor to recipient. To complete the life cycle of *H. canis,* circulating gamonts need to pass through the tick in which the sporozoites, the infective stage of the parasite, are produced in oocysts. However, it is not known if merozoites from tissue stages may circulate in the dogs' blood and be contagious to other dogs. Therefore, it is reasonable to avoid using dogs infected with *H. canis* or *H. americanum* as blood donors.

Hepatozoon americanum

Etiology and epidemiology

Hepatozoon americanum was first documented in 1978 in a coyote from Texas followed by dogs in several south-central and southeastern states. The North American parasite was initially thought to be *H canis* due to morphologic similarities of gamont stages.[40–42] In 1997, *H. americanum* was recognized as a novel parasite and causative agent of American canine hepatozoonosis (ACH) based on several characteristics including morphology of asexual stages (meronts), tissue tropism, and clinical manifestations in canine hosts.[42–46] Salient clinical features of ACH are due to the inflammation occurring in the striated muscle tissue in response to *H. americanum* presence and merogonic cycles.[45,47–51] Dogs become infected with *H. americanum* by ingesting infected Gulf Coast ticks containing sporulated oocysts of *H. americanum.* Ingestion of infected ticks occurs through self-grooming, grooming other animals, or preying or scavenging on animals with ticks on them.[42,43,52]

Autochthonous cases of ACH generally occur in areas where Gulf Coast ticks are known to be long established, which include states spanning westward from Texas to North Carolina, particularly coastal states.[40,42,53,54] However, the aggressive and hardy tick species is now established in several landlocked Midwestern and southern states, and in Atlantic states as far northeast as Delaware. ACH is an emerging disease that may become enzootic in these more inland and northern regions where Gulf Coast ticks have extended in geographic range.[54–59] Dogs infected with *H. americanum* have also been documented in states where *A. maculatum* is not known to be endemic, likely due to displacement or travel of infected dogs.[23,60]

H americanum readily transmits transstadially from infected *A maculatum* larvae to nymphs, nymphs to adults, and larvae to adults.[43,49] However, the natural prevalence of *H americanum* in field-caught *A. maculatum* in ACH enzootic areas seems to be low.[61,62] Coyotes (*Canis latrans*) may serve as reservoirs of infection to Gulf Coast ticks in south-central states, as some focal survey studies have shown a high prevalence of infection.[17,63,64] Although rodents and rabbits are infected with other *Hepatozoon* species in nature, and experimentally can serve as paratenic hosts of *H. americanum, H. americanum* has not yet been identified in wildlife other than coyotes.[17,52,54,63–66] Transplacental transmission of *H. americanum* from infected dam to puppies, unlike in *H. canis* infection, does not seem to occur.[28]

Pathogenesis

Reproducing meronts exhibit blastophore formation, and induce host cell encystment via production of mucopolysaccharide layers, presumably to protect intracellular parasites from immunologic attack.[47,67] The cysts are aptly dubbed "onion skin cysts" because the mucopolysaccharide strata resemble the concentric layers of an onion in stained histologic sections (**Fig. 3**).[42,51,68] The pathogenesis of ACH is attributed to merozoites erupting out of host cells, breaching protective mucopolysaccharide cyst layers, and inciting inflammation in striated muscle. Local influxes of inflammatory cells are recruited, often leading to pyogranuloma formation where intact cysts once were (**Fig. 4**).[50] Intact cysts can remain dormant for years, but will periodically

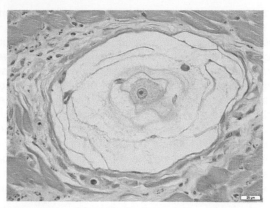

Fig. 3. Characteristic onion skin cyst in the skeletal muscle of a dog infected with *Hepatozoon americanum* (hematoxylin-eosin stain).

reactivate to cause clinical relapse.[50,53] Glomerulonephritis and amyloidosis may occur in chronically infected dogs, likely due to prolonged inflammation.[67]

Bony proliferation, particularly along the periosteum of long bones commonly occurs in patients with ACH. The mechanism behind this pathologic condition is not clear but may be associated with the tremendous inflammation occurring proximally in skeletal muscle tissue, or possibly humoral factors.[69] Osteal changes associated with ACH are more commonly observed in younger dogs.[67]

Clinical signs
Severity of ACH in many dogs suggests that domestic dogs are not well-adapted hosts of *H. americanum,* but more likely accidental hosts.[50,67] Dogs of varying ages are diagnosed with ACH and suffer severe clinical manifestations, indicating that age does not seem to influence how well or poorly dogs tolerate infection. Unlike *H. canis* infection, concurrent infection or immunosuppression does not seem to lead to increased severity of clinical disease caused by *H. americanum.*[42,67] In experimental infections, dogs present with clinical signs of ACH approximately 4 to 5 weeks

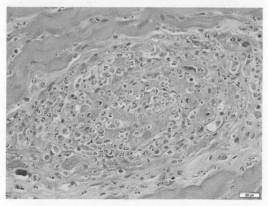

Fig. 4. Pyogranuloma in the skeletal muscle of a dog infected with *Hepatozoon americanum.* Zoites are present in numerous leukocytes and displacing nuclei (hematoxylin-eosin stain).

after ingesting *H. americanum* oocysts, although muscle lesions can be observed by histopathology as soon as 3 weeks postinfection.[48]

Clinical features of ACH include altered gait, bilateral mucopurulent ocular discharge and decreased tear production, cachexia, generalized weakness, inability to rise, lethargy, muscle atrophy, myositis, painfulness, pyrexia, and reluctance to move (**Fig. 5**). Clinical signs can mimic those of discospondylitis or meningitis due to pain, stiffness, and neck guarding. Pyrexia may abate and then episodically recur corresponding with parasite merogony cycles. Dogs often maintain a fairly normal appetite, but will continue to lose weight due to the increased caloric demands of severe, persistent inflammation. In chronically infected dogs with glomerulonephritis or amyloidosis, polydipsia and polyuria may be noted; nephrotic syndrome and thromboembolism may ensue. Other less commonly observed clinical signs of ACH include abnormal lung sounds, cough, diarrhea, lymphadenomegaly, and pale mucous membranes.[42,50,53,70,71]

Laboratory findings

Complete blood cell count analysis will often reveal neutrophilic leukocytosis, which is sometimes profound. Mild-to-moderate anemia, normocytic normochromic and nonregenerative, is another frequent abnormality on blood work. Platelet counts are often normal to elevated. Thrombocytopenia is more rarely detected, and usually in dogs with ACH and concurrent tick-borne diseases, including babesiosis, ehrlichiosis, and Rocky Mountain spotted fever.[67]

Aberrations on serum chemistry panels are often seen in patients with ACH. A mild increase in ALP is typical, possibly attributable to new bone formation. Decreased glucose concentration is observed, but this is not a true hypoglycemia, rather an in vitro result of glucose utilization by elevated leukocyte numbers. Low albumin is commonly observed, possibly caused by decreased protein intake, prolonged inflammation, or renal disease. Blood urea nitrogen (BUN) is often decreased. The concomitance of apparent hypoglycemia, decreased albumin and BUN, and elevated ALP in serum may give clinicians the erroneous impression of liver failure. However, fasting and postprandial bile acids in patients with ACH are most often normal to very slightly elevated. Despite myositis, CK is typically normal. Hyperglobulinemia is also uncommon.[42,67,71]

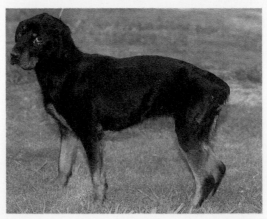

Fig. 5. Dog naturally infected with *Hepatozoon americanum* and displaying clinical signs including mucopurulent ocular discharge and areas of marked muscle atrophy. (Image courtesy of Dr. Nancy Vincent-Johnson.)

Plain radiography will show bony changes in most dogs with ACH. The bone lesions morphologically resemble those of hypertrophic osteopathy and can vary from subtle irregular exostoses to thick layers forming pseudocortices parallel to the original cortex. The lesions associated with *H americanum* infection are the most prominent on the diaphysis of long bones, and to a lesser degree on flat and irregular bones.[50,53,67,71]

Diagnosis

History of tick exposure, geographic region, clinical signs, blood count abnormalities (in particular profound neutrophilia), and bony lesions on radiographs can all help aid in the diagnosis of dogs with ACH. Muscle biopsy, although invasive, is considered the gold-standard method for diagnosing *H. americanum* infections. Biopsy specimens (approximately 2 × 2 cm) are taken from the biceps femoris or semitendinous muscles under general anesthesia. Although the parasite is widely distributed in striated muscle, false-negative results may occur when biopsy specimens do not contain parasite stages or characteristic lesions (see **Figs. 3** and **4**); to increase sensitivity, 2 to 3 muscle biopsy specimens can be taken.[51,53,71]

Unlike in *H canis* infections, gamonts of *H. americanum* are very rarely found in stained blood films. Less than 0.1% of leukocytes on peripheral blood smears will contain *H. americanum* gamonts (**Fig. 6**). Examination of buffy coat smears may increase likelihood for microscopic observation of *H. americanum* gamonts.[42,53,67,71] Molecular methods have been developed for detecting *H. americanum* DNA in whole blood but may lack sensitivity in early or chronic phases of disease when gamonts in circulation are few to absent, leading to false-negative results.[23,60] A real-time PCR is commercially available to veterinary practitioners seeking to test dogs for *Hepatozoon* spp. A negative PCR test result should not alone rule out *H. americanum* infection; it is recommended that muscle biopsy be performed in clinically suspicious dogs when PCR results are negative.[60]

Treatment and prognosis

Currently recommended treatments for ACH are not curative, because all *H. americanum* tissue stages cannot be eliminated, but they will result in remission of clinical signs, and offer infected dogs quality of life and longevity.[42,50,67,72,73] Patients with ACH are initially treated with either a triple combination of trimethoprim-sulfadiazine

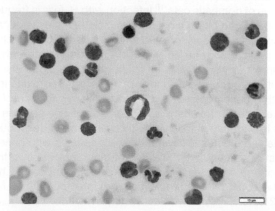

Fig. 6. Rare gamont of *Hepatozoon americanum* in a neutrophil on a blood smear from a dog with ACH (Giemsa stain).

(15 mg/kg twice a day), clindamycin (10 mg/kg 3 times a day), and pyrimethamine (0.25 mg/kg once daily), often abbreviated as TCP, or ponazuril (10 mg/kg 2 times a day) orally for 14 days. Response to either initial parasiticidal treatment is often remarkable, with clinical signs including fever and pain resolving within 1 week. Supplemental nonsteroidal anti-inflammatory drugs (NSAIDs) may be given for fever and pain control until the parasiticide begins to take effect, or as needed depending on clinical condition.[72,73]

To stave off relapse, it is necessary to follow TCP or ponazuril treatment with decoquinate (10–20 mg/kg by mouth twice a day) continuously for 2 years, which seems to arrest parasite zoites as they are released from meronts. Unfortunately, mild relapse can still occur even with decoquinate therapy. If relapse occurs, it is recommended to repeat the initial parasiticidal treatment and continue follow-up treatment with decoquinate. Once relapses begin to occur they tend to become more frequent, and with every episode there is increased risk of developing complications from amyloidosis, cachexia, glomerulonephropathy, and vasculitis.[71–74]

Prevention

Protecting dogs from ACH can be achieved through an integrative pest management approach combining the use of oral or topical acaricides in dogs, environmental acaricides, and removal of attached ticks when observed. In addition, limiting predation or scavenging opportunities for dogs will prevent dogs from ingesting infected ticks parasitizing other animals or infected tissues from possible paratenic hosts.[42,52,53,67,71]

Feline Hepatozoonosis

Domestic cat hepatozoonsis has been reported in Asia, Africa, Europe, and North and South America. Three species of Hepatozoon, Hepatozoon felis, Hepatozoon silvestris, and H. canis, have been described to infect domestic cats (see **Table 1**).[2] The description of clinical findings associated with these species is based on a small number of reported cases published in the veterinary scientific literature.[75–78] The arthropod vectors of H. felis and H. silvestris are currently unknown. Transplacental transmission from the queen to its offspring during pregnancy and also transmission by prey on other possible mammal hosts have been suspected for H. felis.

Leucocytozoon felis domestici later renamed H. felis was reported for the first time from a domestic cat in India in 1908.[79] Hepatozoon felis develops mainly in skeletal and cardiac muscles of domestic cats.[18] Infection with H. felis is frequently subclinical, and its detection in stained blood smears or muscle biopsies is occasionally an incidental finding. Clinical findings associated with H. felis infection include anemia, and increased serum muscle enzyme activities of CK and lactate dehydrogenase.[75] A cat from Austria infected with H. felis in which other infectious diseases were ruled out presented with a poor body condition, lethargy, anorexia, icterus, a painful abdomen, fever, thrombocytopenia, and leukopenia.[76] H. felis and H. felis-like infections have been reported in a variety of nondomestic feline species as well as other carnivores, and it is currently not clear whether all of these descriptions refer to only 1 species, or if these are actually several different species with genetic similarities.[1]

Epidemiologic surveys conducted by PCR of blood have shown that H. felis infection is frequent in some countries. Fifteen percent of 80 apparently healthy cats from Cape Verde off the coast of Western Africa were infected with H. felis.[80] In another study 36% of 152 cats surveyed in Israel were positive for H. felis, and a significant association was found between infection and outdoor access but not with gender, age, or feline immunodeficiency virus (FIV) infection. Of 282 cats examined for

Hepatozoon spp infection in Greece, 26% were positive by blood PCR for *H. felis* and 9 of them (13%) showed gamonts by blood smear microscopy.[81] Coinfection with another disease agent may worsen *H. felis* infection and allow the parasite to increase its proliferation and dissemination in the cat tissues. Coinfections with *H. felis* have been reported in several surveys and clinical reports of *H. felis* infection.[18,82] Coinfections described in a study of cats with a travel history from Germany included leishmaniosis, hemotrophic mycoplasmosis, FIV, and feline leukemia virus (FeLV).[78]

Hepatozoon silvestris was initially described in a wild cat species (*Felis silvestris*) in Bosnia and Herzegovina in 2017 and was detected also by PCR in the blood of a domestic cat in Italy in the same year.[2,83] *H silvestris* was reported thereafter to be associated with a fatal lymphoplasmacytic and histiocytic myocarditis in a cat from Switzerland that presented with weakness and anorexia and died shortly after presentation to a veterinary clinic.[77]

Hepatozoon canis has been reported to infect domestic cats based on PCR surveys and molecular detection of the parasite DNA in blood in several countries including Israel, Spain, Italy, and Brazil. However, no distinct clinical signs have been associated so far with *H canis* infection of domestic cats.[2,18,84]

Diagnosis of feline hepatozoonsis is possible by detection of *Hepatozoon* spp gamonts in blood smears, detection of meront stages in tissues by histopathology, or by PCR of blood or tissues.[18] The gamonts of *H. felis* are elongated spherical structures about 10.5 by 4.7 μm in size surrounded by a membrane and possess an acentric rounded nucleus (**Fig. 7**). The meront developmental stages in tissues are mostly found in *H. felis* and *H. silvestris* infections in skeletal and myocardial muscles; however, meronts have also been reported in other tissues including the spleen, pancreas, and lungs.[18,83] Meronts seen on histopathology are round to oval with a mean length and width of 39 by 35 μm for *H. felis* and surrounded by a thick membrane and containing developing or fully mature merozoites.[18]

No controlled experiments have been published on the treatment of feline hepatozoonosis, and the drugs used in some published cases of *Hepatozoon* spp infection are not approved for cats and their use was off-label. Imidocarb dipropionate at 6 mg/kg injected subcutaneously twice with an interval of 14 days in combination with doxycycline monohydrate at 5 mg/kg orally for 4 weeks has been reported to be effective in a cat that recovered from *H. felis* infection.[76] Another cat that recovered

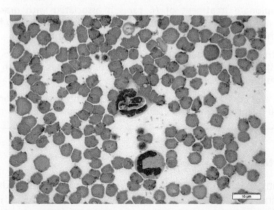

Fig. 7. Gamont of *Hepatozoon felis* in the blood of a cat coinfected with *Mycoplasma hemofelis* (May Grunwald-Giemsa stain).

clinically was treated with primaquine, an antimalarial drug, at 2 mg/kg orally once and oxytetracycline at 50 mg/kg twice daily.[85]

Although no vectors of feline *Hepatozoon* species have been described, it is possible that ectoparasites such as ticks, fleas, or other arthropod vectors may transmit hepatozoonosis, and it is therefore recommended to use ectoparasite preventives licensed for cats against fleas and ticks. Hunting of rodents or other animals by cats should also be prevented because it has been shown that other *Hepatozoon* spp are transmitted to their hosts by consuming infected small mammals.

Public health importance

The zoonotic risk of human infection with canine and feline *Hepatozoon* spp, although not known, is likely low due to route of infection, which is the ingestion of infected vectors rather than the blood feeding of infected arthropods. Still, caution should be exercised when removing ticks from infested dogs and cats because known zoonotic blood-borne pathogens may be present within ticks.

SUMMARY

Comparison of the *Hepatozoon* species that infect dogs and cats shows that they vary in their main target organs and the patterns of disease that they induce. *H. canis* targets the hemolymphoid organs, subclinical infections are widely prevalent in much of the world, and the parasite rarely causes overt disease in dogs, whereas *H. americanum* typically causes severe myositis with prevalent clinical disease, and so far infections in dogs are limited to the United States. The feline *Hepatozoon* species target skeletal muscles and the myocardium like *H. americanum;* however, they seem to be less virulent except for sporadic cases of severe disease. Currently used drugs against hepatozoonosis are effective in ameliorating clinical disease but not in eliminating infection, and more effective drugs are needed for treating these diseases effectively.

CLINICS CARE POINTS

- Detection of *H. canis* gamonts in the blood of dogs with clinical disease by blood smear microscopy is frequent, whereas finding similar-looking gamonts in the blood of dogs with *H americanum* infection is rare.

- Imidocarb dipropionate treatment of *H. canis* is associated with gradual decrease in parasitemia but not with parasite elimination, and dogs may continue to be blood PCR positive after clinical improvement and long medical treatment.

- Coinfections with other pathogens are frequent in *H. canis*-infected dogs and are often associated with their clinical condition and laboratory outcomes. A search to detect and treat coinfections is imperative.

- Blood PCR of *H. americanum* may be negative in dogs with overt ACH, and diagnosis may then be achieved by muscle biopsies of affected skeletal muscles.

CASE DESCRIPTION

"Cowboy," a 2-year-old castrated male Corgi from Midwest City, Oklahoma, was presented to a veterinarian with a 3-week history of lameness and lethargy. The owner said that he seemed stiff and reluctant to move, and over the past several days would only eat and drink if his bowls were brought to him. The veterinarian noted a bilateral mucopurulent ocular discharge, which the owner said began 1 week prior. Physical examination revealed the dog had an elevated body temperature of 104.2°F (40.1°C); appeared painful with palpation of head, neck, limb, and trunk muscles; and had a body condition score of 4/9 with moderate generalized muscle atrophy apparent. Result of ophthalmic examination was normal. Complete blood cell count revealed neutrophilia (26,400 cells/μL), and serum chemistry indicated decreased BUN (8 mg/dL) and elevated ALP (132 U/L) levels. Multiple blood smears were negative for microorganisms. No ectoparasites were observed on Cowboy, he was current on all vaccinations, received monthly heartworm preventive, and had no travel history outside of Oklahoma. Cowboy is an indoor dog but is allowed to run around and explore on the family farm. The veterinarian suspected hepatozoonosis based on geographic region, clinical signs, and laboratory findings and sent blood to a diagnostic laboratory for confirmation by PCR. The blood PCR result was negative. Muscle biopsy was performed on Cowboy under anesthesia to sample 3 areas with notable atrophy. Histopathologic examination revealed lesions found throughout the muscle biopsy samples from Cowboy (**Fig. 8**).

Based on the muscle biopsy demonstrating parasitic cysts compatible with *H americanum* infection, Cowboy was diagnosed with American canine hepatozoonosis.

TREATMENT

Cowboy was begun on a regimen of ponazuril (10 mg/kg, by mouth, every 12 hours for 14 days) and an NSAID for pain. The owner indicated that Cowboy had improved greatly in just 1 week, and seemed completely back to normal activity after the 14-day course of ponazuril. After the ponazuril treatment, Cowboy was started on long-term decoquinate therapy (15 mg/kg, by mouth, every 12 hours with food). After approximately 3 months, the owner thought that Cowboy was healed and decided to stop giving the twice-daily decoquinate. One week after the treatment was ceased, the condition relapsed and Cowboy was again presented to the veterinarian. Physical examination findings and laboratory results were similar to those at initial presentation.

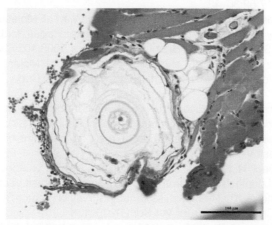

Fig. 8. (Case report) Onion skin cyst found in muscle biopsy sample from Cowboy (hematoxylin-eosin stain). (Photomicrograph courtesy of Drs. Rory Chien and Anthony Confer, Oklahoma State University's College of Veterinary Medicine and the Oklahoma Animal Disease Diagnostic Laboratory Summer 2018 (Vol. 17) E-NEWS alert.)

Another regimen of ponazuril was administered, followed by uninterrupted decoquinate therapy. After 1 year, Cowboy has not relapsed.

SUMMARY

This case illustrates that diagnosis of ACH is not straight forward and that geographic region, clinical signs, and laboratory findings are key to identifying patients. The veterinarian suspected ACH in Cowboy, despite negative blood smears and a negative result of PCR of blood; muscle biopsy confirmed his suspicion. Cowboy responded very well to treatment, but the follow-up decoquinate treatment must be continued long-term to prevent relapse. After 1 year, the condition has not relapsed.

DISCLOSURE

The authors declare that they have no conflict of interest related to any of the topics presented in this publication.

REFERENCES

1. Baneth G. Perspectives on canine and feline hepatozoonosis. Vet Parasitol 2011; 181:3–11.
2. Giannelli A, Latrofa MS, Nachum-Biala Y, et al. Three different *Hepatozoon* species in domestic cats from southern Italy. Ticks Tick Borne Dis 2017;8:721–4.
3. Modrý D, Beck R, Hrazdilová K, et al. A Review of methods for detection of *Hepatozoon* infection in carnivores and arthropod Vectors. Vector Borne Zoonotic Dis 2017;17:66–72.
4. James SP. On a parasite found in the white corpuscles of the blood of dogs. Sci Mem Off Med Sanit Dep Gov India 1905;14:1–12.
5. Heylen D, Day M, Schunack B, et al. A community approach of pathogens and their arthropod vectors (ticks and fleas) in dogs of African Sub-Sahara. Parasit Vectors 2021;14:576.
6. Aktas M, Ozubek S. A survey of canine haemoprotozoan parasites from Turkey, including molecular evidence of an unnamed *Babesia*. Comp Immunol Microbiol Infect Dis 2017;52:36–42.
7. Rubini AS, dos Santos Paduan K, Von Ah Lopes V, et al. Molecular and parasitological survey of *Hepatozoon canis* (Apicomplexa: Hepatozoidae) in dogs from rural area of Sao Paulo state, Brazil. Parasitol Res 2008;102:895–9.
8. Díaz-Sánchez AA, Hofmann-Lehmann R, Meli ML, et al. Molecular detection and characterization of *Hepatozoon canis* in stray dogs from Cuba. Parasitol Int 2021; 80:102200.
9. Iatta R, Sazmand A, Nguyen VL, et al. Vector-borne pathogens in dogs of different regions of Iran and Pakistan. Parasitol Res 2021;120:4219–28.
10. Abd Rani PA, Irwin PJ, Coleman GT, et al. A survey of canine tick-borne diseases in India. Parasit Vectors 2011;4:141.
11. Dordio AM, Beck R, Nunes T, et al. Molecular survey of vector-borne diseases in two groups of domestic dogs from Lisbon, Portugal. Parasit Vectors 2021;14:163.
12. Battisti E, Zanet S, Khalili S, et al. Molecular Survey on Vector-Borne Pathogens in Alpine Wild Carnivorans. Front Vet Sci 2020;7:1.
13. Hodžić A, Georges I, Postl M, et al. Molecular survey of tick-borne pathogens reveals a high prevalence and low genetic variability of *Hepatozoon canis* in free-ranging grey wolves (*Canis lupus*) in Germany. Ticks Tick Borne Dis 2020;11: 101389.

14. Mitková B, Hrazdilová K, D'Amico G, et al. Eurasian golden jackal as host of canine vector-borne protists. Parasit Vectors 2017;10(1):183.
15. Viljoen S, O'Riain MJ, Penzhorn BL, et al. Black-backed jackals (*Canis mesomelas*) from semi-arid rangelands in South Africa harbour *Hepatozoon canis* and a *Theileria* species but apparently not *Babesia rossi*. Vet Parasitol Reg Stud Rep 2021;24:100559.
16. Netherlands EC, Stroebel C, du Preez LH, et al. Molecular confirmation of high prevalence of species of *Hepatozoon* infection in free-ranging African wild dogs (*Lycaon pictus*) in the Kruger National Park, South Africa. Int J Parasitol Parasites Wildl 2021;14:335–40.
17. Starkey LA, Panciera RJ, Paras K, et al. Genetic diversity of *Hepatozoon* spp. in coyotes from the south-central United States. J Parasitol 2013;99:375–8.
18. Baneth G, Sheiner A, Eyal O, et al. Redescription of *Hepatozoon felis* (Apicomplexa: Hepatozoidae) based on phylogenetic analysis, tissue and blood form morphology, and possible transplacental transmission. Parasit Vectors 2013; 6:102.
19. Iatta R, Natale A, Ravagnan S, et al. Zoonotic and vector-borne pathogens in tigers from a wildlife safari park, Italy. Int J Parasitol Parasites Wildl 2020;12:1–7.
20. Criado-Fornelio A, Martín-Pérez T, Verdú-Expósito C, et al. Molecular epidemiology of parasitic protozoa and *Ehrlichia canis* in wildlife in Madrid (central Spain). Parasitol Res 2018;117:2291–8.
21. Ortuño M, Nachum-Biala Y, García-Bocanegra I, et al. An epidemiological study in wild carnivores from Spanish Mediterranean ecosystems reveals association between *Leishmania infantum*, *Babesia* spp. and *Hepatozoon* spp. infection and new hosts for *Hepatozoon martis*, *Hepatozoon canis* and *Sarcocystis* spp. Transbound Emerg Dis 2021;10:1111.
22. da Silva MRL, Fornazari F, Demoner LC, et al. *Didelphis albiventris* naturally infected with *Hepatozoon canis* in southeastern Brazil. Ticks Tick Borne Dis 2017;8:878–81.
23. Allen KE, Li Y, Kaltenboeck B, et al. Diversity of *Hepatozoon* species in naturally infected dogs in the southern United States. Vet Parasitol 2008;154:220–5.
24. Scott JD, Pesapane RR. Detection of *Anaplasma phagocytophilum*, *Babesia odocoilei*, *Babesia* sp., *Borrelia burgdorferi* sensu lato, and *Hepatozoon canis* in *Ixodes scapularis* ticks collected in eastern Canada. Pathogens 2021;10:1265.
25. Baneth G, Samish M, Shkap V. Life cycle of *Hepatozoon canis* (Apicomplexa: Adeleorina: Hepatozoidae) in the tick *Rhipicephalus sanguineus* and domestic dog (*Canis familiaris*). J Parasitol 2007;93:283–99.
26. Rubini AS, Paduan KS, Martins TF, et al. Acquisition and transmission of *Hepatozoon canis* (Apicomplexa: Hepatozoidae) by the tick *Amblyomma ovale* (Acari: Ixodidae). Vet Parasitol 2009;164:324–7.
27. Giannelli A, Lia RP, Annoscia G, et al. *Rhipicephalus turanicus*, a new vector of *Hepatozoon canis*. Parasitology 2017;144:730–7.
28. Murata T, Inoue M, Tateyama S, et al. Vertical transmission of *Hepatozoon canis* in dogs. J Vet Med Sci 1993;55:867–8.
29. Baneth G, Weigler B. Retrospective case-control study of hepatozoonosis in dogs in Israel. J Vet Intern Med 1997;11:365–70.
30. Karagenc TI, Pasa S, Kirli G, et al. A parasitological, molecular and serological survey of *Hepatozoon canis* infection in dogs around the Aegean coast of Turkey. Vet Parasitol 2006;135:113–9.
31. Kontos V, Koutinas A. Canine hepatozoonosis: a review of 11 naturally occurring cases. Bull Hell Vet Med Soc 1990;41:73–81.

32. Vezzani D, Scodellaro CF, Eiras DF. Hematological and epidemiological characterization of *Hepatozoon canis* infection in dogs from Buenos Aires, Argentina. Vet Parasitol Reg Stud Rep 2017;8:90–3.

33. Baneth G, Harmelin A, Presentey BZ. *Hepatozoon canis* infection in two dogs. J Am Vet Med Assoc 1995;206:1891–4.

34. Chhabra S, Uppal SK, Singla LD. Retrospective study of clinical and hematological aspects associated with dogs naturally infected by *Hepatozoon canis* in Ludhiana, Punjab, India. Asian Pac J Trop Biomed 2013;3:483–6.

35. Thongsahuan S, Chethanond U, Wasiksiri S, et al. Hematological profile of blood parasitic infected dogs in southern Thailand. Vet World 2020;13:2388–94.

36. Aktas M, Özübek S, Altay K, et al. A molecular and parasitological survey of *Hepatozoon canis* in domestic dogs in Turkey. Vet Parasitol 2015;209:264–7.

37. Sasanelli M, Paradies P, Greco B, et al. Failure of imidocarb dipropionate to eliminate *Hepatozoon canis* in naturally infected dogs based on parasitological and molecular evaluation methods. Vet Parasitol 2010;171:194–9.

38. De Tommasi AS, Giannelli A, de Caprariis D, et al. Failure of imidocarb dipropionate and toltrazuril/emodepside plus clindamycin in treating *Hepatozoon canis* infection. Vet Parasitol 2014;200:242–5.

39. Voyvoda H, Pasa S, Uner A. Clinical *Hepatozoon canis* infection in a dog in Turkey. J Small Anim Pract 2004;45:613–7.

40. Craig TM, Smallwood JE, Knauer KW, et al. *Hepatozoon canis* infection in dogs: clinical, radiographic, and hematologic findings. J Am Vet Med Assoc 1978;173:967–72.

41. Davis DS, Robinson RM, Craig TM. Naturally occurring hepatozoonosis in a coyote. J Wildl Dis 1978;14:244–6.

42. Vincent-Johnson NA, Macintire DK, Lindsay DS, et al. A new *Hepatozoon* species from dogs: description of the causative agent of canine hepatozoonosis in North America. J Parasitol 1997;83:1165–72.

43. Mathew JS, Ewing SA, Panciera RJ, et al. Experimental transmission of *Hepatozoon americanum* Vincent-Johnson et al., 1997 to dogs by the Gulf Coast tick, *Amblyomma maculatum* Koch. Vet Parasitol 1998;80:1–14.

44. Mathew JS, Van Den Bussche RA, Ewing SA, et al. Phylogenetic relationships of *Hepatozoon* (Apicomplexa: Adeleorina) based on molecular, morphologic, and life-cycle characters. J Parasitol 2000;86:366–72.

45. Panciera RJ, Mathew JS, Cummings CA, et al. Comparison of tissue stages of *Hepatozoon americanum* in the dog using immunohistochemical and routine histologic methods. Vet Pathol 2001;38:422–6.

46. Ewing SA, Mathew JS, Panciera RJ. Transmission of *Hepatozoon americanum* (Apicomplexa: Adeleorina) by ixodids (Acari: Ixodidae). J Med Entomol 2002;39:631–4.

47. Panciera RJ, Ewing SA, Mathew JS, et al. Observations on tissue stages of *Hepatozoon americanum* in 19 naturally infected dogs. Vet Parasitol 1998;78:265–76.

48. Panciera RJ, Ewing SA, Mathew JS, et al. Canine hepatozoonosis: comparison of lesions and parasites in skeletal muscle of dogs experimentally or naturally infected with *Hepatozoon americanum*. Vet Parasitol 1999;82:261–72.

49. Ewing SA, DuBois JG, Mathew JS, et al. Larval Gulf Coast ticks (*Amblyomma maculatum*) [Acari: Ixodidae] as host for *Hepatozoon americanum* [Apicomplexa: Adeleorina]. Vet Parasitol 2002;103:43–51.

50. Ewing SA, Panciera RJ. American canine hepatozoonosis. Clin Microbiol Rev 2003;16:688–97.

51. Cummings CA, Panciera RJ, Kocan KM, et al. Characterization of stages of *Hepatozoon americanum* and of parasitized canine host cells. Vet Pathol 2005;42: 788–96.

52. Johnson EM, Panciera RJ, Allen KE, et al. Alternate pathway of infection with *Hepatozoon americanum* and the epidemiologic importance of predation. J Vet Intern Med 2009;23:1315–8.

53. Potter TM, Macintire DK. Hepatozoon americanum: an emerging disease in the south-central/southeastern United States. J Vet Emerg Crit Care (San Antonio) 2010;20:70–6.

54. Paddock CD, Goddard J. The evolving medical and veterinary importance of the Gulf Coast tick (Acari: Ixodidae). J Med Entomol 2015;52:230–52.

55. Phillips VC, Zieman EA, Kim CH, et al. Documentation of the expansion of the Gulf Coast Tick (Amblyomma maculatum) and Rickettsia parkeri: first Report in Illinois. J Parasitol 2020;106:9–13.

56. Maestas LP, Reeser SR, McGay PJ, et al. Surveillance for Amblyomma maculatum (Acari: Ixodidae) and Rickettsia parkeri (Rickettsiales: Rickettsiaceae) in the state of Delaware, and their public health implications. J Med Entomol 2020;57:979–83.

57. Lockwood BH, Stasiak I, Pfaff MA, et al. Widespread distribution of ticks and selected tick-borne pathogens in Kentucky (USA). Ticks Tick Borne Dis 2018;9: 738–41.

58. Portugal JS 3rd, Goddard J. Evaluation of human attachment by larval Amblyomma maculatum (Acari: Ixodidae). J Med Entomol 2016;53:451–3.

59. Sonenshine DE. Range expansion of tick disease vectors in North America: implications for spread of tick-borne disease. Int J Environ Res Public Health 2018; 15:478.

60. Li Y, Wang C, Allen KE, et al. Diagnosis of canine Hepatozoon spp. infection by quantitative PCR. Vet Parasitol 2008;157:50–8.

61. Parkins ND, Stokes JV, Gavron NA, et al. Scarcity of Hepatozoon americanum in Gulf Coast tick vectors and potential for cultivating the protozoan. Vet Parasitol Reg Stud Rep 2020;21:100421.

62. Saleh MN, Allen KE, Lineberry MW, et al. Ticks infesting dogs and cats in North America: biology, geographic distribution, and pathogen transmission. Vet Parasitol 2021;294:109392.

63. Kocan AA, Breshears M, Cummings C, et al. Naturally occurring hepatozoonosis in coyotes from Oklahoma. J Wildl Dis 1999;35:86–9.

64. Kocan AA, Cummings CA, Panciera RJ, et al. Naturally occurring and experimentally transmitted *Hepatozoon americanum* in coyotes from Oklahoma. J Wildl Dis 2000;36:149–65.

65. Johnson EM, Allen KE, Panciera RJ, et al. Field survey of rodents for *Hepatozoon* infections in an endemic focus of American canine hepatozoonosis. Vet Parasitol 2007;150:27–165.

66. Johnson EM, Allen KE, Breshears MA, et al. Experimental transmission of *Hepatozoon americanum* to rodents. Vet Parasitol 2008;151:164–9.

67. Vincent-Johnson NA. American canine hepatozoonosis. Vet Clin North Am Small Anim Pract 2003;33:905–20.

68. Droleskey RE, Mercer SH, DeLoach JR, et al. Ultrastructure of *Hepatozoon canis* in the dog. Vet Parasitol 1993;50:83–99.

69. Panciera RJ, Mathew JS, Ewing SA, et al. Skeletal lesions of canine hepatozoonosis caused by *Hepatozoon americanum*. Vet Pathol 2000;37:225–30.

70. Macintire DK, Vincent-Johnson N, Dillon AR, et al. Hepatozoonosis in dogs: 22 cases (1989-1994). J Am Vet Med Assoc 1997;210:916–22.

71. Baneth G, Vincent-Johnson NA. Hepatozoonosis. In: Shaw S, editor. Arthropod-borne infectious diseases of the dog and cat. Boca Raton, FL: CRC Press; 2016. p. 109–24.

72. Macintire DK, Vincent-Johnson NA, Kane CW, et al. Treatment of dogs infected with Hepatozoon americanum: 53 cases (1989-1998). J Am Vet Med Assoc 2001;218:77–82.

73. Companion Animal Parasite Council. American canine hepatozoons. is 2013. Available at: https://capcvet.org/guidelines/american-canine-hepatozoonosis/. Accessed January 29, 2022.

74. Allen KE, Little SE, Johnson EM, et al. Treatment of Hepatozoon americanum infection: review of the literature and experimental evaluation of efficacy. Vet Ther 2010;11:E1–8.

75. Baneth G, Aroch I, Tal N, et al. Hepatozoon species infection in domestic cats: a retrospective study. Vet Parasitol 1998;79:123–33.

76. Basso W, Görner D, Globokar M, et al. First autochthonous case of clinical Hepatozoon felis infection in a domestic cat in Central Europe. Parasitol Int 2019;72: 101945.

77. Kegler K, Nufer U, Alic A, et al. Fatal infection with emerging apicomplexan parasite Hepatozoon silvestris in a domestic cat. Parasit Vectors 2018;11:428.

78. Schäfer I, Kohn B, Volkmann M, et al. Retrospective evaluation of vector-borne pathogens in cats living in Germany (2012-2020). Parasit Vectors 2021;14:123.

79. Patton WS. The haemogregarines of mammals and reptiles. Parasitology 1908;1: 318–21.

80. Pereira C, Maia JP, Marcos R, et al. Molecular detection of Hepatozoon felis in cats from Maio Island, Republic of Cape Verde and global distribution of feline hepatozoonosis. Parasit Vectors 2019;12:294.

81. Morelli S, Diakou A, Traversa D, et al. First record of Hepatozoon spp. in domestic cats in Greece. Ticks Tick Borne Dis 2021;12:101580.

82. Attipa C, Neofytou K, Yiapanis C, et al. Follow-up monitoring in a cat with leishmaniosis and coinfections with Hepatozoon felis and 'Candidatus Mycoplasma haemominutum. JFMS Open Rep 2017;3.

83. Hodžić A, Alić A, Prašović S, et al. Hepatozoon silvestris sp. nov.: morphological and molecular characterization of a new species of Hepatozoon (Adeleorina: Hepatozoidae) from the European wild cat (Felis silvestris silvestris). Parasitology 2017;144:650–61.

84. Díaz-Regañón D, Villaescusa A, Ayllón T, et al. Molecular detection of Hepatozoon spp. and Cytauxzoon sp. in domestic and stray cats from Madrid, Spain. Parasit Vectors 2017;10:112.

85. Van Amstel S. Hepatozoönose in 'n kat. J S Afr Vet Assoc 1979;50:215–6.

Leishmaniasis

Gad Baneth, DVM, PhD[a],*, Laia Solano-Gallego, DVM, PhD[b]

KEYWORDS

- *Leishmania infantum* • Canine leishmaniasis • Feline leishmaniasis • Co-infection
- Allopurinol • Meglumine antimoniate • Miltefosine • Topical insecticides

KEY POINTS

- Leishmaniasis is one of the most important zoonotic diseases in large areas of Europe, Asia, Africa, and Latin America.
- Dogs are considered the main reservoir hosts of *Leishmania infantum* for humans.
- Visceral leishmaniasis of humans and canine leishmaniasis caused by *L. infantum* are potentially fatal if not treated.
- Canine leishmaniasis causes a spectrum of disease patterns and may affect cutaneous, renal, ocular, skeletal muscle, and hemolymphatic target organs.
- Dogs and cats infected by *L. infantum* may suffer similar diseases.

INTRODUCTION

The leishmanlases are a group of diseases caused by protozoa of the genus *Leishmania* and transmitted mostly by the bite of phlebotomine sand fly vectors. There are more than 20 zoonotic *Leishmania* species that infect animals and humans. Dogs are infected by at least 13 *Leishmania* species and cats have been reported to be infected by at least 6 species.[1–4] This review focuses on *Leishmania infantum*, the main *Leishmania* species associated with severe disease in dogs and cats in Europe, Asia, Africa, and the Americas.

Leishmania (order: Kinetoplastida, family: Trypanosmatidae) are diphasic parasites whose amastigote stage is found intracellularly in host macrophages and its flagellated promastigote stage develops in the sand fly gut extracellularly. Canine and feline leishmaniasis caused by *L. infantum* are endemic in regions whereby vector sand flies are present and transmit infection.[1,5]

[a] The Koret School of Veterinary Medicine, The Hebrew University of Jerusalem, PO Box 12, Rehovot 7610001, Israel; [b] Departament de Medicina i Cirurgia Animal, Facultat de Veterinària, Universitat Autònoma de Barcelona, Bellaterra, Spain
* Corresponding author.
E-mail address: gad.baneth@mail.huji.ac.il

Vet Clin Small Anim 52 (2022) 1359–1375
https://doi.org/10.1016/j.cvsm.2022.06.012
0195-5616/22/© 2022 Elsevier Inc. All rights reserved.

CANINE LEISHMANIASIS
Epidemiology

Dogs are considered the main reservoir for human *L. infantum* infection and canine leishmaniasis is a major zoonosis endemic in more than 70 countries in an area that spans Southern Europe, Northern Africa, the Middle East, Central Asia, China, and South America.[1] *L. infantum* has also emerged in dogs in the USA and Canada, whereby transmission is thought to be mainly transplacental, rather than by sand flies.[6] The travel and importation of infected dogs and cats make the disease an important concern in endemic and nonendemic areas.[5,7]

Leishmania infection may give rise to a chronic and severe disease that can eventually be fatal in dogs and cats. However, only a small fraction of the infected animals in endemic areas develop the clinical disease while a larger part of the exposed population is subclinically infected. Longitudinal studies of natural infection with *L. infantum* have shown that some subclinically infected animals eventually develop clinical disease; however, the majority remain subclinically infected or resolve infection.[8–11] It has been estimated based on serologic surveys that 2.5 million dogs are infected with *L. infantum* in Portugal, Spain, France, and Italy. Furthermore, several million dogs are infected in South America and other endemic regions. Genetic evidence suggests that the introduction of *L. infantum* to the Americas occurred by infected dogs during the Spanish and Portuguese colonization.[12,13]

Pathogenesis

Leishmania spp. are transmitted to the skin of animals and humans when an infected female sand fly bites the host, takes a blood meal, and transmits the promastigote stage of the parasite. Promastigotes are then phagocytized by macrophages. They transform and replicate within cytoplasmic vesicles within the macrophages as amastigotes. *L. infantum* amastigotes migrate in macrophages from the skin to the local draining lymph node, and then disseminate to the spleen, bone marrow, and internal organs whereby they invade other cells.[14] After an incubation period, parasites travel back to the host skin whereby they are available for being taken up in the blood meals of feeding female sand flies. The amastigotes in the blood meal develop in the gut of a suitable sand-fly vector. They then move from the hindgut toward the fly's pharynx and are introduced into the skin of a new host when the sand fly feeds again.[9,14]

The outcome of canine infection following the infecting sand fly bite depends on the balance between the parasite virulence and infectious dose, and the immediate and long-term immune responses mounted by the infected animal host. An effective cell-mediated immune response associated with γ-interferon and reactive oxygen species production that facilitates the activation of macrophages and killing of the intracellular *Leishmania* parasites has been shown to be protective and enables infected animals to control infection. In contrast, a response that predominantly involves the secretion of interleukin 4 (IL4) and evolution of B-cell lymphocytes into plasma cells with increased IgG production and hyperglobulinemia is associated with uncontrolled infection and progression to clinical disease. T lymphocytes from dogs with chronic disease increasingly express the programmed death-1 (PD-1) cell-surface receptor and demonstrate decreased lymphocyte proliferation when stimulated with *L. infantum* antigen. These lead to a phenomenon termed T cell exhaustion in which there is a reduction in γ-interferon secretion and minimal to absent *Leishmania*-specific lymphocyte proliferation.[15,16] Hypergammaglobulinemia and high parasite load in canine leishmaniasis are associated with the formation of circulating immune complexes which are deposited in the kidneys and other organs and induce immune-complex glomerulonephritis with proteinuria. Loss of albumin through damaged glomeruli in the urine, and an inflammatory response that decreases the production of albumin, a negative acute-phase protein, by the liver, are the reasons for the subsequent serum hypoalbuminemia. Renal disease, which is considered the main cause of death in dogs with leishmaniasis, develops gradually over time. The time of onset and severity of renal disease varies between individual infected animals. Renal disease is frequently not evident in the early stages of infection.[17]

Overall, the progression of L. infantum infection to clinical disease in dogs is marked by a depression in cell-mediated immunity and an excessive humoral response.[16] Dogs that are resistant to the development of disease may develop low and sometimes intermittent and borderline antibody levels and remain subclinically infected. Dogs affected by clinical disease and subclinically infected dogs are both infectious to sand flies, and therefore constitute reservoirs.[18] A factor that may enhance transmission of L. infantum is that clinically affected dogs were found to be more attractive to sand flies in search of blood meals than uninfected dogs.[19] Naturally infected dogs and cats may develop initial signs of clinical disease after a variable subclinical incubation period of at least 3 months (for dogs), or remain subclinically infected for their lifetime.[8,20] In other cases, animals succumb to disease long after infection often due to immune-suppression by another condition such as malignant neoplasia, endocrine disease or concurrent infectious disease. A retrospective study from the University of Barcelona in Spain found that the age distribution of the disease in dogs is bimodal with a peak of prevalence at 2 to 4 years and a secondary peak from the age of 7 years.[21] The early peak likely represents dogs susceptible to the development of clinical disease while the second peak includes older dogs that may have been harboring infection subclinically for a long time and whose immune response may have been weakened by concurrent disease conditions. Age has also been associated with differences in clinicopathological findings and disease severity in canine leishmaniasis. Young dogs less than 3 years old were found to develop systemic signs with renal and hematologic abnormalities less frequently than older dogs, while dermatologic signs were more common in young and adult dogs, compared with old dogs older than 8 years.[22]

Susceptibility or resistance to canine leishmaniasis is influenced by the host's genetics. Examples of this include the overrepresentation in canine leishmaniasis surveys of breeds that originated from nonendemic countries for leishmaniasis such as the Boxer, Rottweiler, Doberman Pinscher, and German shepherd.[21,23] In comparison, severe disease is rare and significantly lower than among other breeds such as Ibizan hounds from the endemic Balearic Islands of Spain.[24] Studies have shown that Ibizan hounds produce a predominantly cellular immune response against L. infantum infection.[24,25] Genetic studies have found that disease tends to develop more frequently in dogs with certain genotypic markers. However, it is clear that many genetic loci and genes contribute to susceptibility or resistance to the disease, and their relative contributions are difficult to infer. A dog leukocyte antigen (DLA) class II DLA-DRB1 genotype, which is a dog major histocompatibility complex (MHC) class II allele, was linked to an increased risk of being infected in an endemic area in Brazil.[26] Other studies have linked the polymorphism of the canine Slc11a1(NRAMP1) gene which encodes an iron transporter protein involved in the control of intraphagosomal replication of parasites and macrophage activation, and inferred that susceptible dogs have mutations in this gene.[27]

Infection with additional vector-borne disease agents has been shown to impact the risk of developing canine leishmaniasis and the progression to clinical disease.[28,29] In a longitudinal study of 214 hunting dogs in the USA, dogs infected with 3 or more tick-borne diseases were eleven times more likely to be associated with progression to clinical leishmaniasis than dogs with no tick-borne disease. In addition, dogs with exposure to both tick-borne diseases and *Leishmania* spp. were five times more likely to die.[29] Other studies have found an association between canine leishmaniasis and canine ehrlichiosis caused by *Ehrlichia canis*. Dogs with this coinfection can develop higher skin *Leishmania* parasite loads than dogs solely infected with *Leishmania* spp.[28,30,31]

Clinical Signs

The history of dogs with canine leishmaniasis often includes weight loss, weakness, skin lesions, ocular abnormalities, epistaxis, and signs of renal disease such as polyuria and polydipsia. On physical examination, the main clinical signs found in canine leishmaniasis are dermal lesions, lymphadenomegaly, splenomegaly, ocular lesions, muscle atrophy, and poor body condition. Dogs with leishmaniasis may also present with vomiting, diarrhea, gastrointestinal disease, tongue lesions, melena, rhinitis, neurologic abnormalities, onychogryphosis (abnormal nail growth), and lameness. Fever is found in less than 20% of canine leishmaniasis cases which usually presents as a chronic disease. Sixteen to 80% of the dogs with clinical leishmaniasis have ocular or periocular lesions including uveitis and keratoconjunctivitis.[32–34]

A variety of skin lesions are found in dogs with leishmaniasis.[35] The most common is exfoliative dermatitis (**Fig. 1**), which can be generalized or localized over the face, ears, tail, and limbs. Ulcerative dermatitis is frequently found over bony prominences. Nodular dermatitis and pustular dermatitis are occasionally reported, and a mild form of papular dermatitis has also been described in dogs that have a strong cell-mediated immunity to *L. infantum* infection (**Fig. 2**).[25,36,37]

Laboratory Findings

Canine leishmaniasis is a systemic disease that affects multiple systems and organs and causes pathology which induces alterations in hematological, serum biochemistry, and urine test parameters. Anemia, which is usually mild to moderate normocytic normochromic and nonregenerative, is a common finding in dogs with leishmaniasis. About 67% of the dogs admitted for veterinary care due to the disease are anemic, and 26% have lymphopenia while 24% have leukocytosis.[33] Thrombocytopenia is apparently not common with about 6% prevalence in a study that ruled out other conditions causing decreased platelet concentrations such as *Ehrlichia canis* infection.

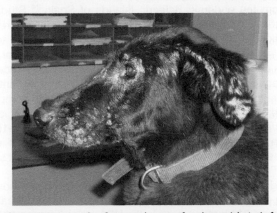

Fig. 1. Exfoliative dermatitis over the face and ears of a dog with *L. infantum* infection.

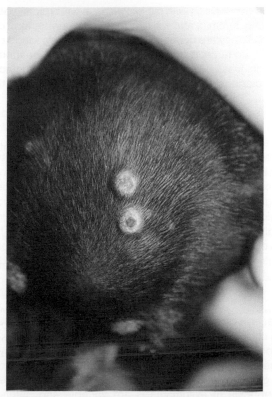

Fig. 2. Papular dermatitis due to *L. Infantum* on the head of a seven-month-old Pinscher. Note the typical crater forms with central crust and indurated margins. (*Courtesy* Dr. Laura Ordeix (Dermatology Service, Fundació Hospital Clínic Veterinari-UAB).)

The most common serum biochemistry alterations in dogs with leishmaniasis are hyperproteinemia with elevated gamma-globulins in 73%, increased beta-globulins in 68%, and hypoalbuminemia in 55%, producing a decreased albumin/globulin ratio in 78% of the affected dogs.[33] Other serum biochemistry parameters including cholesterol levels and alanine aminotransferase (ALT) activity are less frequently elevated. Azotemia with increases in urea and creatinine levels is found in dogs with advanced kidney disease due to *L. infantum* infection. Proteinuria with increased urine protein to creatinine ratio (UPC) was found in 48% of dogs affected clinically by leishmaniasis whose urine was tested.[33]

The levels of some acute-phase proteins can be used as markers for the severity of inflammation in canine leishmaniasis and for following the response to treatment.[38,39] C-reactive protein (CRP), ferritin, and haptoglobin increase in canine leishmaniasis, whereas the negative acute-phase protein paraoxonase 1 (PON1) decreases in clinical disease. Albumin which is also considered a negative acute-phase protein also decreases during disease irrespective of kidney disease and urinary loss.[38]

Clinical Evaluation of Dogs Suspected of Leishmaniasis

Evaluation of dogs suspected of leishmaniasis includes a thorough physical examination, complete blood count (CBC), serum biochemistry, and urinalysis. Due to the common ocular involvement in the disease, a thorough ophthalmologic examination is needed in infected dogs. Dogs with clinical disease will typically be hyperglobuline-mic, hypoalbuminemic, anemic, and will frequently have proteinuria due to glomerular loss of albumin, even if they are not azotemic. If proteinuria is found on a dipstick test, quantification by the urine protein/creatinine (UPC) ratio is needed to evaluate the magnitude of protein loss. Specific laboratory tests for the detection of infection described in the diagnosis section are indicated to confirm the suspicion of leishmaniasis.

A clinical staging system presented by the LeishVet association divides the canine disease into 4 clinical stages based on clinical signs, clinicopathological abnormalities, and level of antileishmanial antibodies.[40] These 4 clinical stages include stage I-mild disease, stage II-moderate disease, stage III-severe disease, and stage IV-very severe disease. The severity of the disease is mainly based on the degree of renal disease. A good example of stage I-mild disease is papular dermatitis (see **Fig. 2**) as the sole clinical sign without any evidence of systemic disease including the absence of clinicopathological abnormalities. Most sick dogs which are diagnosed with leishmaniasis in Mediterranean basin countries are classified as having stage II-moderate disease or stage III-severe disease while stage IV is less common.[40] Staging is helpful for decisions regarding the most suitable treatment and for determining prognosis.

Diagnosis

Canine leishmaniasis is often illusive and challenging to diagnose because of the variety of presenting clinical signs and clinical pathologic abnormalities, and the frequent occurrence of subclinical infection. Subclinically infected dogs may have no clinical pathologic changes and remain subclinically infected for long periods of time or develop changes gradually as they progress toward clinical disease. The indications for pursuing a diagnosis of leishmaniasis are variable and differing presentations may require the use of different tests. The presentation of dogs with clinical signs or clinical-pathological abnormalities compatible with the disease is perhaps the most common reason for seeking the diagnosis of the disease. However, the detection of subclinical infection in blood donors or testing dogs from endemic areas for importation to certain countries such as Australia and South Africa, are also indications for testing. Follow-up of dogs during disease treatment and after recovery, and testing of dogs before vaccination against leishmaniasis or as part of a health check, are additional reasons for testing for this infection. Some diagnostic assays such as cytologic detection of amastigotes in tissues will only be positive in dogs with high *Leishmania* parasite loads, as often found in animals with clinical disease, while other tests such as quantitative serology are more likely to be positive than cytologic tests that directly demonstrate the presence of the organism in dogs with lower parasite loads, including some subclinically infected animals.[40,41]

Cytologic examination of aspirates from the bone marrow, spleen, lymph nodes or skin, or touch impressions from the skin and other tissues can be used to detect *Leishmania* amastigotes. Slides can be stained by a Romanoswsky-type stain such as May Grunwald-Giemsa or quick commercial stains and viewed by light microscopy. The *Leishmania* amastigote stage is detected in the cytoplasm of macrophages and more rarely in neutrophils, and may also be viewed outside cells as an artifactual result of cell damage that can occur while making cytologic preparations.[42,43] Amastigote forms are about 1 to 4 μm long by 1 to 2 μm wide and contain a prominent nucleus and a rod-like kinetoplast structure (**Fig. 3**). The detection of the parasite by cytology is often unrewarding due to the possibility of a low number of visible tissue amastigotes even in dogs with full-blown clinical disease.

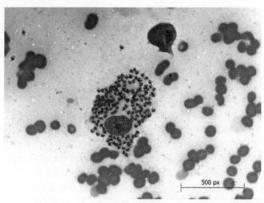

Fig. 3. Cytology of a skin lesion from the cat in **Fig. 4** showing a macrophage laden with *L. infantum* amastigotes in its cytoplasm as well as free amastigotes seen in the hemodiluted background. Diff-quick staining. (*Courtesy* Dr. Laura Ordeix (Dermatology Service, Fundació Hospital Clínic Veterinari-UAB).)

Histopathology of tissues from dogs with leishmaniasis often shows granulomatous, pyogranulomatous, or lymphoplasmocellular inflammatory patterns compatible with the disease; however, the definitive detection of *Leishmania* amastigotes in biopsy sections of the skin or other infected organs is frequently difficult. In such cases, *Leishmania* immunohistochemical staining can be used to detect and verify the presence of parasite in the tissue.[43–45]

Serology is a major diagnostic technique regularly used for the diagnosis of canine leishmaniasis.[32] Several serologic methods are used for the detection of anti-*Leishmania* antibodies. These include the enzyme-linked immunosorbent assay (ELISA), indirect immunofluorescence assay (IFA), direct agglutination test (DAT), and western blotting. ELISA and IFA are the most frequently used techniques for diagnostic and research purposes. Recombinant antigens such as rK39 and k26 are also used to detect antibodies in dogs.[46] Rapid kits for the serologic evaluation of canine leishmaniasis are commercially available and provide qualitative positive or negative results. Increased sensitivity and specificity are obtained with quantitative serologic laboratory methods such as the IFA and ELISA. However, while dogs with a clinical disease are almost always seroreactive, dogs with subclinical infection are less frequently seroreactive. Therefore, serology is not the optimal assay for detecting subclinical infection.[47]

Serologic cross-reactivity with other infectious organisms and especially with trypanosomatids such as *Trypanosoma cruzi* are a problem in areas whereby canine trypanosomiasis is common, particularly in areas of Latin America and Texas.[48,49] Serologic cross-reactivity is also found between different species of *Leishmania* which infect dogs, and antibodies formed against *Leishmania tropica*, *Leishmania major*, *Leishmania braziliensis* and *Leishmania amazonensis* are reactive with *L. infantum* antigen.[50,51] This may present difficulties in regions whereby several species of *Leishmania* cause clinical disease in dogs such as the Middle East (*L. major, L. tropica* and *L. infantum*) and South America (*L. braziliensis, L. amazonensis, Leishmania mexicana,* and *L. infantum*).

PCR to detect parasite DNA in tissues allows specific detection of *Leishmania* spp. Different PCR assays with a variety of parasite target sequences of genomic loci or kinetoplast DNA (kDNA) are used for the diagnosis of infection. kDNA PCR assays are more sensitive than genomic DNA assays which target parts of the *Leishmania* ribosomal operon DNA such as the internal transcribed spacer (ITS) region. Nevertheless, ITS-PCR is able to identify the infecting *Leishmania* species while kDNA PCR is only indicative of *Leishmania* infection without species identification.[52] The preferred and most sensitive sampling sites for *Leishmania* PCR are the lymph nodes, bone marrow, spleen, and skin, while PCR of blood or urine are less sensitive and may be negative also in cases of overt clinical disease.[32,53] Conjunctival swab PCR is a sensitive noninvasive technique which can be used in surveys and when invasive sampling of bone marrow, lymph nodes or spleen is risky.[54,55]

The LeishVet guidelines for the practical management of canine leishmaniasis recommend using quantitative serology as the main diagnostic test in dogs with clinical signs suspected of leishmaniasis, or with hematological and serum biochemistry abnormalities compatible with the disease.[32] Moderate to high antileishmanial antibody levels with clinical findings compatible with the disease are considered sufficient to reach a diagnosis of canine leishmaniasis. PCR, cytology, and histopathology demonstrating the presence of the parasite are ancillary tests that can aid in the diagnostic process of dogs with the suspected disease in the case of uncertain serologic results.[32] Combining serology and PCR may facilitate the diagnosis of subclinical infection in apparently healthy dogs and blood donors.

Treatment

Medical treatment varies according to the clinical stage of the infected dog.[40] Treatment of canine leishmaniasis is prolonged and although it is frequently successful in achieving clinical cure, if the affected dog is not in a progressive stage of the disease, complete elimination of the parasite is often not accomplished. Treatment requires long-term monitoring to follow the dog's response and detect possible relapse, ascertain that renal disease, if present or develops during treatment, does not deteriorate, and that possible side effects of the drugs do not cause harm.

Allopurinol is the main drug used for the treatment of canine leishmaniasis. It is administered orally and acts by interfering with the purine pathway and the parasite's RNA synthesis. Allopurinol is given as long-term treatment of at least 6 months and usually a year or more (**Table 1**). The pentavalent antimony meglumine antimoniate (Glucantime) which inhibits leishmanial glycolysis and fatty acid oxidation and is injected subcutaneously is frequently used in combination with allopurinol for the first 4 weeks of treatment. Alternatively, miltefosine (Milteforan), can be used orally for the first month of treatment in combination with allopurinol instead of meglumine antimoniate. Monotherapy with meglumine antimoniate or miltefosine has not been shown to produce consistent long-term suppression of parasite loads in dogs and may result in disease relapse within 6 months to 1 year.[56,57] Other second-line drugs such as paramomycin and marbofloxacin have been shown to have antileishmanial effects.[58] The standard treatment protocol in Europe for dogs in the stable clinical condition is allopurinol at 10 mg/kg every 12 hours per-os (P.O), in combination with meglumine antimoniate at 100 mg/kg injected subcutaneously every 24 hours for 28 days, or in combination with miltefosine at 2 mg/kg P.O. every 24 hours for 28 days.[58] Dogs with severe clinical condition, particularly those with progressive renal disease due to leishmaniasis, may be treated with allopurinol alone. Long-term treatment of canine leishmaniasis is deemed a success and discontinued when all the following 3 conditions are met: (1) disappearance of clinical signs; (2) normalization of the hematology, blood biochemistry profile, and urinalysis; and (3) quantitative serology has decreased to below the cut-off value.[32]

A follow-up study of 1 year with 37 dogs that were treated with the combined allopurinol and meglumine antimoniate protocol, of which 32 dogs were in LeishVet stage

Table 1
The main antiprotozoal drugs used for the treatment of canine and feline leishmaniasis

Drug Name	Dose for Dogs	Dose for Cats
Allopurinol	10 mg/kg q 12 hr orally for 6–12 mo or more, until clinical signs disappear, clinicopathological findings return to reference values and quantitative serology reaches the cut-off value.[58]	10 mg/kg q 12 hr or 20 mg/kg q 24 h for at least 6 mo 3
Meglumine antimoniate	100 mg/kg injected subcutaneously q 24 hr for 28 d. Usually used during the first 4 weeks of the dog's treatment in combination with allopurinol administered as above.[58]	20–50 mg/kg q 24 hr subcutaneously for 30 d, alone or combined with allopurinol treatment.[3]
Miltefosine	2 mg/kg orally q 24 hr for 28 d. Usually used during the first 4 weeks of the dog's treatment in combination with allopurinol administered as above.[58]	

II and 5 in stage III, found that all dogs showed improvement in their clinical status and clinicopathological abnormalities within 30 days of treatment. There was also a substantial but incomplete drop in their blood parasite loads and antibody levels in the first 6 months of treatment. Nevertheless, despite the marked clinical improvement of most dogs, only 5 (16%) were eligible for stopping treatment at the end of 1 year of therapy.[53] In another study that included 23 dogs in LeishVet stage II treated and followed-up for 2 to 9 years, survival was generally long, although antibody levels remained positive in most dogs after 1 year of treatment. Three dogs from this study had a clinical relapse with high antibody levels and parasitemia, 8 dogs had immune-mediated lesions, such as uveitis, arthritis, and cutaneous vasculitis, and In all of these cases, the dogs had persistently high anti-*Leishmania* antibody levels at diagnosis and during follow-up. Three dogs in this study developed xanthine urolithiasis which was likely associated with their allopurinol treatment.[59]

Treated dogs can remain carriers of leishmaniasis and be infectious to sand flies and therefore dogs during and after therapy should be treated with topical insecticides to prevent transmission to other animals and to humans.[60] Owners of dogs should receive a thorough explanation about the disease, its zoonotic potential, and the prognosis of their dog.

The main adverse effects of the drugs recommended for the treatment of canine leishmaniasis include gastrointestinal signs for miltefosine, local inflammation and pain in the injection site, and potential nephrotoxicity for meglumine antimoniate, and xanthine urolithiasis and renal mineralization for allopurinol.[58]

Resistance to antileishmanial drugs including pentavalent antimonials and miltefosine has been extensively reported in humans. Disease relapse of dogs with canine leishmaniasis during allopurinol treatment has been described and was associated with allopurinol resistance of *L. infantum* isolated from these animals.[61,62] Sporadic cases of *L. infantum* isolates from dogs resistant to other drugs have been reported but clinical relapses have not been consistently described in these dogs.[63,64]

Ancillary therapy for canine leishmaniasis includes treatment with domperidone (Leishguard) which is registered in some European countries for prophylaxis of the disease.[65] Domperidone is a dopamine D2 receptor antagonist with immunostimulant properties via the stimulation of prolactin secretion which acts as a proinflammatory agent. It is claimed to reduce the probability of progression to clinical disease by stimulating cellular immunity. A dietary supplement of nucleotides and active hexose also has been assessed as an additional adjunctive for the management of sick dogs as well as the treatment of subclinically infected dogs to prevent disease progression.[66,67]

Follow-up during the treatment of canine leishmaniasis varies according to the dogs' clinical status. Dogs in stable condition and no renal disease can be monitored 1 month after the beginning of treatment with a physical examination, CBC, serum biochemistry, and urinalysis, and then if no deterioration is noted, every 3 to 4 months during the first year of treatment. Repeated serology with a quantitative assay is recommended 3 and 6 months after the beginning of treatment, and then every 6 to 12 months. A marked increase in the antibody levels of dogs during or after the end of therapy, often precedes disease relapse, and requires additional testing and consideration of repeated treatment, or the use of additional drugs and an increase in allopurinol dose in dogs under treatment.

Prevention

Transmission of L. infantum from infected dogs to vector sand flies and subsequently to naïve dogs can be greatly reduced by insecticides that prevent and repel sand fly bites. Topical insecticides containing pyrethroids in collars, spot-on formulations, and sprays, have been shown to effectively reduce Leishmania transmission. Slow release deltamethrin and flumethrin collars and long acting spot on drops containing permethrin with imidacloprid or permethrin with fipronil have been reported to significantly reduce the number of sand fly bites to dogs under experimental transmission and also to decrease transmission of infection in field studies.[68–70] The use of commercial topical insecticides proven to prevent L. infantum transmission is, therefore, currently considered as the most effective mean of protecting dogs from Leishmania infection.[71]

Commercial vaccines against canine leishmaniasis have been approved for the protection of dogs in Europe and Brazil. Overall, vaccination decreases the likelihood of clinical disease development in dogs but is less successful in entirely preventing the establishment of infection.[72] The currently marketed vaccines, Letifend in Europe and LeishTec in Brazil are based on Leishmania recombinant proteins. The Letifend consists of a chimerical protein (protein Q) formed by 5 antigenic fragments from 4 L. infantum proteins with no adjuvant, whereas the LeishTec includes recombinant protein A2 from Leishmania donovani and saponin as adjuvant. Two vaccines that are no longer produced include the Leishmune based on the fucose-mannose ligand (FML) of L. donovani and a saponin adjuvant, and the CaniLeish composed of purified excreted–secreted proteins of L. infantum adjuvanted with Quilaja saponaria saponin. Additional studies are needed for the evaluation of current vaccines and development of future vaccines against canine leishmaniasis.[72,73]

Feline leishmaniasis

Cats have been reported to be infected with at least 6 species of the genus Leishmania in different parts of the word including L. infantum, L. major, L. tropica, L. mexicana, L. braziliensis, and L. amazonensis.[3,4,74] Infection with L. infantum in cats has been described mostly from areas whereby the disease is prevalent in dogs, although clinical disease seems to be less frequent than in canines.[3,74] A study of 249 stray cats from Madrid in Spain found 4.8% seroreactivity for L. infantum and a significant association with feline immunodeficiency (FIV) infection. Only 2 of the seroreactive stray cats had clinical signs compatible with feline leishmaniasis.[75] A nationwide study of L. infantum infection in 2659 cats from Italy found an overall prevalence of 3.9% by

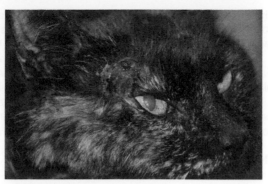

Fig. 4. Ulcerative cutaneous lesion due to squamous cell carcinoma and *L. infantum* infection in an FIV-positive cat. (*Courtesy* Dr. Laura Ordeix (Dermatology Service, Fundació Hospital Clínic Veterinari-UAB).)

combined serology and PCR with a higher infection rate of 10.5% in warmer southern Italy.[76] The risk of *L. infantum* infection in cats was associated with being older than 18 months, intact and positive for FIV.[3,76,77] Naturally infected cats are infectious to sand flies and have been speculated to be a source of infection for dogs and humans[78–80]

The clinical findings in feline leishmaniasis due to *L. infantum* are usually similar to those found in dogs with the disease. The most common clinical signs include lymphadenomegaly, skin lesions with ulcerative (**Fig. 4**), crusting, exfoliative or nodular dermatitis, ocular lesions with uveitis and conjunctivitis, gingivostomatitis, poor body condition, rhinitis and signs of renal disease. The main clinicopathological alterations are hyperproteinemia with hypergammaglobulinemia, anemia, proteinuria, and azotemia. About 50% of the cats with leishmaniasis suffer from other disease conditions such as coinfections with FIV or Feline leukemia virus (FeLV), hemotrophic *Mycoplasma* infection, malignant neoplasia, endocrine diseases, and treatment with immune-suppressive drugs.[3,77]

The diagnosis of feline leishmaniasis is performed for dogs by cytology and histopathology, serology, and PCR. Using more than one diagnostic technique is often needed to confirm the diagnosis.[77] Treatment of feline leishmaniasis may include allopurinol at 10 mg/kg q 12 hr or 20 mg/kg q 24 hr for at least 6 months (see **Table 1**). Meglumine antimoniate has also been used for cats at 20 to 50 mg/kg q 24 hr subcutaneously for 30 days, alone or combined with allopurinol treatment.[3,77] The median survival time for cats with leishmaniasis treated with antileishmanial drugs described in a case series from Spain was 17 months. Cats with concomitant diseases had a mean survival of 13 months, whereas cats with no complicating diseases had a mean survival of 41 months.[77]

Testing is recommended for feline blood donors living in or originating from a *Leishmania* endemic area. Cats can be protected from infection by the use of topical insecticides licensed for use in felines. Most of the pyrethroid-based topical insecticides licensed for dogs are toxic for cats. A flumethrin and imidacloprid collar licensed for cats was effective in decreasing *L. infantum* infection in a field trial.[81]

Public Health Importance

Human visceral leishmaniasis due to *L. infantum* is a severe and potentially fatal disease. Dogs are well-known peridomestic reservoirs for this disease and cats may also serve as reservoirs for humans through transmission by sand flies. In southern Europe whereby human visceral leishmaniasis is usually sporadic and the ratio between clinically affected people and infected dogs is high, ownership of diseased animals is often not perceived as associated with increased risk to humans. However, studies in Brazil and Iran have reported that increased prevalence of leishmaniasis in the canine population, poor socioeconomic conditions, and dog ownership are risk factors for human leishmaniasis.[82–85] Therefore, in areas whereby sand-fly vectors of leishmaniasis are present and transmission of the disease occurs, dogs and cats should be protected against sand fly-bites by topical insecticides and animal owners should be educated about the risks of this disease.

CLINICS CARE POINTS

- Leishmaniasis should be suspected in dogs and cats with compatible skin lesions, ocular lesions, renal disease, lymphadenomegaly, splenomegaly, unexplained hyperglobulinemia, epistaxis, and a variety of other clinical abnormalities.
- Dogs and cats presenting with renal disease, ocular lesions, or other pathologies caused by *L. infantum* in the absence of characteristic skin lesions should not be overlooked.
- Subclinical infection with *L. infantum* is more common than clinical disease in endemic areas.
- *Leishmania infantum* can be transmitted by blood transfusion. Blood donors from endemic areas and kennels whereby disease is present need to be tested for infection.
- Transmission of canine leishmaniasis in North American kennels and hunting dogs is mainly transplacental rather than vector borne.
- Quantitative serology is considered the most useful method for the detection of leishmaniasis in dogs and cats with suspected clinical disease.
- PCR of blood is frequently negative in dogs with clinical disease. Bone marrow, lymph node, spleen, conjunctiva, and skin samples are more likely to yield a positive PCR.
- Treatment of leishmaniasis is long-term and should not be stopped before clinical signs disappear, hematology and serum biochemistry abnormalities normalize, and quantitative serology becomes negative.
- The most effective way to prevent canine infection is protection with topical insecticides tested and approved for the prevention of leishmaniasis.

DISCLOSURE

The authors declare that they have no conflict of interest related to any of the topics presented in this publication.

REFERENCES

1. Dantas-Torres F, Solano-Gallego L, Baneth G, et al. Canine leishmaniosis in the old and new worlds: unveiled similarities and differences. Trends Parasitol 2012;28:531–8.
2. Iatta R, Mendoza-Roldan JA, Latrofa MS, et al. *Leishmania tarentolae* and *Leishmania infantum* in humans, dogs and cats in the Pelagie archipelago, southern Italy. PLoS Negl Trop Dis 2021;15:e0009817.
3. Pennisi MG, Cardoso L, Baneth G, et al. LeishVet update and recommendations on feline leishmaniosis. Parasit Vectors 2015;8:302.

4. Paşa S, Tetik Vardarlı A, Erol N, et al. Detection of *Leishmania major* and *Leishmania tropica* in domestic cats in the Ege Region of Turkey. Vet Parasitol 2015; 212:389–92.

5. Schäfer I, Volkmann M, Beelitz P, et al. Retrospective evaluation of vector-borne infections in dogs imported from the Mediterranean region and southeastern Europe (2007-2015). Parasit Vectors 2019;12:30.

6. Toepp AJ, Schaut RG, Scott BD, et al. *Leishmania* incidence and prevalence in U.S. hunting hounds maintained via vertical transmission. Vet Parasitol Reg Stud Rep 2017;10:75–81.

7. Schäfer I, Kohn B, Volkmann M, et al. Retrospective evaluation of vector-borne pathogens in cats living in Germany (2012-2020). Parasit Vectors 2021;14:123.

8. Oliva G, Scalone A, Foglia Manzillo V, et al. Incidence and time course of *Leishmania infantum* infections examined by parasitological, serologic, and nested-PCR techniques in a cohort of naive dogs exposed to three consecutive transmission seasons. J Clin Microbiol 2006;44:1318–22.

9. Baneth G, Koutinas AF, Solano-Gallego L, et al. Canine leishmaniosis - new concepts and insights on an expanding zoonosis: part one. Trends Parasitol 2008;24: 324–30.

10. Solano-Gallego L, Llull J, Ramis A, et al. Longitudinal study of dogs living in an area of Spain highly endemic for leishmaniasis by serologic analysis and the leishmanin skin test. Am J Trop Med Hyg 2005;72:815–8.

11. Grimaldi G Jr, Teva A, Santos CB, et al. The effect of removing potentially infectious dogs on the numbers of canine *Leishmania infantum* infections in an endemic area with high transmission rates. Am J Trop Med Hyg 2012;86:966–71.

12. Momen H, Pacheco RS, Cupolillo E, et al. Molecular evidence for the importation of Old World *Leishmania* into the Americas. Biol Res 1993;26:249–55.

13. Maurício IL, Stothard JR, Miles MA. The strange case of *Leishmania chagasi*. Parasitol Today 2000;16:188–9.

14. Serafim TD, Iniguez E, Oliveira F. *Leishmania infantum*. Trends Parasitol 2020; 36:80–1.

15. Solano-Gallego L, Montserrrat-Sangrà S, Ordeix L, et al. *Leishmania infantum*-specific production of IFN-γ and IL-10 in stimulated blood from dogs with clinical leishmaniosis. Parasit Vectors 2016;9:317.

16. Toepp AJ, Petersen CA. The balancing act: Immunology of leishmaniosis. Res Vet Sci 2020;130:19–25.

17. Koutinas AF, Koutinas CK. Pathologic mechanisms underlying the clinical findings in canine leishmaniasis due to *Leishmania infantum/chagasi*. Vet Pathol 2014;51:527–38.

18. Laurenti MD, Rossi CN, da Matta VL, et al. Asymptomatic dogs are highly competent to transmit *Leishmania (Leishmania) infantum chagasi* to the natural vector. Vet Parasitol 2013;196:296–300.

19. Chelbi I, Maghraoui K, Zhioua S, et al. Enhanced attraction of sand fly vectors of *Leishmania infantum* to dogs infected with zoonotic visceral leishmaniasis. PLoS Negl Trop Dis 2021;15:e0009647.

20. Otranto D, Paradies P, de Caprariis D, et al. Toward diagnosing *Leishmania infantum* infection in asymptomatic dogs in an area where leishmaniasis is endemic. Clin Vaccin Immunol 2009;16:337–43.

21. Miranda S, Roura X, Picado A, et al. Characterization of sex, age, and breed for a population of canine leishmaniosis diseased dogs. Res Vet Sci 2008;85:35–8.

22. Cabré M, Planellas M, Ordeix L, et al. Is signalment associated with clinicopathological findings in dogs with leishmaniosis? Vet Rec 2021;189:e451.

23. Gharbi M, Jaouadi K, Mezghani D, et al. Symptoms of canine leishmaniosis in Tunisian dogs. Bull Soc Pathol Exot 2018;111:51–5.

24. Solano-Gallego L, Llull J, Ramos G, et al. The Ibizian hound presents a predominantly cellular immune response against natural *Leishmania* infection. Vet Parasitol 2000;90:37–45.

25. Burnham AC, Ordeix L, Alcover MM, et al. Exploring the relationship between susceptibility to canine leishmaniosis and anti-*Phlebotomus perniciosus* saliva antibodies in Ibizan hounds and dogs of other breeds in Mallorca, Spain. Parasit Vectors 2020;13:129.

26. Quinnell RJ, Kennedy LJ, Barnes A, et al. Susceptibility to visceral leishmaniasis in the domestic dog is associated with MHC class II polymorphism. Immunogenetics 2003;55:23–8.

27. Sanchez-Robert E, Altet L, Utzet-Sadurni M, et al. Slc11a1 (formerly Nramp1) and susceptibility to canine visceral leishmaniasis. Vet Res 2008;39:36.

28. Mekuzas Y, Gradoni L, Oliva G, et al. *Ehrlichia canis* and *Leishmania infantum* co-infection: a 3-year longitudinal study in naturally exposed dogs. Clin Microbiol Infect 2009;15(Suppl 2):30–1.

29. Toepp AJ, Monteiro GRG, Coutinho JFV, et al. Comorbid infections induce progression of visceral leishmaniasis. Parasit Vectors 2019;12:54.

30. Attipa C, Solano-Gallego L, Papasouliotis K, et al. Association between canine leishmaniosis and *Ehrlichia canis* co-infection: a prospective case-control study. Parasit Vectors 2018;11:184.

31. Andrade GB, Barreto WT, Santos LL, et al. Pathology of dogs in Campo Grande, MS, Brazil naturally co-infected with *Leishmania infantum* and *Ehrlichia canis*. Rev Bras Parasitol Vet 2014;23:509–15.

32. Solano-Gallego L, Miró G, Koutinas A, et al. LeishVet guidelines for the practical management of canine leishmaniosis. Parasit Vectors 2011;4:86.

33. Meléndez-Lazo A, Ordeix L, Planellas M, et al. Clinicopathological findings in sick dogs naturally infected with *Leishmania infantum*: Comparison of five different clinical classification systems. Res Vet Sci 2018;117:18–27.

34. Oliveira CS, Ratzlaff FR, Pötter L, et al. Clinical and pathological aspects of canine cutaneous leishmaniasis: A meta-analysis. Acta Parasitol 2019;64:916–22.

35. Saridomichelakis MN, Koutinas AF. Cutaneous involvement in canine leishmaniosis due to *Leishmania infantum* (syn. *L. chagasi*). Vet Dermatol 2014;25:61–71,e22.

36. Colombo S, Abramo F, Borio S, et al. Pustular dermatitis in dogs affected by leishmaniosis: 22 cases. Vet Dermatol 2016;27:9.e4.

37. Lombardo G, Pennisi MG, Lupo T, et al. Papular dermatitis due to *Leishmania infantum* infection in seventeen dogs: diagnostic features, extent of the infection and treatment outcome. Parasit Vectors 2014;7:120.

38. Ceron JJ, Pardo-Marin L, Caldin M, et al. Use of acute phase proteins for the clinical assessment and management of canine leishmaniosis: general recommendations. BMC Vet Res 2018;14:196.

39. Daza González MA, Fragío Arnold C, Fermín Rodríguez M, et al. Effect of two treatments on changes in serum acute phase protein concentrations in dogs with clinical leishmaniosis. Vet J 2019;245:22–8.

40. Solano-Gallego L, Cardoso L, Pennisi MG, et al. Diagnostic Challenges in the era of canine *Leishmania infantum* vaccines. Trends Parasitol 2017;33:706–17.

41. Moreira MA, Luvizotto MC, Garcia JF, et al. Comparison of parasitological, immunological and molecular methods for the diagnosis of leishmaniasis in dogs with different clinical signs. Vet Parasitol 2007;145:245–52.

42. Oliveira GA, Sarmento VAS, Costa EWDS, et al. Detection of *Leishmania infantum* amastigotes in neutrophil from peripheral blood in a naturally infected dog. Rev Bras Parasitol Vet 2021;30:e004821.

43. Paltrinieri S, Gradoni L, Roura X, et al. Laboratory tests for diagnosing and monitoring canine leishmaniasis. Vet Clin Pathol 2016;45:552–78.

44. Ordeix L, Dalmau A, Osso M, et al. Histological and parasitological distinctive findings in clinically-lesioned and normal-looking skin of dogs with different clinical stages of leishmaniosis. Parasit Vectors 2017;10:121.

45. Kost WO, Pereira SA, Figueiredo FB, et al. Frequency of detection and load of amastigotes in the pancreas of *Leishmania infantum*-seroreactive dogs: clinical signs and histological changes. Parasit Vectors 2021;14:321.

46. Porrozzi R, Santos da Costa MV, Teva A, et al. Comparative evaluation of enzyme-linked immunosorbent assays based on crude and recombinant leishmanial antigens for serodiagnosis of symptomatic and asymptomatic *Leishmania infantum* visceral infections in dogs. Clin Vaccin Immunol 2007;14:544–8.

47. Mettler M, Grimm F, Capelli G, et al. Evaluation of enzyme-linked immunosorbent assays, an immunofluorescent-antibody test, and two rapid tests (immunochromatographic-dipstick and gel tests) for serological diagnosis of symptomatic and asymptomatic *Leishmania* infections in dogs. J Clin Microbiol 2005;43: 5515–9.

48. Duprey ZH, Steurer FJ, Rooney JA, et al. Canine visceral leishmaniasis, United States and Canada, 2000-2003. Emerg Infect Dis 2006;12:440–6.

49. Meyers AC, Edwards EE, Sanders JP, et al. Fatal Chagas myocarditis in government working dogs in the southern United States: Cross-reactivity and differential diagnoses in five cases across six months. Vet Parasitol Reg Stud Rep 2021;24: 100545.

50. Baneth G, Yasur-Landau D, Gilad M, et al. Canine leishmaniosis caused by *Leishmania major* and *Leishmania tropica*: comparative findings and serology. Parasit Vectors 2017;10:113.

51. Paz GF, Rugani JMN, Marcelino AP, et al. Implications of the use of serological and molecular methods to detect infection by *Leishmania* spp. in urban pet dogs. Acta Trop 2018;182:198–201.

52. Talmi-Frank D, Nasereddin A, Schnur LF, et al. Detection and identification of old world *Leishmania* by high resolution melt analysis. PLoS Negl Trop Dis 2010;4: e581.

53. Solano-Gallego L, Di Filippo L, Ordeix L. Early reduction of *Leishmania infantum*-specific antibodies and blood parasitemia during treatment in dogs with moderate or severe disease. Parasit Vectors 2016;9:235.

54. Strauss-Ayali D, Jaffe CL, Burshtain O, et al. Polymerase chain reaction using noninvasively obtained samples, for the detection of *Leishmania infantum* DNA in dogs. J Infect Dis 2004;189:1729–33.

55. Di Muccio T, Veronesi F, Antognoni MT, et al. Diagnostic value of conjunctival swab sampling associated with nested PCR for different categories of dogs naturally exposed to *Leishmania infantum* infection. J Clin Microbiol 2012;50:2651–9.

56. Slappendel RJ, Teske E. The effect of intravenous or subcutaneous administration of meglumine antimonate (Glucantime) in dogs with leishmaniasis. A randomized clinical trial. Vet Q 1997;19:10–3.

57. Manna L, Gravino AE, Picillo E, et al. *Leishmania* DNA quantification by real-time PCR in naturally infected dogs treated with miltefosine. Ann N Y Acad Sci 2008; 1149:358–60.

58. Miró G, Petersen C, Cardoso L, et al. Novel areas for prevention and control of canine leishmaniosis. Trends Parasitol 2017;33:718–30.

59. Torres M, Bardagí M, Roura X, et al. Long term follow-up of dogs diagnosed with leishmaniosis (clinical stage II) and treated with meglumine antimoniate and allopurinol. Vet J 2011;188:346–51.

60. Miró G, Gálvez R, Fraile C, et al. Infectivity to *Phlebotomus perniciosus* of dogs naturally parasitized with *Leishmania infantum* after different treatments. Parasit Vectors 2011;4:52.

61. Yasur-Landau D, Jaffe CL, David L, et al. Allopurinol Resistance in *Leishmania infantum* from dogs with disease relapse. PLoS Negl Trop Dis 2016;10:e0004341.

62. Yasur-Landau D, Jaffe CL, David L, et al. Resistance of *Leishmania infantum* to allopurinol is associated with chromosome and gene copy number variations including decrease in the S-adenosylmethionine synthetase (METK) gene copy number. Int J Parasitol Drugs Drug Resist 2018;8:403–10.

63. Maia C, Nunes M, Marques M, et al. In vitro drug susceptibility of *Leishmania infantum* isolated from humans and dogs. Exp Parasitol 2013;135:36–41.

64. Gonçalves G, Campos MP, Gonçalves AS, et al. Increased *Leishmania infantum* resistance to miltefosine and amphotericin B after treatment of a dog with miltefosine and allopurinol. Parasit Vectors 2021;14:599.

65. Sabaté D, Llinás J, Homedes J, et al. A single-centre, open-label, controlled, randomized clinical trial to assess the preventive efficacy of a domperidone-based treatment programme against clinical canine leishmaniasis in a high prevalence area. Prev Vet Med 2014;115:56–63.

66. Segarra S, Miró G, Montoya A, et al. Prevention of disease progression in *Leishmania infantum*-infected dogs with dietary nucleotides and active hexose correlated compound. Parasit Vectors 2018;11:103.

67. Segarra S. Nutritional modulation of the immune response mediated by nucleotides in canine leishmaniosis. Microorganisms 2021;16(9):2601.

68. Brianti E, Napoli E, Gaglio G, et al. Field evaluation of two different treatment approaches and their ability to control fleas and prevent canine leishmaniosis in a highly endemic area. PLoS Negl Trop Dis 2016;10:e0004987.

69. Gálvez R, Montoya A, Fontal F, et al. Controlling phlebotomine sand flies to prevent canine *Leishmania infantum* infection: A case of knowing your enemy. Res Vet Sci 2018;121:94–103.

70. Yimam Y, Mohebali M. Effectiveness of insecticide-impregnated dog collars in reducing incidence rate of canine visceral leishmaniasis: A systematic review and meta-analysis. PLoS One 2020;15:e0238601.

71. Dantas-Torres F, Nogueira FDS, Menz I, et al. Vaccination against canine leishmaniasis in Brazil. Int J Parasitol 2020;50:171–6.

72. Velez R, Gállego M. Commercially approved vaccines for canine leishmaniosis: a review of available data on their safety and efficacy. Trop Med Int Health 2020;25:540–57.

73. Calzetta L, Pistocchini E, Ritondo BL, et al. Immunoprophylaxis pharmacotherapy against canine leishmaniosis: A systematic review and meta-analysis on the efficacy of vaccines approved in European Union. Vaccine 2020;38:6695–703.

74. Rivas AK, Alcover M, Martínez-Orellana P, et al. Clinical and diagnostic aspects of feline cutaneous leishmaniosis in Venezuela. Parasit Vectors 2018;11:141.

75. Montoya A, García M, Gálvez R, et al. Implications of zoonotic and vector-borne parasites to free-roaming cats in central Spain. Vet Parasitol 2018;251:125–30.

76. Iatta R, Furlanello T, Colella V, et al. A nationwide survey of *Leishmania infantum* infection in cats and associated risk factors in Italy. PLoS Negl Trop Dis 2019;13: e0007594.
77. Fernandez-Gallego A, Feo Bernabe L, Dalmau A, et al. Feline leishmaniosis: diagnosis, treatment and outcome in 16 cats. J Feline Med Surg 2020;22: 993–1007.
78. Asfaram S, Fakhar M, Teshnizi SH. Is the cat an important reservoir host for visceral leishmaniasis? A systematic review with meta-analysis. J Venom Anim Toxins Incl Trop Dis 2019;25:e20190012.
79. Batista JF, Magalhães Neto FDCR, Lopes KSPDP, et al. Transmission of *Leishmania infantum* from cats to dogs. Rev Bras Parasitol Vet 2020;29:e017820.
80. Vioti G, da Silva MD, Galvis-Ovallos F, et al. Xenodiagnosis in four domestic cats naturally infected by *Leishmania infantum*. Transbound Emerg Dis 2021. https:// doi.org/10.1111/tbed.14216.
81. Brianti E, Falsone L, Napoli E, et al. Prevention of feline leishmaniosis with an imidacloprid 10%/flumethrin 4.5% polymer matrix collar. Parasit Vectors 2017; 10:334.
82. Gavgani AS, Mohite H, Edrissian GH, et al. Domestic dog ownership in Iran is a risk factor for human infection with *Leishmania infantum*. Am J Trop Med Hyg 2002;67:511–5.
83. Margonari C, Freitas CR, Ribeiro RC, et al. Epidemiology of visceral leishmaniasis through spatial analysis, in Belo Horizonte municipality, state of Minas Gerais, Brazil. Mem Inst Oswaldo Cruz 2006;101:31–8.
84. da Silva Santana Cruz C, Soeiro Barbosa D, Oliveira VC, et al. Factors associated with human visceral leishmaniasis cases during urban epidemics in Brazil: a systematic review. Parasitology 2021;148:639–47.
85. Matsumoto PSS, Hiramoto RM, Pereira VBR, et al. Impact of the dog population and household environment for the maintenance of natural foci of *Leishmania infantum* transmission to human and animal hosts in endemic areas for visceral leishmaniasis in Sao Paulo state, Brazil. PLoS One 2021;16:e0256534.

UNITED STATES POSTAL SERVICE® Statement of Ownership, Management, and Circulation
(All Periodicals Publications Except Requester Publications)

1. Publication Title	2. Publication Number	3. Filing Date
VETERINARY CLINICS: SMALL ANIMAL PRACTICE	003 – 150	9/18/2022

4. Issue Frequency	5. Number of Issues Published Annually	6. Annual Subscription Price
JAN, MAR, MAY, JUL, SEP, NOV	6	$365.00

7. Complete Mailing Address of Known Office of Publication (Not printer) (Street, city, county, state, and ZIP+4®)

ELSEVIER INC.
230 Park Avenue, Suite 800
New York, NY 10169

Contact Person
Malathi Samayan
Telephone (Include area code)
91-44-4299-4507

8. Complete Mailing Address of Headquarters or General Business Office of Publisher (Not printer)

ELSEVIER INC.
230 Park Avenue, Suite 800
New York, NY 10169

9. Full Names and Complete Mailing Addresses of Publisher, Editor, and Managing Editor (Do not leave blank)

Publisher (Name and complete mailing address)

DOLORES MELONI, ELSEVIER INC.
1600 JOHN F KENNEDY BLVD. SUITE 1800
PHILADELPHIA, PA 19103-2899

Editor (Name and complete mailing address)

STACY EASTMAN, ELSEVIER INC.
1600 JOHN F KENNEDY BLVD. SUITE 1800
PHILADELPHIA, PA 19103-2899

Managing Editor (Name and complete mailing address)

PATRICK MANLEY, ELSEVIER INC.
1600 JOHN F KENNEDY BLVD. SUITE 1800
PHILADELPHIA, PA 19103-2899

10. Owner (Do not leave blank. If the publication is owned by a corporation, give the name and address of the corporation immediately followed by the names and addresses of all stockholders owning or holding 1 percent or more of the total amount of stock. If not owned by a corporation, give the names and addresses of the individual owners. If owned by a partnership or other unincorporated firm, give its name and address as well as those of each individual owner. If the publication is published by a nonprofit organization, give its name and address.)

Full Name	Complete Mailing Address
WHOLLY OWNED SUBSIDIARY OF REED/ELSEVIER, US HOLDINGS	1600 JOHN F KENNEDY BLVD. SUITE 1800 PHILADELPHIA, PA 19103-2899

11. Known Bondholders, Mortgagees, and Other Security Holders Owning or Holding 1 Percent or More of Total Amount of Bonds, Mortgages, or Other Securities. If none, check box ▶ ☐ None

Full Name	Complete Mailing Address
N/A	

12. Tax Status (For completion by nonprofit organizations authorized to mail at nonprofit rates) (Check one)
The purpose, function, and nonprofit status of this organization and the exempt status for federal income tax purposes:
☒ Has Not Changed During Preceding 12 Months
☐ Has Changed During Preceding 12 Months (Publisher must submit explanation of change with this statement)

PS Form 3526, July 2014 [Page 1 of 4 (see instructions page 4)] PSN: 7530-01-000-9931   PRIVACY NOTICE: See our privacy policy on www.usps.com.

---

13. Publication Title	14. Issue Date for Circulation Data Below
VETERINARY CLINICS: SMALL ANIMAL PRACTICE	JULY 2022

15. Extent and Nature of Circulation			Average No. Copies Each Issue During Preceding 12 Months	No. Copies of Single Issue Published Nearest to Filing Date
a. Total Number of Copies (Net press run)			544	511
b. Paid Circulation (By Mail and Outside the Mail)	(1)	Mailed Outside-County Paid Subscriptions Stated on PS Form 3541 (Include paid distribution above nominal rate, advertiser's proof copies, and exchange copies)	345	329
	(2)	Mailed In-County Paid Subscriptions Stated on PS Form 3541 (Include paid distribution above nominal rate, advertiser's proof copies, and exchange copies)	0	0
	(3)	Paid Distribution Outside the Mails Including Sales Through Dealers and Carriers, Street Vendors, Counter Sales, and Other Paid Distribution Outside USPS®	135	135
	(4)	Paid Distribution by Other Classes of Mail Through the USPS (e.g., First-Class Mail®)	0	0
c. Total Paid Distribution (Sum of 15b (1), (2), (3), and (4))		▶	480	464
d. Free or Nominal Rate Distribution (By Mail and Outside the Mail)	(1)	Free or Nominal Rate Outside-County Copies included on PS Form 3541	48	31
	(2)	Free or Nominal Rate In-County Copies Included on PS Form 3541	0	0
	(3)	Free or Nominal Rate Copies Mailed at Other Classes Through the USPS (e.g. First-Class Mail)	0	0
	(4)	Free or Nominal Rate Distribution Outside the Mail (Carriers or other means)	0	0
e. Total Free or Nominal Rate Distribution (Sum of 15d (1), (2), (3) and (4))		▶	48	31
f. Total Distribution (Sum of 15c and 15e)		▶	528	495
g. Copies not Distributed (See Instructions to Publishers #4 (page #3))		▶	16	16
h. Total (Sum of 15f and g)		▶	544	511
i. Percent Paid (15c divided by 15f times 100)		▶	90.9%	93.7%

* If you are claiming electronic copies, go to line 16 on page 3. If you are not claiming electronic copies, skip to line 17 on page 3.

16. Electronic Copy Circulation		Average No. Copies Each Issue During Preceding 12 Months	No. Copies of Single Issue Published Nearest to Filing Date
a. Paid Electronic Copies	▶		
b. Total Paid Print Copies (Line 15c) + Paid Electronic Copies (Line 16a)	▶		
c. Total Print Distribution (Line 15f) + Paid Electronic Copies (Line 16a)	▶		
d. Percent Paid (Both Print & Electronic Copies) (16b divided by 16c × 100)	▶		

☒ I certify that 50% of all my distributed copies (electronic and print) are paid above a nominal price.

17. Publication of Statement of Ownership

☒ If the publication is a general publication, publication of this statement is required. Will be printed in the __NOVEMBER 2022__ issue of this publication.   ☐ Publication not required.

18. Signature and Title of Editor, Publisher, Business Manager, or Owner	Date
Malathi Samayan - Distribution Controller *Malathi Samayan*	9/18/2022

I certify that all information furnished on this form is true and complete. I understand that anyone who furnishes false or misleading information on this form or who omits material or information requested on the form may be subject to criminal sanctions (including fines and imprisonment) and/or civil sanctions (including civil penalties).

PS Form 3526, July 2014 (Page 3 of 4)   PRIVACY NOTICE: See our privacy policy on www.usps.com

Moving?

Make sure your subscription moves with you!

To notify us of your new address, find your **Clinics Account Number** (located on your mailing label above your name), and contact customer service at:

Email: journalscustomerservice-usa@elsevier.com

800-654-2452 (subscribers in the U.S. & Canada)
314-447-8871 (subscribers outside of the U.S. & Canada)

Fax number: 314-447-8029

Elsevier Health Sciences Division
Subscription Customer Service
3251 Riverport Lane
Maryland Heights, MO 63043

*To ensure uninterrupted delivery of your subscription,
please notify us at least 4 weeks in advance of move.

Printed and bound by CPI Group (UK) Ltd, Croydon, CR0 4YY

03/10/2024

01040468-0007